In Clinical Practice

Taking a practical approach to clinical medicine, this series of smaller reference books is designed for the trainee physician, primary care physician, nurse practitioner and other general medical professionals to understand each topic covered. The coverage is comprehensive but concise and is designed to act as a primary reference tool for subjects across the field of medicine.

More information about this series at http://www.springer.com/series/13483

Marco Matucci-Cerinic
Christopher P. Denton
Editors

Practical Management of Systemic Sclerosis in Clinical Practice

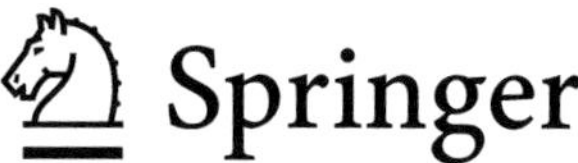

Editors
Marco Matucci-Cerinic
University of Florence
Firenze, FI
Italy

Christopher P. Denton
University College London
Royal Free Hospital
London
UK

ISSN 2199-6652 ISSN 2199-6660 (electronic)
In Clinical Practice
ISBN 978-3-030-53735-7 ISBN 978-3-030-53736-4 (eBook)
https://doi.org/10.1007/978-3-030-53736-4

© Springer Nature Switzerland AG 2021
This work is subject to copyright. All rights are reserved by the Publisher, whether the whole or part of the material is concerned, specifically the rights of translation, reprinting, reuse of illustrations, recitation, broadcasting, reproduction on microfilms or in any other physical way, and transmission or information storage and retrieval, electronic adaptation, computer software, or by similar or dissimilar methodology now known or hereafter developed.
The use of general descriptive names, registered names, trademarks, service marks, etc. in this publication does not imply, even in the absence of a specific statement, that such names are exempt from the relevant protective laws and regulations and therefore free for general use.
The publisher, the authors, and the editors are safe to assume that the advice and information in this book are believed to be true and accurate at the date of publication. Neither the publisher nor the authors or the editors give a warranty, expressed or implied, with respect to the material contained herein or for any errors or omissions that may have been made. The publisher remains neutral with regard to jurisdictional claims in published maps and institutional affiliations.

This Springer imprint is published by the registered company Springer Nature Switzerland AG
The registered company address is: Gewerbestrasse 11, 6330 Cham, Switzerland

Contents

Chapter 1
Major Scleroderma Emergencies

Voon H. Ong and Christopher P. Denton

Introduction

Of the immune-mediated rheumatic diseases, SSc has the highest case-specific mortality and substantial non-lethal complications. This is largely related to the significant burden from major organ complications in particular cardiopulmonary involvement. However, some of the complications may present as acute emergencies as listed in Table 1.1. Briefly, acute emergencies in SSc can be broadly classified as acute decompensation of existing organ disease, acute emergencies specific to SSc and other medical and surgical emergencies in SSc including opportunistic infections. Key aspects of these emergencies are covered in other chapters. These include pulmonary hypertension, critical digital ischaemia, hypertensive renal crisis, gastrointestinal disease, issues related to pregnancy and cardiac involvement. Importantly, complications related to overlap disease that may affect a fifth of SSc patients need to be carefully evaluated [1]. The objectives of

V. H. Ong (✉) · C. P. Denton
Centre for Rheumatology and Connective Tissue Diseases, UCL Division of Medicine, London, UK
e-mail: v.ong@ucl.ac.uk; c.denton@ucl.ac.uk

© Springer Nature Switzerland AG 2021
M. Matucci-Cerinic, C. P. Denton (eds.), *Practical Management of Systemic Sclerosis in Clinical Practice*, In Clinical Practice,
https://doi.org/10.1007/978-3-030-53736-4_1

Table 1.1 Spectrum of key acute emergencies in SSc

SSc-specific emergencies	Digital ischaemia and gangrene
	Hypertensive renal crisis
	GI haemorrhage (gastric antral vascular ectasia)
	Pseudo-obstruction
Decompensation of SSc complications	Worsening of pulmonary hypertension
	Progressive myocardial disease
	Exacerbation of interstitial lung fibrosis
	Malabsorption with nutritional weight loss
Non-SSc acute emergency	Opportunistic infections
	Overlap syndromes[a]
	Pregnancy-related complications[b]
	Peripheral vascular disease

[a]Overlap syndromes include inflammatory muscle disease, inflammatory arthritis, systemic lupus erythematosus, vasculitis
[b]Pregnancy-related issues include pre-eclampsia, premature rupture of the membrane and placenta abruptio GI:Gastrointestinal

this module are to illustrate with case vignettes the major emergencies of SSc of commonly encountered symptoms affecting these patients as a life-threatening event requiring urgent intervention. The complexity of multiorgan involvement in these cases often requires multidisciplinary coordination including rheumatological review and immediate patient's referral to appropriate specialties to ensure adequate joint management.

Case History 1

The first case describes an acute vascular crisis with an uncommon cause and highlights the need to consider a broad differential diagnoses for a common vascular manifestation of SSc complication.

A 62 year old lady with established anti-topoisomerase I antibody associated limited cutaneous systemic sclerosis with mild interstitial lung disease (FVC 79% DLCO 68%) presented with severe pain across all toes with a dry ulcer over her right second toe with dependent oedema up to the knees (Fig. 1.1a, b). Her current vasodilator treatment includes Losartan 100 mg daily and Diltiazem 360 mg in divided doses. She has had cardiac stenting for ischemic heart disease 3 years ago and she is maintained on Aspirin 75 mg daily with isosorbide mononitrate 10 mg daily and Clopidogrel was recently discontinued as part of investigation for haematuria. Although she has had episodic digital ulcers affecting her fingers requiring intravenous prostacyclin infusions, she has never had ulcers affecting her lower limbs. More proximal causes of distal limb gangrene should be evaluated with Doppler imaging and Echocardiogram in particular for valvular abnormalities [2, 3]. Echocardiogram showed only mild aortic stenosis with mean gradient of 9 mmHg with no other major valvular abnormalities. Bilateral lower limb arterial tree assessment showed patent superficial femoral, popliteal, anterior and posterior tibial and peroneal arteries bilaterally with normal triphasic waveforms. Vascular opinion was sought and large vessel cause of gangrene was excluded. She was commenced on intravenous prostacyclin infusion.

Hb 7.4 g/L: platelet 445 x 10^9/L RDW 15.1% [11–16] with positive markers for haemolysis with reticulocytes 171 × 10^9/L(50–150) haptoglobin <0.2 g/L (0.3–1.9) LDH 383 U/L (135–214). Peripheral blood film showed agglutination and polychromasia. DAT was strongly positive with anti-CD3d and negative for IgG. Total Bilirubin 9 umol/L (<21), direct bilirubin 5 umol/L (<5) CRP 2 mg/L (<5) ESR 15 mm/h.

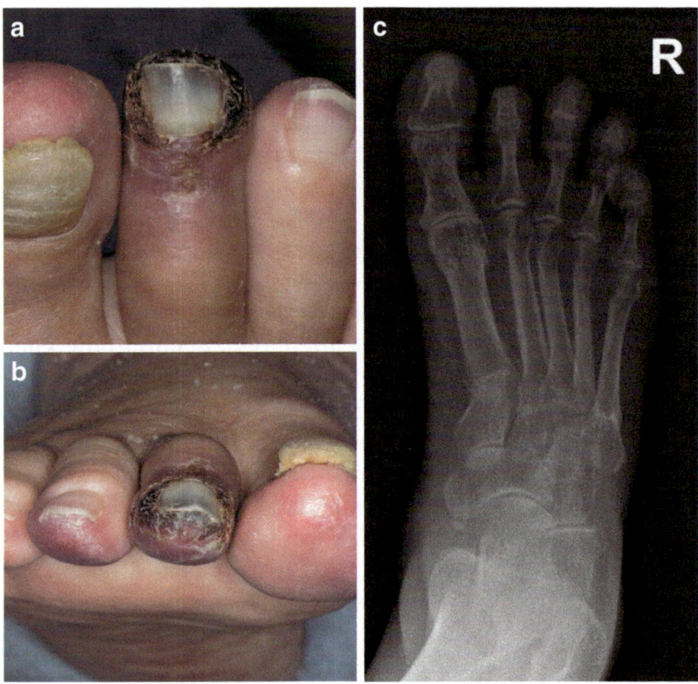

FIGURE 1.1 Critical digital ischaemia in systemic sclerosis with cryoglobulinaemia. Gangrenous right second toe tip (**a**, **b**). Autoamputation of the affected to at the level of DIP was evident radiologically 6 months post-onset of the gangrenous ulcer (**c**). There was no cortical thinning or osteolysis to suggest osteomyelitis. There was incidental fifth metatarsal base fracture (**c**)

Paraprotein 5 g/L and immunofixation showed immunoglobulin M (IgM) kappa paraprotein.

Cryoglobulin screen showed Type 1 monoclonal IgM kappa cryoglobulin. Iron 6 umol/L (11–36) TIBC 65 umol/L (53–85) transferrin 9.2% (20–40) ferritin 43 ug/L. It is noteworthy that haematuria may reflect the haemoglobinuria related to ongoing haemolysis that occurs during the course of the disease [4]. She was commenced on oral Prednisolone 50 mg daily (1 mg/kg) for autoimmune haemolytic anaemia (AIHA).

Type 1 cryoglobulinaemia is associated exclusively with B cell proliferative diseases mainly monoclonal gammopathy of undetermined significance and less commonly Waldenström macroglobulinaemia and multiple myeloma [5, 6] whereby the sera of these patients contain monoclonal IgM, and more rarely IgG, or IgA cryoglobulins. In almost half of the patients, type I cryoglobulinemia is characterized by severe cutaneous involvement with a lower frequency of glomerulonephritis compared to other types of cryoglobulinemia. Hyperviscosity syndrome contributing to vascular crisis may also occur in due to high concentration of monoclonal cryoglobulins owing to the concomitant lymphoproliferative disorder. Specifically, cutaneous involvement is characterized by presence of symptoms related to cold exposure such as acrocyanosis, livedo, urticaria, cold-induced necrotic purpura, or as in this case with painful ulcers and gangrene of the extremities.

This patient underwent bone marrow aspirate and trephine. Smears were unremarkable. Flow cytometry identified at least 10% population of kappa restricted CD5 negative B cells. MYD88 mutation was negative. The trephine did not show an obvious abnormal lymphoid or plasmacytic infiltrate. Aspirate morphology showed normocellular particles and trails. Trilineage haematopoiesis was seen with normal granulopoiesis and no abnormal infiltrate. Erythropoiesis was normoblastic. Megakaryocytes were seen in adequate numbers with normal morphology. Low levels plasma cells (2%) were seen but these were clustered around the particles.

PET CT did not show any hypermetabolic or pathological lymphadenopathy.

The low frequency and its considerable diverse clinical heterogeneity meant that there is a lack of evidence-based standardised therapies for AIHA. However, only aggressive and prompt treatment can induce a rapid response of dysproteinaemic state and reduce the organ damage caused by cryoglobulin. In light of her progressive gangrene, she also received plasma exchange to transiently remove cryoglobulins from her circulation although a decrease of serum cryoglobulins was shown to occur in only half the patients and plasma exchange does not prevent formation of new cryoglobulins [7]. Alkylating agents such as cyclophosphamide, bortezomib (a proteasome inhibitor) and rituximab-based regimens are the main therapeutic options to eliminate the B cell clones that produce cryoglobulins. In our patient, prompt start of an integrated therapeutic approach with prostanoid infusion, plasmapheresis, and chemotherapy halted further progression of the occlusive vasculopathy with resultant autoamputation of the affected toe (Fig. 1.1c).

In some cases, these patients may also require ongoing plasmapheresis to control the vascular manifestations of the disease that occur in the presence of even small amounts of monoclonal immunoglobulin that may persists despite effective treatment of the malignancy. Despite these therapeutic measures, these patients may experience ongoing problems, especially skin-related symptoms.

Whilst acute vascular digital crisis and anaemia in SSc are often attributable to associated complications of the disease itself, there are few reported cases of AIHA in SSc and coexisting overlap diseases including lupus, antiphospholipid syndrome and cryoglobulinaemia should be considered as differential diagnoses [8–10].

Case History 2

The second case describes a patient with worsening exertional dyspnoea and reflects the complexity of multiorgan involvement in SSc and important considerations are required to evaluate carefully the individual components of organ-based disease and potential complications.

50 year old lady with established limited SSc diagnosed 20 years ago and she developed pulmonary arterial hypertension 2 years ago that is well controlled on Macitentan 10 mg twice daily and Sildenafil 50 mg thrice daily. Her other medications include Ramipril 10 mg daily, Omeprazole 20 mg daily. She harbours anti centromere (ACA) and anti-Ro-52, -La antibodies. She is a never-smoker.

She presented with increasing exertional breathlessness climbing incline on stairs and hills (Functional Class III) with NT-proBNP 1174 ng/L with troponin 11 ng/L. Cardiac MRI demonstrated right ventricular dilatation with biatrial dilatation (LA 30 cm^2 and RA 31 cm^2) with increased T1 and T2 uptake with patchy septal gadolinium enhancement and preserved left ventricular function. In summary, this tissue characterization is suggestive of progressive myocardial disease. A 24 hour tape showed 2000 ventricular ectopics with first degree heart block with no non-sustained ventricular tachycardia.

A year before the current presentation, she developed an acute episode of pleurisy treated as pneumonia although sputum cultures were negative and shortly after this, she developed acute renal injury with increased protein creatinine ratio 831 mg/mmol (<30) with normal albumin 35 g/L (35–50). Subsequent renal biopsy demonstrated membranous glomerulonephritis. She also developed increasing paraethesiae over left hand and right foot that was confirmed as sensory axonal neuropathy on EMG. She was commenced on mycophenolate but discontinued due to an acute episode of pleuritic chest pain with breathlessness. This was substituted with Azathioprine. It was noted that she had mild lymphopaenia 0.16 × 109/L (1.0–4.0), elevated ESR 63 mm/h and platelets 130 × 10^9 (140–400) with C3 0.77 g/L (0.9–1.8). dsDNA 7.5 IU/mL (<10) Crithidia lucillae antibody negative.

Serial lung function investigations (Table 1.2) showed a reduction in forced vital capacity (FVC) from 81 to 65 (15–25% reduction of baseline) suggesting interstitial changes with markedly impaired gas transfer. The latter is out of keeping with her recent stable haemodynamics with pulmonary

Table 1.2 Serial lung function for Case 2

	2019	2018	2017
FVC %(value)	67 (2.76)	65 (2.66)	81 (2.95)
DLCO % (value)	25 (2.32)	35 (2.58)	32 (3.0)
KCO % (value)	33 (0.53)	42 (0.67)	46 (0.73)

vascular resistance (PVR) well controlled with high cardiac output (CO) possibly driven by active inflammatory disease (right heart catheter assessment: mean pulmonary arterial (PA) pressure mean 43 mmHg, pulmonary capillary wedge pressure 8 mmHg, CO 9.7 L/min cardiac index 5.4 L/min/M^2 PVR 289 ARU dynes/s/cm PA saturation 64% systemic saturation 86% on finger oximetry but 98% in wedge position), 6 min walk test stable 427 but below 500 several years ago suggesting the possibility of additional pathology such as pulmonary veno-occlusive disease (PVOD) or other lung disease.

Two serial HRCT Chest were compared (Figs. 1.2 and 1.3). There is diffuse ground glass attenuation with centrilobular predominance sparing the periphery. The latter does not favour hypersensitivity pneumonitis. In addition there are cystic appearances and these have enlarged over time (Fig. 1.2). There is dilated pulmonary artery (Fig. 1.3). There is no pleural or pericardial effusion. The CT approach to diag-

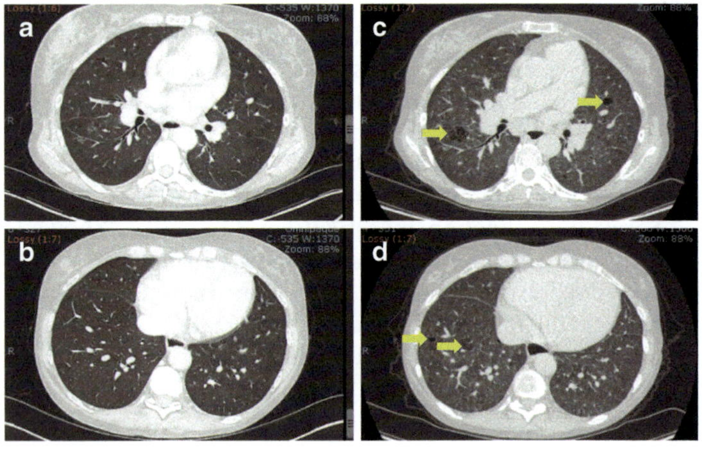

Figure 1.2 Progression of parenchymal lung disease in systemic sclerosis. There is centrilobular ground-glass opacification in both lungs with more extensive cystic lung disease (yellow arrows) over 2 year period (Panels **a** and **b** (2017) and **c** and **d** (2019) respectively). There is dilatation of the oesophagus with food debris

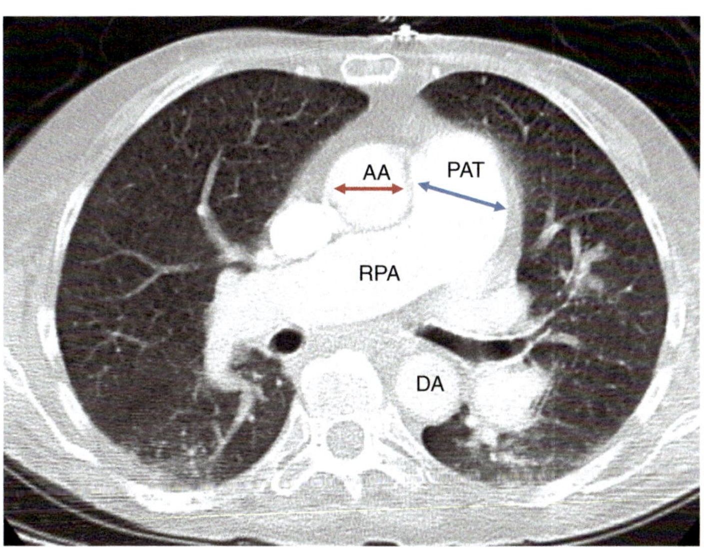

FIGURE 1.3 Features of pulmonary hypertension on contrast CT scan of the chest. Enlarged pulmonary arterial trunk (PAT) is larger than that of the ascending aorta (AA) at the same level. Right pulmonary artery (RPA) is also dilated. Descending aorta (DA) also shown

nosis of PH begins with identifying an enlarged pulmonary artery diameter greater than 29 mm, which is usually larger than that of the ascending aorta at the same level [11]. This diameter must be measured in the axial plane at the bifurcation, orthogonal to the long axis of the pulmonary artery. A variety of parenchymal changes in PH has been described. These include mosaic attenuation in PH due to regional differences in lung perfusion, in addition to diffuse bilateral centrilobular ground-glass opacities (increased lung parenchyma attenuation without obscuration of the underlying vasculature or airways) but without interlobular septal thickening to suggest PVOD. As a subtype of PAH group I, PVOD is an important consideration as there is an unexpectedly high incidence of PVOD in patients with SSc-PH-ILD and it is an unrecognised contributor to the dismal prognosis of these patients. It is critical to distinguish PVOD from PAH as treating PVOD with vasodilators may lead to fatal pulmonary oedema and death. However, this patient is tolerating Macitentan with well preserved saturations thus the diagnosis of PVOD is less likely.

Interstitial lung fibrosis is a major complication in SSc particularly among those with anti-Scl70 antibody. Those with ACA limited SSc is less likely to develop ILD with cumulative incidence of clinically significant lung fibrosis is 8.5% at later stage of disease [12]. Acute exacerbation of lung fibrosis have been described in SSc-ILD in particular those with overlap diseases [13, 14] although the mechanisms related to acute exacerbation in connective tissue diseases-related ILD are unclear but these few factors like intrinsic factor leading to progression of underlying disease, infection and role of gastro-oesophageal reflux disease with microaspiration may be relevant. Accepting this is a rare entity, management of this disease is largely empirical with recent evidence that early institution of disease modifying agents including biological agents Rituximab may improve survival. In this case, in the context of lupus with presence of Ro antibody, a distinct subtype of interstitial lung disease—lymphocytic interstitial pneumonia (LIP) should be considered [15]. Alternatively, the cysts on HRCT could be due to emphysema in never-smokers in SSc-ILD [16, 17].

Another possible cause of acute deterioration is worsening of PAH. PAH is a progressive disease with the majority of patients succumb as a result of right ventricular (RV) failure. As PAH progresses, the RV must adapt to increases in PVR and afterload [18]. Despite structural remodeling, the RV eventually cannot adapt to the increased afterload resulting in right heart failure. These patients need to be carefully managed to reverse the inciting event and optimise fluid balance, haemodynamics, and RV function and this is best managed by a multidisciplinary team with experience in managing patients with PAH [19]. Any reversible causes of acute decompensation should be appropriately addressed. Patients should be carefully monitored, as RV failure can eventually lead to multiorgan failure through decreased perfusion to other organs. Fluid balance must be carefully managed in patients with PAH as both hypovolaemia and hypervolaemia can have damaging effects to patients. It is important to note that over-diuresis could lead to a greater worsening of CO further impacting end-organ perfusion.

It is also noteworthy that SSc patients demonstrate peculiar vulnerability to infectious complications in part to intrinsic disease-related immune dysregulation, disease-related factors (such as ILD) and in part to the immunosuppressive treatments including biological therapies. The lung is among the most frequent sites of infection in SSc in particular among those with severe ILD or reflux/aspiration and they are susceptible to developing pneumonia sustained both by common pathogens such as anaerobic bacteria and by opportunistic microorganisms., as well as routine bacterial and viral respiratory pathogens. Oesophageal involvement, like dysmotility disorder or reflux, can also be associated to lung infections. In SSc, the most frequent causes of death not directly related to SSc are infections, pneumonia [20]. Furthermore, many drugs used in SSc treatment, such as cyclophosphamide, mycophenolate and rituximab have been associated to a raised risk of developing infections, mostly bacterial or mycotic pneumonia [21]. Thus, when patients with SSc manifest new respiratory symptoms, especially if treated with immunosuppressive drugs, both routine and opportunistic lung infections should be considered for appropriate diagnostic and therapeutic intervention [22]. It is noteworthy that repeated immune-mediated stimuli from recurrent lung infections has been postulated to be a trigger for pleuropulmonary fibroelastosis (PPFE), a recently described entity characterized by a combination of fibrosis involving the visceral pleura and fibroelastotic changes predominating in the subpleural lung parenchyma have been reported in SSc and may contribute to worsening of respiratory symptoms in SSc-ILD [23, 24]. However, there are no CT appearances to suggest PPFE in this case.

In light of her overlap lupus features with renal disease, neuropathy with likely LIP features on HRCT and possibly myocardial disease, this patient was managed with rituximab and clinical and biochemical parameters related to each of the affected organs will be carefully evaluated for response over time.

Summary

Although SSc is often associated with major organ involvement, serious and potentially life-threatening acute emergencies may occur in the context of acute decompensation or acute exacerbation of chronic complication of SSc. Non-SSc related complications in particular opportunistic infections and overlap immune-mediated overlap disease should be carefully considered as well.

References

1. Pakozdi A, Nihtyanova S, Moinzadeh P, Ong VH, Black CM, Denton CP. Clinical and serological hallmarks of systemic sclerosis overlap syndromes. J Rheumatol. 2011;38(11):2406–9.
2. Jivegard L, Arfvidsson B, Frid I, Haljamae H, Holm J. Cardiac output in patients with acute lower limb ischaemia of presumed embolic origin--a predictor of severity and outcome? Eur J Vasc Surg. 1990;4(4):401–7.
3. Conte MS, Bradbury AW, Kolh P, White JV, Dick F, Fitridge R, et al. Global vascular guidelines on the management of chronic limb-threatening ischemia. J Vasc Surg. 2019;69(6s):3S-125S.e40.
4. Swiecicki PL, Hegerova LT, Gertz MA. Cold agglutinin disease. Blood. 2013;122(7):1114–21.
5. Neel A, Perrin F, Decaux O, Dejoie T, Tessoulin B, Halliez M, et al. Long-term outcome of monoclonal (type 1) cryoglobulinemia. Am J Hematol. 2014;89(2):156–61.
6. Terrier B, Karras A, Kahn JE, Le Guenno G, Marie I, Benarous L, et al. The spectrum of type I cryoglobulinemia vasculitis: new insights based on 64 cases. Medicine. 2013;92(2):61–8.

7. Roccatello D, Saadoun D, Ramos-Casals M, Tzioufas AG, Fervenza FC, Cacoub P, et al. Cryoglobulinaemia. Nat Rev Dis Primers. 2018;4(1):11.
8. Katsumata K. A case of systemic sclerosis complicated by autoimmune hemolytic anemia. Mod Rheumatol. 2006;16(3):191–5.
9. Lugassy G, Reitblatt T, Ducach A, Oren S. Severe autoimmune hemolytic anemia with cold agglutinin and sclerodermic features--favorable response to danazol. Ann Hematol. 1993;67(3):143–4.
10. Oshima M, Maeda H, Morimoto K, Doi M, Kuwabara M. Low-titer cold agglutinin disease with systemic sclerosis. Inter Med. 2004;43(2):139–42.
11. Frazier AA, Galvin JR, Franks TJ, Rosado-De-Christenson ML. From the archives of the AFIP: pulmonary vasculature: hypertension and infarction. Radiographics. 2000;20(2):491–524. quiz 30-1, 32
12. Nihtyanova SI, Sari A, Harvey JC, Leslie A, Derrett-Smith EC, Fonseca C, et al. Using autoantibodies and cutaneous subset to develop outcome-based disease classification in systemic sclerosis. Arthr Rheumatol. 2019.
13. Tomiyama F, Watanabe R, Ishii T, Kamogawa Y, Fujita Y, Shirota Y, et al. High prevalence of acute exacerbation of interstitial lung disease in Japanese patients with systemic sclerosis. Tohoku J Exp Med. 2016;239(4):297–305.
14. Park IN, Kim DS, Shim TS, Lim CM, Lee SD, Koh Y, et al. Acute exacerbation of interstitial pneumonia other than idiopathic pulmonary fibrosis. Chest. 2007;132(1):214–20.
15. Garcia D, Young L. Lymphocytic interstitial pneumonia as a manifestation of SLE and secondary Sjogren's syndrome. BMJ Case Reports. 2013;2013:bcr2013009598.
16. Antoniou KM, Margaritopoulos GA, Goh NS, Karagiannis K, Desai SR, Nicholson AG, et al. Combined pulmonary fibrosis and emphysema in scleroderma-related lung disease has a major confounding effect on lung physiology and screening for pulmonary hypertension. Arthr Rheumatol. 2016;68(4):1004–12.
17. Yamakawa H, Takemura T, Iwasawa T, Yamanaka Y, Ikeda S, Sekine A, et al. Emphysematous change with scleroderma-associated interstitial lung disease: the potential contribution of vasculopathy? BMC Pulm Med. 2018;18(1):25.
18. Vonk Noordegraaf A, Galie N. The role of the right ventricle in pulmonary arterial hypertension. Eur Resp Review. 2011;20(122):243–53.

19. Price LC, Dimopoulos K, Marino P, Alonso-Gonzalez R, McCabe C, Kemnpy A, et al. The CRASH report: emergency management dilemmas facing acute physicians in patients with pulmonary arterial hypertension. Thorax. 2017;72(11):1035–45.
20. Tyndall AJ, Bannert B, Vonk M, Airo P, Cozzi F, Carreira PE, et al. Causes and risk factors for death in systemic sclerosis: a study from the EULAR scleroderma trials and research (EUSTAR) database. Ann Rheum Dis. 2010;69(10):1809–15.
21. Omair MA, Alahmadi A, Johnson SR. Safety and effectiveness of mycophenolate in systemic sclerosis. A systematic review. PLoS One. 2015;10(5):e0124205.
22. Solomon JJ, Olson AL, Fischer A, Bull T, Brown KK, Raghu G. Scleroderma lung disease. Eur Respir Rev. 2013;22(127):6–19.
23. Chua F, Desai SR, Nicholson AG, Devaraj A, Renzoni E, Rice A, et al. Pleuroparenchymal Fibroelastosis. A review of clinical, radiological, and pathological characteristics. Ann Am Thorac Soc. 2019;16(11):1351–9.
24. Enomoto Y, Nakamura Y, Colby TV, Johkoh T, Sumikawa H, Nishimoto K, et al. Radiologic pleuroparenchymal fibroelastosis-like lesion in connective tissue disease-related interstitial lung disease. PLoS One. 2017;12(6):e0180283.

Chapter 2
Scleroderma Renal Crisis

Marie Hudson, Cybele Ghossein, and John Varga

Introduction

The kidneys can be affected in patients with systemic sclerosis (SSc) in multiple ways. While renal involvement can be indolent and relatively benign, scleroderma renal crisis (SRC), the most dramatic form of renal involvement that occurs in up to 10% of patients with diffuse cutaneous SSc, commonly has an abrupt onset and progressive course, and is associated with poor outcomes and high mortality.

Case #1 Classic Case of SRC

Diane is a 55-year old woman who developed Raynaud's phenomenon and puffy fingers approximately 2 years ago. At

M. Hudson (✉)
Jewish General Hospital, Lady Davis Institute, McGill University, Montreal, QC, Canada
e-mail: marie.hudson@mcgill.ca

C. Ghossein · J. Varga
Scleroderma Program, Feinberg School of Medicine, Northwestern University, Chicago, IL, USA
e-mail: Cybele.ghossein@nm.org; j-varga@northwestern.edu

© Springer Nature Switzerland AG 2021
M. Matucci-Cerinic, C. P. Denton (eds.), *Practical Management of Systemic Sclerosis in Clinical Practice*, In Clinical Practice,
https://doi.org/10.1007/978-3-030-53736-4_2

that time, she was found to have a high titre speckled ANA and positive anti-RNA polymerase III antibodies. Her baseline blood pressure was normal (130/70 mmHg) as was her creatinine (75 umol/L or 0.85 mg/dL). She noted progressive thickening of her skin involving the fingers, hands, forearms, face, chest, thighs and feet. A diagnosis of SSc was made, and her modified Rodnan skin score (MRSS) was 23. Treatment with mycophenolate (1 gm bid) was initiated. Three months prior to her admission, she complained of joint pain, and was started on low-dose prednisone (7.5 mg/day). She presented to the clinic without an appointment complaining of general unwellness and shortness of breath over the last 2 weeks. In the clinic, her blood pressure was 180/90 mmHg. Blood tests were remarkable for new anemia (hemoglobin 95 g/L) and an elevated creatinine (145 umol/L or 1.64 mg/dL). How should this patient be managed?

Scleroderma renal crisis (SRC) is characterized by new onset malignant hypertension and acute kidney injury. Risk factors for SRC include early SSc (less than 5 years), rapidly progressive skin disease and the presence of anti-RNA polymerase III antibody. When anti-RNA polymerase III testing is not available, a speckled, and at times nucleolar, immunofluorescence staining pattern in the absence of other known fine specificities may be a clue. Other risk factors for SRC include male sex, tendon friction rubs and exposure to nephrotoxic drugs, including non-steroidal anti-inflammatory drugs and calcineurin inhibitors. Exposure to glucocorticoids, even at low doses, is commonly reported as a risk factor [1]. Whether the association of SRC and glucocorticoid exposure is causal or instead represents the presence of active disease remains uncertain; nevertheless, glucocorticoids remain relatively contra-indicated in SSc patients with risk factors for SRC. It is interesting to note that the conditioning regimen used in most autologous hematopoietic stem cell transplant (AHSCT) protocols includes high-dose glucocorticoids, prompting the *prophylactic* use of ACE inhibitors in this setting. Although AHSCT might be a possible risk factor for SRC, the role of prophylactic ACE inhibitors in this setting remains uncertain.

Patients presenting with signs and symptoms of SRC should be immediately referred to a monitored setting (such as an emergency room or an intensive care unit) for continuous blood pressure monitoring, and assessed for evidence of acute kidney injury (AKI). The Kidney Disease Improving Global Outcomes (KDIGO) definition of AKI is as follows [2]:

- Increase in serum creatinine by >26.5 umol/L (> 0.3 mg/dL) within 48 h.
- Increase in serum creatinine to >1.5 times baseline, known or presumed to have occurred within the prior 7 days.
- Urine volume < 0.5 mL/kg/h for 6 h.

Evaluation

Urinalysis and urine microscopy are essential to rule out alternative explanations for new onset hypertension and AKI. In particular, hematuria, dysmorphic red blood cells and casts could suggest vasculitis or glomerulonephritis. Target organ dysfunction could manifest as encephalopathy, seizures, heart failure, pericardial effusion and retinopathy. A cardiac echocardiogram and ophthalmoscopic exam, the latter preferably performed by an ophthalmologist, are therefore also part of the basic work up. Appropriate testing for thrombotic microangiopathy should be performed.

The indications for kidney biopsy (Fig. 2.1) in an SSc patient presenting with classic hypertensive SRC remain uncertain. Although kidney biopsy for SRC may be useful prognostically [3], this must be balanced with the risks of

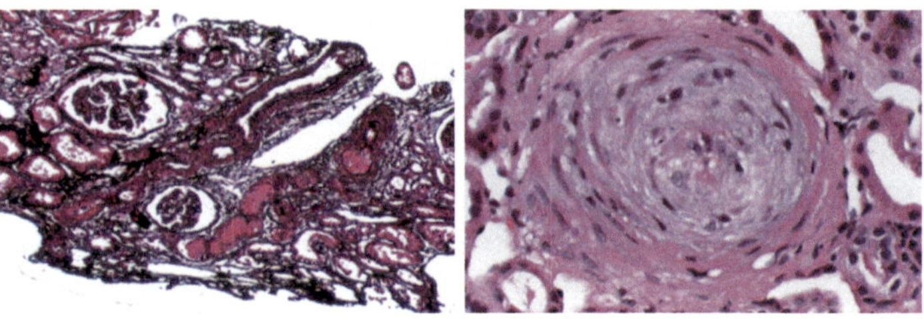

FIGURE 2.1 Renal biopsy findings of SRC

Diagnosis	Assess target organ damage	Treatment goals	If goals are not reached	Long-term management
• SRC is an emergency • Refer to a monitored setting (emergency room, intensive care unit) • Involve renal and critical care specialists	• Assess for thrombotic microangiopathy, encephalopathy, heart failure, pericarditis • Treat with anti-epileptics,diuretics and other symptomatic treatments as needed	• Achieve blood pressure control in 48-72 hours • Begin captopril at a dose of 6.25 to12.5 mg, escalate in 12.5 to 25 mg increments every 4-8 hours until the blood pressure is controlled or a maximum dose of 300 to 450 mg/day is attained • May need intra-venous therapy with agents such as nicardipine for rapid and titratable blood pressure control	• Add additional anti-hypertensive agents • Consider adding endothelin inhibitor • Consider complement inhibition (eg. eculizumab) if thrombotic microangiopathy is present • Consider dialysis if patient develops uremia, oligo-anuria or hyperkalemia	• Maintain background ACE inhibitor • Consider renal transplant if there is no renal recovery after 1-2 years

FIGURE 2.2 Management of scleroderma renal crisis

bleeding in the setting of uncontrolled hypertension and anemia. Unexplained AKI in a normotensive SSc patient, however, is an indication for a kidney biopsy. Approximately 10% of cases of SRC are not associated with hypertension.

Management (Fig. 2.2)

Initial management for suspected SRC consists of ACE inhibition using a short-acting agent such as captopril. If the patient is unable to take oral medications, intravenous enalaprilat could be used, although it is not preferred because of a long duration of action (up to 36 h). In our experience, combination therapy with intravenous nicardipine is helpful to control blood pressure as the dose of oral ACE inhibitor is titrated to maximal tolerated dose. There are no standard guidelines on the target for blood pressure control; however, restoring the patient's baseline blood pressure should be the goal. Of note, since hypertension in SRC is acute, commonly used targets for controlling chronic hypertension are not applicable. In fact, in SRC, we generally aim to normalize the blood pressure rapidly (over 2–3 days) with the goal of preserving renal function.

It is not unusual to note a rise in creatinine as ACE inhibitors are up-titrated. This increase can reflect hemodynamic changes as a result of ACE inhibition, as well as worsening SRC or an alternative cause of AKI. We recommend a coordinated team approach with rheumatologists and nephrologists in the management of SRC.

If blood pressure goals are not achieved with ACE inhibitors and calcium channel blockers, additional antihypertensive medication should be added. Although angiotensin receptor blockers (ARB) might be expected to be effective in patients with SRC, there are multiple caveats. First, they have not been adequately evaluated as monotherapy in this setting. Second, they should not replace ACE inhibitors because, unlike ACE inhibitors, they do not inhibit the degradation of bradykinin, which are potent vasodilators. Third, studies in other diseases have suggested that patients treated with both an ACE inhibitor and ARB are at higher risk of adverse events compared with those treated with only one agent. Endothelin inhibitors have been used in the setting of SRC, although results with bosentan, a non-selective endothelin-1 receptor antagonist, have so far been disappointing [4]. There is an ongoing trial with zibotentan, a selective endothelin-A antagonist (NCT02047708). Since SRC can be associated with a thrombotic microangiopathy and in view of recent evidence of the potential role of complement activation in other thrombotic microangiopathies such as atypical hemolytic uremic syndrome, the complement inhibitor eculizumab has been used in some cases of SRC [5]; however the proper role of anti-complement therapy in the treatment of SRC remains to be established. Although there are theoretical advantages for using direct renin antagonists, the published evidence remains sparse. Beta blockers should be avoided because of the risk of reducing cardiac output and triggering "renal" Raynaud's.

Patients with SRC require close monitoring for blood pressure, creatinine and urine output until blood pressure is adequately controlled, kidney function stabilizes, and signs of microangiopathy and target organ dysfunction resolve. Improvement in renal function can continue for up to 1–2 years following an episode of SRC. Hence, decisions regarding kidney transplantation should be deferred until that time.

Life-long use of ACE inhibitors after SRC is usually recommended, even in the absence of hypertension. However, the data on the use of ACE inhibition post-transplant is sparse and insufficient to make a reliable recommendation.

Case #2 Isolated Systemic Hypertension

Jay is a 55-year old African-American man with a 2-year history of Raynaud's phenomenon, sclerodactyly, gastro-esophageal reflux and a positive anti-centromere antibody. His only medication is a proton pump inhibitor. At his yearly appointment, he reported feeling well, but was noted to have newly elevated blood pressure (150/90). Laboratory investigations including hemoglobin, platelets and creatinine (90 umol/L or 1.02 mg/dL) were all normal and not changed from his baseline. How should newly diagnosed isolated hypertension be managed in this patient with limited cutaneous SSc?

SSc patients presenting with hypertension need to be carefully assessed and risk stratified. Although this patient has some risk factors for SRC (male sex and relatively early disease), his limited cutaneous involvement and serology (anti-centromere antibody) put him at low risk. In particular, anti-centromere antibody positivity appears to be "protective" for SRC. Nevertheless, a thorough work up, including evaluation of family history of hypertensive disease, urinalysis and investigation for hemolysis, are indicated for this patient. Creatinine should be monitored. If hypertension persists, without evidence of AKI or other signs and symptoms of SRC, we would diagnose essential hypertension. Of note, a recent study suggested that hypertension (as well as proteinuria and chronic kidney disease) at the time of SSc diagnosis may be risk factors for SRC [6]. Thus, continued vigilance is warranted over time.

Treatment of essential hypertension in SSc remains a challenge. The obvious dilemma is whether new "isolated" hypertension in a patient with SSc could in fact herald the onset of SRC, and whether initiating treatment with an ACE inhibitor could abort a crisis. However, while definitive answers are lacking, some studies suggested that exposure to ACE inhibitors in SSc prior to SRC may not be protective, and may in fact be harmful [7]. We therefore recommend a calcium channel blocker (which may also have benefit on Raynaud's phenomenon) for patients with SSc and new onset isolated hypertension. We also recommend avoiding beta-blockers, which may worsen Raynaud's and exacerbate "renal" Raynaud's, and diuretics, because fluid shifts have been proposed as potential triggers for SRC.

Some advocate the use of ACE inhibitors in early SSc to prophylax against SRC (Fig. 2.3). There is no data at this time to support the role of prophylactic ACE inhibition for SSc patients without indications for ACE inhibition (eg. hypertension or chronic kidney disease with proteinuria [which is not uncommon in SSc] [8]). Therefore, we do not recommend prophylactic ACE inhibitors at this time.

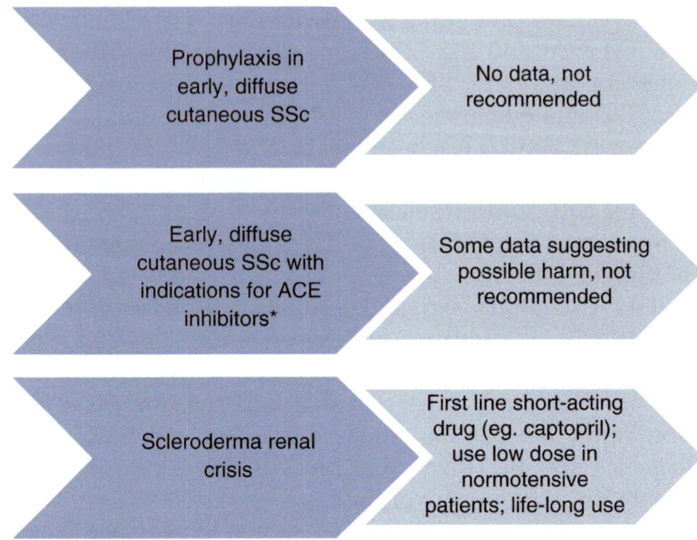

FIGURE 2.3 ACE inhibitors in systemic sclerosis

Acknowledgements We would like to acknowledge Dr. Agnes Fogo from the Department of Pathology, Vanderbilt University Medical Center, Nashville, TN, for kindly allowing us to reproduce images of renal biopsies of SRC.

References

1. DeMarco PJ, Weisman MH, Seibold JR, Furst DE, Wong WK, Hurwitz EL, et al. Predictors and outcomes of scleroderma renal crisis: the high-dose versus low-dose D-penicillamine in early diffuse systemic sclerosis trial. Arthritis Rheum. 2002;46(11):2983–9.
2. Kellum J, Lameire N, Aspelin P, Barsoum R, Burdmann E, Goldstein S. Kidney disease: improving global outcomes (KDIGO) acute kidney injury work group. KDIGO clinical practice guideline for acute kidney injury. Kidney Int. 2012;2(1):1–138.
3. Batal I, Domsic RT, Shafer A, Medsger TA Jr, Kiss LP, Randhawa P, et al. Renal biopsy findings predicting outcome in scleroderma renal crisis. Hum Pathol. 2009;40(3):332–40.

4. Bérezné A, Hendy A, Karras A, Marie I, Huart A, Ficheux M, et al. Bosentan in scleroderma renal crisis: a National Open Label Prospective Study [abtract]. Arthr Rheumatol. 2017;69 (suppl 10).
5. Thomas CP, Nester CM, Phan AC, Sharma M, Steele AL, Lenert PS. Eculizumab for rescue of thrombotic microangiopathy in PM-Scl antibody-positive autoimmune overlap syndrome. Clin Kidney J. 2015;8(6):698–701.
6. Gordon SM, Stitt RS, Nee R, Bailey WT, Little DJ, Knight KR, et al. Risk factors for future scleroderma renal crisis at systemic sclerosis diagnosis. J Rheumatol. 2019;46(1):85–92.
7. Hudson M, Baron M, Tatibouet S, Furst DE, Khanna D. International scleroderma renal crisis study I. exposure to ACE inhibitors prior to the onset of scleroderma renal crisis-results from the international scleroderma renal crisis survey. Semin Arthritis Rheum. 2014;43(5):666–72.
8. Steen VD, Syzd A, Johnson JP, Greenberg A, Medsger TA Jr. Kidney disease other than renal crisis in patients with diffuse scleroderma. J Rheumatol. 2005;32(4):649–55.

Chapter 3
Anemia and Thrombocytopenia

Gianluca Bagnato and Daniel E. Furst

Outline

Anemia and thrombocytopenia are relevant findings in the clinical assessment of systemic sclerosis patients and several mechanism of actions are involved in the determination of these complications. Studies on the prevalence of anemia in SSc suggest that its prevalence is 25–40% [1], with higher prevalence in those with early diffuse disease [2] and in Caucasians [3]. Anemia has been included in the 5-item prediction rule for 2 and 5 year mortality in SSc patients with early diffuse disease. Even moderate anemia (Hb < 10 mg/

G. Bagnato
Leeds Institute of Rheumatic and Musculoskeletal Medicine, University of Leeds, Leeds, West Yorkshire, UK
e-mail: g.bagato@leeds.ac.iuk

D. E. Furst (✉)
University of California in Los Angeles, Los Angeles, CA, USA

University of Washington, Seattle, WA, USA

University of Florence, Florence, Italy
e-mail: dan@furst.us.com

© Springer Nature Switzerland AG 2021

M. Matucci-Cerinic, C. P. Denton (eds.), *Practical Management of Systemic Sclerosis in Clinical Practice*, In Clinical Practice,
https://doi.org/10.1007/978-3-030-53736-4_3

dL) represents an independent risk factor for mortality (HR 1.88/4.57) [2, 4, 5].

In another aspect of SSc,the PHAROS registry study highlighted that, in SSc patients at risk to develop pulmonary arterial hypertension (PAH), anemia was strongly associated with higher mortality [6], while another prospective study suggested that anemia is the only laboratory risk factor associated with the development of PAH [7].

Anemia of chronic illness is commonly observed in systemic sclerosis, but several other disease-specific vascular complications can exacerbate it, as noted above, including scleroderma renal crisis. Other causes of anemia, less frequent and less well-defined in SSc, such as autoimmune and drug-induced anemia, will also be discussed.

The most common complications characterized by the association between anemia and thrombocytopenia, such as scleroderma renal crisis, thrombotic thrombocytopenic purpura and atypical haemolytic uremic syndrome will be analysed and compared, providing points for differential diagnosis and treatment.

In addition other conditions associated with the simultaneous presence of anemia and thrombocytopenia will be discussed.

Nutritional Deficit Anemia

Iron-deficiency has been documented in 16.4/18.35% patients with systemic sclerosis [8]. Gastric antral vascular ectasia (GAVE, watermelon stomach) is one of the most frequent causes of this nutritional-related type of anemia in SSc patients. It is mostly prevalent in early diffuse cutaneous systemic sclerosis with rapid skin progression and a distinct antibody profile (anti-RNA polymerase III positivity) [9].

GAVE is represented by chronic gastrointestinal bleeding and iron deficiency anemia and it corresponds to a characteristic endoscopic finding of longitudinal rows of sacculated and dilated mucosal vessels in the antrum of the stomach.

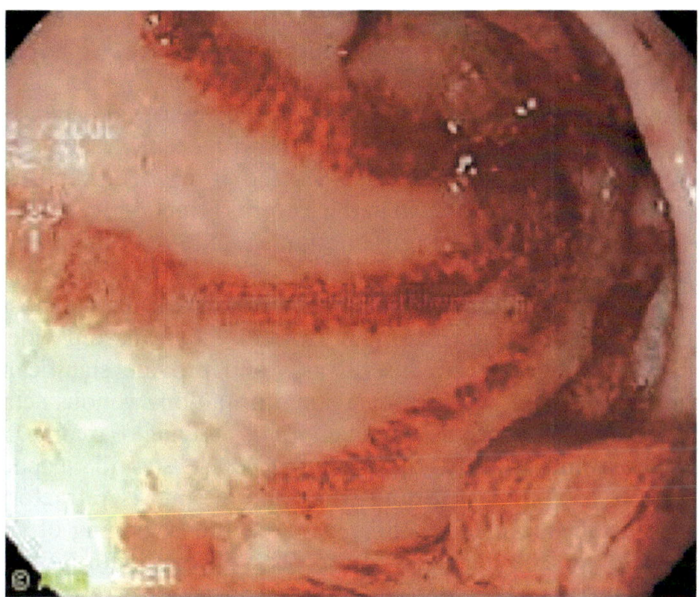

FIGURE 3.1 Watermelon stomach. An endoscopic view of a Gastric Antral Vascular Ectasia (GAVE). Note the longitudinal rows of vessels in the stomach resembling the stripes of a watermelon. "Courtesy of PathologyOutline.com"

This is said to resemble the stripes on a watermelon [10] (Fig. 3.1).

Several hypotheses have been proposed to explain the pathogenesis of GAVE. One possibility is the prolapse of the antral mucosa due to alterations in the connection between the distal gastric mucosa and the adjacent muscularis externa or in peristalsis. More recently it has been suggested that GAVE is a possible disease-specific vascular manifestation of systemic sclerosis, according to the evidence that up to 60% of GAVE patients have skin telangiectasias. A third theory supports a link between GAVE and autoimmunity suggesting a possible cross-reactivity with specific proteins in the gastric mucosa and submucosa.

Most of the patients present either with symptomatic iron deficiency anemia (weakness, fatigue, or dyspnea) or asymptomatic anemia (with laboratory findings like low hemoglobin and mean corpuscular volume). Patients affected by diffuse systemic sclerosis can present with occult fecal blood, hematochezia, or hematemesis. Indeed, it has been reported that GAVE can occur also in the lower GI tract or even in the rectum [11], so clinical presentation should direct the appropriate GI tract to study first.

Digestive endoscopy is the gold standard for the diagnosis of GAVE and enteroscopy, red blood cell scan, and video capsule endoscopy are useful aids and provide significant help to differentiate it from AV malformations, venous ectasia, gastric telangiectasia, hemangioma, and angiosarcoma.

Most importantly, the rheumatologist should suspect GAVE in a clinical setting when the anemia is refractory. Given that the mean of time between the beginning of the disease and the diagnosis of GAVE is 3 years, with a mean hemoglobin of 8.2 g/dL, a high index of suspicion, especially in patients with early disease, is important.

Because more than 90% of SSc patients have gastrointestinal disturbances, such as malabsorption and small intestinal bacterial overgrowth (SIBO), other nutritional deficits (vitamin B12, folic acid) should be considered as possible causes of nutrient-related anemia.

Recent data confirm that up to 70% of SSc patients might be considered as vitamin B12-deficient and half of them show a severe deficiency (<200 pg/mL) [12]. Notably a case report strongly linked the subcutaneous administration of vitamin B12 with sclerodermoid reaction at the site of injection [13], compatible with the histology of localized scleroderma. Few case reports detail of the occurrence of pernicious anemia in systemic sclerosis [14].

Of note, multifactorial causes of anemia should be always considered since data confirm that different causes of anemia can coexist in the same patient, such as GAVE and pernicious anemia [15] or more complex case reports of overlap syndromes with pernicious anemia [16]. The presence of a normochromic, normocytic anemia should not stop further lab tests to exclude nutritional deficits or the presence of overlapping causes. Treatment of GAVE can be very challenging and iron supplementation is often not effective; case reports suggest that the combination of methylprednisone and cyclophosphamide, or cyclophosphamide alone, can result in improvement [17, 18]. Autologous stem cell transplantation [19] has also been effective, despite some case reports described the occurrence of GAVE after hematopoietic stem cell transplant (HSCT-GAVE) [20].

Autoimmune Causes of Isolated Anemia and Thrombocytopenia

Compared to the other causes of anemia and thrombocytopenia, evidence for an autoimmune-mediated process are surprisingly scarce in SSc, while frequently reported in overlap syndromes [21] and supported by case reports [22–25]. The diagnosis of autoimmune anemia is based on the presence of signs of haemolysis with reticulocytosis, low haptoglobin, increased lactate dehydrogenase, elevated indirect bilirubin, and a positive direct antiglobulin test (Coombs test).

A case of a SSc patient associated with deficiency of IgA and the C4 component of complement associated with haemolytic anemia further compounds the complexity of the approach necessary to unearth the potential causes of anemia in SSc [26].

The diagnosis of immune thrombocytopenic purpura relies on the exclusion of several known triggers, such as viral infection, lymphoproliferative disorders and genetic diseases. Although it is possible in some settings to identify antiplatelet antibodies, the diagnosis remains clinical. Some cases confirm this association, for example evidence of the presence of anti-platelet antibodies against gpIIb/IIIa in systemic sclerosis [27] and the overlap between autoimmune hepatitis, immune thrombocytopenia and systemic sclerosis [28]. In addition, the occurrence of autoantibody against thrombopoietin receptor has been demonstrated in the serum of a SSc patient with evidence of amegakaryocytic thrombocytopenia [29].

Microangiopathic Anemia and Thrombocytopenia

A microangiopathic heamolytic anemia associated with thrombocytopenia can be one of the peculiar aspects of the scleroderma renal crisis (SRC). SRC can be a life-threatening complication with heterogeneous presentations ranging from a sudden onset of accelerated arterial hypertension and rapidly progressive oliguric renal failure, to less intense elevations in blood pressure and less drastic renal alteration. Rare normotensive SRC has also been documented [30].

In the kidney of a SSc patient with scleroderma renal crisis, the vascular endothelial injury results in obliteration of the renal arcuate and interlobular arteries with consequent reduction in renal blood flow along with hyperplasia of renal juxtaglomerular cells. This sequence of events starts an inappropriate activation of renin and angiotensin leading, therefore, to renal vasoconstriction that eventually causes (frequently malignant) hypertension.

A microangiopathic hemolytic anemia (MAHA) results from fragmentation of red blood cells as they pass through renal vessels occluded by fibrin or platelet thrombi, while thrombocytopenia is the direct consequence of continuous platelet activation and consumption at damaged endothelial sites.

Other thrombotic microangiopathies can present with widespread microvascular thrombosis, thrombocytopenia, and microangiopathic hemolytic anemia (MAHA). These microangiopathies include thrombotic thrombocytopenic purpura (TTP) and hemolytic uremic syndrome (HUS).

HUS is traditionally distinguished as typical (Shiga and Shiga like toxin-associated) and atypical (alternative activation of complement pathway).

Histologically, on renal biopsy, aHUS is indistinguishable from HUS caused by toxin-producing bacteria or TTP.

Indeed, the differential diagnosis between scleroderma renal crisis, thrombotic thrombocytopenic purpura and haemolytic uremic syndrome is probably the most challenging differential in the approach of a SSc patient presenting with thrombocytopenia and haemolytic anemia [31]. Compared to SRC, TTP shows several common clinical presenting features, such as thrombocytopenia, MAHA, elevation of bilirubin and LDH, negative Coombs test and the presence of schistocytes, neurologic dysfunction, thrombotic microangiopathy and acute renal impairment and normal PT and PTT [32, 33].

Relevant differences on the other hand are as follows: hypertension is almost always present in SRC while is possible in TTP, SRC is commonly observed in the diffuse form of SSc while TTP occurs more frequently in the limited form of SSc and most importantly SRC responds to ACEi while TTP requires plasmapheresis.

This difference is mainly based on the pathophysiologic evidence that TTP is due to a reduced or absent activity of the von Willenbrand factor-cleaving protease activity, belonging to the group of a disintegrin and metalloproteinase with thrombospondin motifs (ADAMTS), which can be successfully treated by plasma exchange, in association with antiplatelet agents and anticoagulants, according to platelet count, and steroids. SRC is mainly dependent on aberrant activation of the renin-angiotensin system and thus appropriate therapy directed against this system is the most indicated approach and reduced consistently the rate of mortality for this complication.

Indeed, the exclusion of aHUS remains a critical issue for the multiple similarities with TTP and SRC; the levels of C3 are reduced only in less than half of the cases. It is generally accepted that if ADAMTS13 levels are >5% and the patient is resistant to plasma exchange, then the diagnosis is more likely to be aHUS than TTP. Despite the challenge of diagnosing aHUS, a new monoclonal antibody was recently approved for the treatment of aHUS [34].

Eculizumab is a recombinant, fully humanized monoclonal antibody, with a high binding affinity for C5 thus preventing the formation of C5a and C5a-9 and it has been successfully employed also in patients with SSc [35]. Whether the efficacy of this therapy is due to the activation of complement in misdiagnosed SRC, still remains unclear and this clue offers future direction for research [36].

Drug-Induced Anemia and Thrombocytopenia

Several medications have been associated with the occurrence of anemia and thrombocytopenia in SSc. These include mainly drugs employed for specific SSc-related indications. In SSc patients treated with bosentan for digital ulcers, anemia was the fourth most common adverse event affecting 17.9% of the patients [37]. Similarly but with a lower percentage in the DUAL-1 and DUAL-2 study, in SSc patients treated with macitentan for the management of digital ulcers, anemia occurred in 5–11% of cases [38]. In addition, in a recent pilot study open-label trial in early diffuse systemic sclerosis 3/10 patients exposed to nilotinib, a tyrosine kinase inhibitor, showed anemia [39]. A recent report suggests that gemcitabine might induce an hemolytic uremic syndrome with accelerated hypertension, thrombocytopenia and Raynaud's phenomenon treated successfully with intravenous administration of a calcium channel blocker, oral administration of an angiotensin-converting enzyme inhibitor and angiotensin II receptor blocker plus transfusion of fresh frozen plasma [40].

Several studies support an increased risk of developing SRC with the use of steroids, and up to 60% of patients developing SRC had received steroids before the onset of this renal complication. Another case report linked the onset of scleroderma renal crisis with the use of a combination of tacrolimus and methylprednisolone [41]. Azathioprine is another drug that has been associated with a severe case of pure red cell aplastic anemia in systemic sclerosis patients and further supports a tight CBC monitoring if azathioprine therapy is needed for SSc patients [42].

Reports on cyclosporine use in SSc are contradictory: while some cases of aplastic anemia responded well to anti-thymocyte globulin [43] in association with cyclosporine, this medication was also linked to the development of uremic haemolytic syndrome with anemia and thrombocytopenia [44, 45].

Cases of haemolytic anemia in SSc patients has been reported also with the use of cyclofenil [46]. Of note, some medications have been directly linked to the onset of an immune thrombocytopenia: (1) the ingestion of L-tryptophan [47], used as a muscle-building adjuvant, (2) D-penicillamine [48] and (3) diclofenac [49] therapy have been all associated with an anti-platelet positive IgG immune thrombocytopenia. A case of macrophage activation syndrome has been reported in a SSc patients treated with etanercept [50].

Bone Marrow Insufficiency

In some cases, anemia and thrombocytopenia can be a direct expression of bone marrow dysfunction and some case descriptions report the occurrence of aplastic anemia successfully treated with anti-thymocyte globulin [51]. In addition, it is important to underline that recent case reports suggest the possible occurrence of macrophage activation syndrome in systemic sclerosis [52, 53]. While relatively rare as an haemotologic complication, due to its high mortality rate, this complication should be put high on the differential. Positive outcomes have been reported with etoposide, but larger studies are needed (Table 3.1) [54].

Pregnancy/Post-Partum/Infancy

Isolated reports highlight the relevance of careful CBC monitoring in pregnant patients with SSc and the occurrence of anemia and/or thrombocytopenia further complicates the differential diagnosis [55]. A case of pregnancy-associated

Table 3.1 Causes of anemia and thrombocytopenia

Causes of anemia	Causes of thrombocytopenia
Nutritional deficits (iron, vitamin B12, folic acid)	Microangiopathic/haemolytic (SRC–TTP–HUS)
Microangiopathic/haemolytic (SRC–TTP–aHUS)	Immune (ITP) Drug-induced
Autoimmune (AIHA) Drug-induced	

References: [9, 10, 12, 15, 21, 30, 31, 37–51, 55]
SRC, scleroderma renal crisis; *TTP*, thrombotic thrombocytopenic purpura; *HUS*, haemolytic uremic syndrome; *ITP*, immune thrombotic purpura; *AIHA*, autoimmune haemolytic syndrome

thrombotic thrombocytopenic purpura in a patient with Raynaud's phenomenon and anti-centromere antibodies was successfully treated with plasma exchange and high-dose prednisolone and angiotensin-converting enzyme inhibitor [56]. Additionally, another case reported the occurrence of thrombocytopenia in a pregnant SSc patient with severe preeclampsia [57]. Unfortunately, a severe scleroderma case with onset at 6 months of life [58] with anemia, failure to thrive, recurrent diarrhea, and ascites has been reported as well as the association between localized scleroderma and thrombocytopenia in pediatric age [59].

Conflict of Interest GB-none relevant to this manuscript.
DEF-none relevant to this manuscript.

References

1. Frayha RA, Shulman LE, Stevens MB. Hematological abnormalities in scleroderma. A study of 180 cases. Acta Haematol. 1980;64(1):25–30. https://doi.org/10.1159/000207206.
2. Domsic RT, Nihtyanova SI, Wisniewski SR, et al. Derivation and external validation of a prediction rule for five-year mortality in patients with early diffuse cutaneous systemic sclerosis. Arthritis Rheumatol. 2016;68(4):993–1003. https://doi.org/10.1002/art.39490.

3. Schmajuk G, Bush TM, Burkham J, et al. Characterizing systemic sclerosis in northern California: focus on Asian and Hispanic patients. Clin Exp Rheumatol. 2009;27(3 Suppl 54):22–5.
4. Domsic RT, Nihtyanova SI, Wisniewski SR, et al. Derivation and validation of a prediction rule for two-year mortality in early diffuse cutaneous systemic sclerosis. Arthritis Rheumatol. 2014;66(6):1616–24. https://doi.org/10.1002/art.38381.
5. Wangkaew S, Prasertwitayakij N, Phrommintikul A, et al. Causes of death, survival and risk factors of mortality in Thai patients with early systemic sclerosis: inception cohort study. Rheumatol Int. 2017;37(12):2087–94. https://doi.org/10.1007/s00296-017-3846-7.
6. Hsu VM, Chung L, Hummers LK, et al. Risk factors for mortality and cardiopulmonary hospitalization in systemic sclerosis patients at risk for pulmonary hypertension, in the PHAROS registry. J Rheumatol. 2019;46(2):176–83. https://doi.org/10.3899/jrheum.180018.
7. Coral-Alvarado P, Rojas-Villarraga A, Latorre MC, et al. Risk factors associated with pulmonary arterial hypertension in Colombian patients with systemic sclerosis: review of the literature. J Rheumatol. 2008;35(2):244–50.
8. Ortiz-Santamaria V, Puig C, Soldevillla C, et al. Nutritional support in patients with systemic sclerosis. Reumatol Clin. 2014;10(5):283–7. https://doi.org/10.1016/j.reuma.2013.12.011.
9. Parrado RH, Lemus HN, Coral-Alvarado PX, et al. Gastric antral vascular ectasia in systemic sclerosis: current concepts. Int J Rheumatol. 2015;2015:762546. https://doi.org/10.1155/2015/762546.
10. El-Gendy H, Shohdy KS, Maghraby GG, et al. Gastric antral vascular ectasia in systemic sclerosis: where do we stand? Int J Rheum Dis. 2017;20(12):2133–9. https://doi.org/10.1111/1756-185X.13047.
11. Singh D, Shill M, Kaur H. The watermelon rectum. J Clin Gastroenterol. 2001;33(2):164–6.
12. Tas Kilic D, Akdogan A, Kilic L, et al. Evaluation of vitamin B12 deficiency and associated factors in patients with systemic sclerosis. J Clin Rheumatol. 2018;24(5):250–4. https://doi.org/10.1097/RHU.0000000000000686.
13. Ho J, Rothchild YH, Sengelmann R. Vitamin B12-associated localized scleroderma and its treatment. Dermatol Surg. 2004;30(9):1252–5. https://doi.org/10.1111/j.1524-4725.2004.30387.x.

14. Hirose Y, Yoshida Y, Konda S, et al. Pernicious anemia in a patient with progressive systemic sclerosis. Nihon Ketsueki Gakkai Zasshi. 1977;40(1):1–8.
15. Faure P, Escudie L, Rouquet O, et al. Gastric antral vascular ectasia, systemic sclerosis and pernicious anemia: a non-fortuitous association. Gastroenterol Clin Biol. 2004;28(8–9):814–5.
16. Saad-Dine Y, Macurak RB, Beasley EW, et al. Hashimoto's thyroiditis, pernicious anemia, Sjogren's syndrome, and CRST syndrome -- a case report. J Med Assoc Ga. 1981;70(3):187–9.
17. Matsumoto Y, Hayashi H, Tahara K, et al. Intravenous cyclophosphamide for gastric antral vascular ectasia associated with systemic sclerosis refractory to endoscopic treatment: a case report and review of the pertinent literature. Intern Med. 2019;58(1):135–9. https://doi.org/10.2169/internalmedicine.1431-18.
18. Lorenzi AR, Johnson AH, Davies G, et al. Gastric antral vascular ectasia in systemic sclerosis: complete resolution with methylprednisolone and cyclophosphamide. Ann Rheum Dis. 2001;60(8):796–8.
19. Bhattacharyya A, Sahhar J, Milliken S, et al. Autologous hematopoietic stem cell transplant for systemic sclerosis improves anemia from gastric antral vascular ectasia. J Rheumatol. 2015;42(3):554–5. https://doi.org/10.3899/jrheum.141234.
20. Grant MJ, Horwitz ME. HSCT-GAVE as a manifestation of chronic graft versus host disease: a case report and review of the existing literature. Case Rep Transplant. 2018;2018:2376483–5. https://doi.org/10.1155/2018/2376483.
21. Andrews J, Hall MA. Dermatomyositis-scleroderma overlap syndrome presenting as autoimmune haemolytic anaemia. Rheumatology. 2002;41(8):956–8. https://doi.org/10.1093/rheumatology/41.8.956.
22. Katsumata K. A case of systemic sclerosis complicated by autoimmune hemolytic anemia. Mod Rheumatol. 2006;16(3):191–5. https://doi.org/10.1007/s10165-006-0480-8.
23. Chaves FC, Rodrigo FG, Franco ML, et al. Systemic sclerosis associated with auto-immune haemolytic anaemia. Br J Dermatol. 1970;82(3):298–302.
24. Wanchu A, Sud A, Bambery P. Linear scleroderma and autoimmune hemolytic anaemia. J Assoc Physicians India. 2002;50:441–2.
25. Jordana R, Tolosa C, Selva A, et al. Autoimmune hemolytic anemia and CREST syndrome. Med Clin (Barc). 1990;94(19):740–1.

26. Jones E, Jones JV, Woodbury JF, et al. Scleroderma and hemolytic anemia in a patient with deficiency of IgA and C4: a hitherto undescribed association. J Rheumatol. 1987;14(3):609–12.
27. Czirjak L, Molnar I, Csipo I, et al. Anti-platelet antibodies against gpIIb/IIIa in systemic sclerosis. Clin Exp Rheumatol. 1994;12(5):527–9.
28. Toyoda M, Yokomori H, Kaneko F, et al. Primary biliary cirrhosis-autoimmune hepatitis overlap syndrome concomitant with systemic sclerosis, immune thrombocytopenic purpura. Intern Med. 2009;48(23):2019–23.
29. Katsumata Y, Suzuki T, Kuwana M, et al. Anti-c-Mpl (thrombopoietin receptor) autoantibody-induced amegakaryocytic thrombocytopenia in a patient with systemic sclerosis. Arthritis Rheum. 2003;48(6):1647–51. https://doi.org/10.1002/art.10965.
30. Hoa S, Stern EP, Denton CP, et al. Towards developing criteria for scleroderma renal crisis: a scoping review. Autoimmun Rev. 2017;16(4):407–15. https://doi.org/10.1016/j.autrev.2017.02.012.
31. Keeler E, Fioravanti G, Samuel B, et al. Scleroderma renal crisis or thrombotic thrombocytopenic purpura: seeing through the masquerade. Lab Med. 2015;46(2):e39–44. https://doi.org/10.1309/LM72AM5XFHZYOQCB.
32. Dahlan R, Sontrop JM, Li L, et al. Primary and secondary thrombotic Microangiopathy referred to a single plasma exchange Center for Suspected Thrombotic Thrombocytopenic Purpura: 2000-2011. Am J Nephrol. 2015;41(6):429–37. https://doi.org/10.1159/000437001.
33. Manadan AM, Harris C, Block JA. Thrombotic thrombocytopenic purpura in the setting of systemic sclerosis. Semin Arthritis Rheum. 2005;34(4):683–8. https://doi.org/10.1016/j.semarthrit.2004.08.008.
34. Cavero T, Rabasco C, Lopez A, et al. Eculizumab in secondary atypical haemolytic uraemic syndrome. Nephrol Dial Transplant. 2017;32(3):466–74. https://doi.org/10.1093/ndt/gfw453.
35. Devresse A, Aydin S, Le Quintrec M, et al. Complement activation and effect of eculizumab in scleroderma renal crisis. Medicine (Baltimore). 2016;95(30):e4459. https://doi.org/10.1097/MD.0000000000004459.
36. Uriarte MH, Larrarte C, Rey LB. Scleroderma renal crisis Debute with thrombotic Microangiopathy: a successful case treated with Eculizumab. Case Rep Nephrol. 2018;2018:6051083–4. https://doi.org/10.1155/2018/6051083.

37. Hamaguchi Y, Sumida T, Kawaguchi Y, et al. Safety and tolerability of bosentan for digital ulcers in Japanese patients with systemic sclerosis: prospective, multicenter, open-label study. J Dermatol. 2017;44(1):13–7. https://doi.org/10.1111/1346-8138.13497.
38. Khanna D, Denton CP, Merkel PA, et al. Effect of Macitentan on the development of new ischemic digital ulcers in patients with systemic sclerosis: DUAL-1 and DUAL-2 randomized clinical trials. JAMA. 2016;315(18):1975–88. https://doi.org/10.1001/jama.2016.5258.
39. Gordon JK, Martyanov V, Magro C, et al. Nilotinib (Tasigna) in the treatment of early diffuse systemic sclerosis: an open-label, pilot clinical trial. Arthritis Res Ther. 2015;17:213. https://doi.org/10.1186/s13075-015-0721-3.
40. Yamada Y, Suzuki K, Nobata H, et al. Gemcitabine-induced hemolytic uremic syndrome mimicking scleroderma renal crisis presenting with Raynaud's phenomenon, positive antinuclear antibodies and hypertensive emergency. Intern Med. 2014;53(5):445–8.
41. Nunokawa T, Akazawa M, Yokogawa N, et al. Late-onset scleroderma renal crisis induced by tacrolimus and prednisolone: a case report. Am J Ther. 2014;21(5):e130–3. https://doi.org/10.1097/MJT.0b013e3182583ba1.
42. Suto M, Nagai Y, Hasegawa M, et al. Azathioprine-induced pure red cell aplasia in a systemic sclerosis patient with interstitial pneumonia. J Dermatol. 2011;38(3):285–7. https://doi.org/10.1111/j.1346-8138.2010.01005.x.
43. Suematsu E, Miyamura T, Idutsu K, et al. Efficacy of antithymocyte globulin and cyclosporin a combined therapy in aplastic anemia complicated with limited cutaneous systemic sclerosis. Nihon Rinsho Meneki Gakkai Kaishi. 2005;28(2):99–103.
44. Zachariae H, Hansen HE, Olsen TS. Hemolytic uremic syndrome in a patient with systemic sclerosis treated with cyclosporin a. Acta Derm Venereol. 1992;72(4):307–9.
45. Chen WS, Young AH, Wang HP, et al. Hemolytic uremic syndrome with ischemic glomerulonephropathy and obliterative vasculopathy in a systemic sclerosis patient treated with cyclosporine-a. Rheumatol Int. 2009;29(7):821–4. https://doi.org/10.1007/s00296-008-0826-y.
46. Russell ML, Schachter RK. Cyclofenil-induced hemolytic anemia in scleroderma. Acta Med Scand. 1981;210(5):431–2.

47. Morgan JM, Adams SJ. Scleroderma and autoimmune thrombocytopenia associated with ingestion of L-tryptophan. Br J Dermatol. 1993;128(5):581–3.
48. Natsuda H, Matsui Y, Sakauchi M, et al. Progressive systemic sclerosis complicated with immune thrombocytopenia during D-penicillamine therapy. Intern Med. 1992;31(2):244–5.
49. Epstein M, Vickars L, Stein H. Diclofenac induced immune thrombocytopenia. J Rheumatol. 1990;17(10):1403–4.
50. Sterba G, Sterba Y, Stempel C, et al. Macrophage activation syndrome induced by etanercept in a patient with systemic sclerosis. Isr Med Assoc J. 2010;12(7):443–5.
51. Balaban EP, Sheehan RG, Lipsky PE, et al. Treatment of cutaneous sclerosis and aplastic anemia with antithymocyte globulin. Ann Intern Med. 1987;106(1):56–8.
52. Atteritano M, David A, Bagnato G, et al. Haemophagocytic syndrome in rheumatic patients. A systematic review. Eur Rev Med Pharmacol Sci. 2012;16(10):1414–24.
53. Dhote R, Simon J, Papo T, et al. Reactive hemophagocytic syndrome in adult systemic disease: report of twenty-six cases and literature review. Arthritis Rheum. 2003;49(5):633–9. https://doi.org/10.1002/art.11368.
54. Katsumata Y, Okamoto H, Harigai M, et al. Etoposide ameliorated refractory hemophagocytic syndrome in a patient with systemic sclerosis. Ryumachi. 2002;42(5):820–6.
55. Abudiab M, Krause ML, Fidler ME, et al. Differentiating scleroderma renal crisis from other causes of thrombotic microangiopathy in a postpartum patient. Clin Nephrol. 2013;80(4):293–7. https://doi.org/10.5414/CN107465.
56. Watanabe R, Shirai T, Tajima Y, et al. Pregnancy-associated thrombotic thrombocytopenic purpura with anti-centromere antibody-positive Raynaud's syndrome. Intern Med. 2010;49(12):1229–32.
57. D'Angelo R, Miller R. Pregnancy complicated by severe preeclampsia and thrombocytopenia in a patient with scleroderma. Anesth Analg. 1997;85(4):839–41.
58. Mishra N, Shrestha D, Poudyal RB, et al. Atypical presentation of scleroderma in infancy. Rheumatol Int. 2012;32(4):1069–74. https://doi.org/10.1007/s00296-011-1803-4.
59. Jindal AK, Gupta A, Dogra S, et al. Thrombocytopenia associated with localized scleroderma: report of four pediatric cases and review of the literature. Pediatr Dermatol. 2017;34(4):e174–e78. https://doi.org/10.1111/pde.13159.

Chapter 4
Breathlessness

Celine Ward, Katherine C. Silver, and Richard M. Silver

Breathlessness, or *dyspnea,* is a frequent complaint among patients suffering from systemic sclerosis (SSc, scleroderma) and is often the first indication of significant lung or heart disease. Dyspnea is a "synthetic sensation" often arising from multiple sources of information rather than from stimulation of a single neural receptor. This fact, together with the systemic nature of SSc, mandates a comprehensive and multidisciplinary approach to the evaluation and management of breathlessness in the patient with SSc [1]. The severity of dyspnea varies widely and is often minimized by the patient

C. Ward · R. M. Silver (✉)
Division of Rheumatology & Immunology,
Department of Medicine, Medical University of South Carolina,
Charleston, SC, USA
e-mail: wardce@musc.edu; silverr@musc.edu

K. C. Silver
Division of Rheumatology & Immunology,
Department of Medicine, Medical University of South Carolina,
Charleston, SC, USA

Division of Rheumatology & Immunology,
Department of Pediatrics, Medical University of South Carolina,
Charleston, SC, USA
e-mail: silverk@musc.edu

© Springer Nature Switzerland AG 2021
M. Matucci-Cerinic, C. P. Denton (eds.), *Practical Management of Systemic Sclerosis in Clinical Practice*, In Clinical Practice,
https://doi.org/10.1007/978-3-030-53736-4_4

who reduces the *rate* of work performance, either due to lung or heart disease, or sometimes due to non-cardiopulmonary factors, e.g., fatigue, muscle or joint pain. While standardized tools to quantify dyspnea are used in clinical trials [2], in the office setting it is more practical to assess dyspnea in terms of daily activities, e.g., walking, carrying, climbing stairs, etc., bearing in mind that some patients will have made adaptations to minimize the degree of breathlessness they might experience.

Dyspnea, when present, often signals the presence of significant lung or heart disease. When assessing the complaint of breathlessness, it is important to distinguish *acute* from *chronic* dyspnea as the evaluation and management will differ (Fig. 4.1). For most SSc patients, the onset of dyspnea is more often insidious and chronic in nature. When dyspnea occurs acutely, one should consider pulmonary as well as cardiovascular etiologies that can lead to sudden-onset breathlessness. Pulmonary infectious etiologies, e.g., pneumonia, bronchitis and aspiration, should be considered and ruled out or treated. Other pulmonary causes of acute dyspnea to be considered include: spontaneous pneumothorax in a SSc patient with subpleural blebs and honeycomb lungs; pulmonary embolism in the SSc patient with an underlying hypercoagulable state; and, reflex bronchospasm in the SSc patient with gastroesophageal reflux and aspiration. Cardiovascular causes of acute dyspnea in the SSc patient include pericarditis, rarely cardiac tamponade, acute myocardial ischemia, and acute-onset heart failure [3]. Diagnostic studies will vary according to each clinical setting, but pulmonary etiologies may be discerned with chest radiography, cultures of sputum, blood and/or bronchoalveolar lavage fluid (particularly in the immunocompromised patient), as well as by pulmonary function tests (PFTs) and CT chest scan with pulmonary embolism protocol. For cardiovascular causes of acute dyspnea, diagnostic studies might include EKG, echocardiogram, serum troponin and BNP/NT-proBNP measurements and, in some cases, cardiac catheterization with coronary angiography.

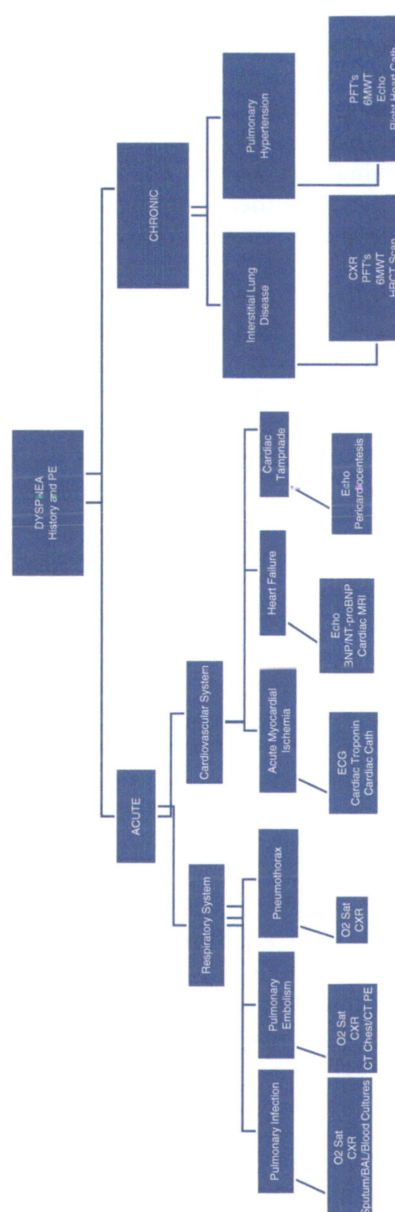

FIGURE 4.1 A diagnostic approach to dyspnea in SSc

For most SSc patients experiencing breathlessness, the onset is insidious and the course is chronic. In the evaluation of the SSc patient with chronic dyspnea, three important etiologies should be considered, keeping in mind that these causes are not mutually exclusive: (1) interstitial lung disease (SSc-ILD); (2) pulmonary arterial hypertension (SSc-PAH); and (3) cardiac disease, either primary SSc heart disease or heart disease secondary to hypertension, aging or other causes.

SSc-ILD most often is characterized as a nonspecific interstitial pneumonia (NSIP) and is the most frequent cause for chronic dyspnea in SSc [1]. Lung biopsy is rarely required for diagnosis. SSc-ILD should be suspected in the patient with dyspnea and fine inspiratory crackles on chest examination. A diagnosis of SSc-ILD is confirmed with the finding of a restrictive PFT pattern along with typical findings on the high resolution computed tomographic (HRCT) chest scan, i.e., relatively symmetric and bilateral ground-glass opacities with associated fine reticulations, often with subpleural sparing, and pulmonary volume loss resulting in traction bronchiectasis.

Pulmonary arterial hypertension (SSc-PAH) is another important cause for chronic dyspnea [4]. Here, PFTs may indicate normal spirometry and normal lung volumes, but the diffusing capacity for carbon monoxide (DL_{CO}) is reduced and the DL_{CO} does not correct when adjusted for alveolar volume (DL/VA). Echocardiography is an essential screening test in any SSc patient who is short of breath. If there are any finding suspicious for PAH, e.g., elevation of right ventricular systolic pressure (RVSP), abnormal size and function of the right ventricle, septal bowing, etc., right heart catheterization (RHC), the gold standard for diagnosing PAH, would be indicated. RHC demonstration of elevated mean pulmonary artery pressure (mPAP >20 mmHg) at rest together with normal pulmonary capillary wedge pressure (PCWP) and high pulmonary vascular resistance (PVR > 3 Wood units) is diagnostic of PAH. If the mean PAP is elevated in the setting of a high PCWP, pulmonary venous hypertension due to diastolic dysfunction or primary SSc heart disease should be suspected. Additional testing to evaluate cardiovascular causes for chronic dyspnea might include serum levels of BNP/NT-proBNP and troponin and, in some cases, cardiac MRI [3].

To illustrate our approach to the SSc patient with *chronic* dyspnea, we present the following two patients, one of whom was found to have SSc-ILD and the other SSc-PAH.

Case One. A 75-year-old female was in her usual state of health until about 4 months prior to presentation when she developed swelling and pain in both hands and feet along with fatigue. Her fingers were "puffy" and she was having difficulty performing activities of daily living. She also reported the new development of color change of her fingers during cold exposure consistent with Raynaud phenomenon. These symptoms were accompanied by cough and dyspnea. Initially, she was evaluated in an Emergency Department and treated with antibiotics when a diagnosis of pneumonia was suspected due to abnormalities on chest x-ray. Upon referral to Rheumatology, she was found to have an oxygen saturation of 96% while breathing room air, and she was noted to have puffy fingers, proximal skin thickening, abnormal nailfold capillaries and anti-Scl70 antibodies consistent with a diagnosis of diffuse cutaneous systemic sclerosis (dcSSc). Pulmonary exam was notable for bibasilar inspiratory crackles. Given the diagnosis of dcSSc with dyspnea and bibasilar crackles, there was a high level of concern for pulmonary involvement. PFTs revealed a forced vital capacity (FVC) of 75% predicted, total lung capacity (TLC) of 70% predicted, and diffusing capacity for carbon monoxide (DL_{CO}) of 57% predicted, which corrected to 97% when adjusted for alveolar volume (DL/VA). On 6-minute walk test (6MWT) the distance walked was moderately reduced and her oxygen saturation (O_2 sat) fell to 93%. HRCT chest scan revealed basilar and peripheral predominant reticular opacities, traction bronchiectasis, consolidation and ground glass opacities without honeycombing, a pattern consistent with nonspecific interstitial pneumonia (NSIP). Additionally, an echocardiogram revealed a normal estimated right ventricular systolic pressure (RVSP) of 26 mmHg. SSc-ILD was diagnosed, and treatment with mycophenolate mofetil (MMF) was instituted. After 4 months of MMF treatment, she was noticeably improved. Cough and dyspnea had resolved. PFTs and 6MWT were repeated as objective measures of response to therapy. 6MWT distance improved and the O_2 sat improved, falling to only 98%. FVC and TLC normalized (98% and 87% predicted, respectively). PFTs also showed an increase in DL_{CO} from 57% to 71% predicted. The excellent outcome in this case is likely attributable to early diagnosis and prompt management with immunosuppressive therapy. Scleroderma Lung Study II and other studies support the use of MMF as initial therapy for SSc-ILD [5, 6]. Other immunosuppressive agents have also been used with varied success, and the addition of anti-fibrotic drug therapy is another consideration.

Case Two. A 70-year-old female presented with a 2-year history of worsening dyspnea on exertion and reduced exercise capacity. She noted increased dyspnea when climbing two flights of stairs or when walking on an incline. She had an 11-year history of limited cutaneous systemic sclerosis (lcSSc) manifested by Raynaud phenomenon, telangiectasias, calcinosis and gastroesophageal reflux disease. An earlier HRCT chest scan had shown mild peripheral, basilar predominant reticulations and ground glass opacification. To evaluate the worsening dyspnea, PFTs were performed and revealed forced vital capacity (FVC) of 85% predicted, forced expiratory volume at 1 sec (FEV1) of 79% predicted, diffusing capacity for carbon monoxide (DL_{CO}) of 52% predicted and a DL_{CO} adjusted for alveolar volume (DL/VA) of 62%. On 6MWT, she walked 460 meters without significant O_2 desaturation (96%). HRCT chest scan showed mild ILD and was unchanged from baseline. Echocardiogram showed an estimated right ventricular systolic pressure (eRVSP) of 39 mmHg. SSc-PAH was suspected on the basis of worsening dyspnea, increased eRVSP on echocardiogram, a declining DL_{CO} that did not correct for alveolar volume. Additionally, serum B-type natriuretic peptide (BNP) was noted to be mildly elevated (120 pg/mL, normal <100 pg/mL). Right heart catheterization was performed and revealed an elevated mean pulmonary artery pressure (mPAP) at rest of 27 mmHg, normal pulmonary capillary wedge pressure (PCWP) of 12 mmHg, and elevated pulmonary vascular resistance (PVR) of 3.97 Wood units, thus confirming a diagnosis of SSc-PAH. Initial combination therapy with tadalafil and ambrisentan was instituted. Dyspnea and exercise capacity improved, and she was able to walk longer distances even on an incline. Serum BNP normalized (84 pg/mL). The excellent outcome in this case is attributable to a high index of suspicion for PAH in a dyspneic lcSSc patient with PFT and echocardiographic findings suggestive of PAH, followed by early confirmation with RHC. Treatment of mildly symptomatic (WHO Functional Class II) PAH patients has been shown to be beneficial [7], and initial combination therapy with tadalafil and ambrisentan, as in this case, has been shown to be superior to monotherapy [8].

References

1. Silver KC, Silver RM. Management of systemic sclerosis-associated interstitial lung disease. In: Mayes MD, editor. Rheumatic disease clinics of N America, Vol. 41, number 3. Philadelphia: Elsevier; 2015. p. 439–58.
2. Parshall MB, Schwartzstein RM, Adams L, et al. An official American Thoracic Society statement: update on the mechanisms, assessment, and management of dyspnea. Am J Respir Crit Care Med. 2012;185(4):435–52.
3. Parks JL, Taylor MH, Parks LP, Silver RM. Systemic sclerosis and the heart. Rheum Dis Clin N Amer. 2014;40:87–102.
4. Sundaram SM, Chung L. An update on systemic sclerosis-associated pulmonary arterial hypertension: a review of the current literature. Curr Rheumatol Rep. 2018;20(2):10. https://doi.org/10.1007/s11926-018-0709-5.
5. Tashkin DP, Roth MD, Clements PJ, et al. Mycophenolate mofetil versus oral cyclophosphamide in scleroderma-related interstitial lung disease: scleroderma lung study II (SLS-II), a double-blind,

parallel group, randomized controlled trial. Lancet Respir Med. 2016;4:708–19.

6. Volkmann ER, Tashkin DP. Treatment of systemic sclerosis-related interstitial lung disease: a review of existing and emerging therapies. Ann Am Thorac Soc. 2016;13(11):2045–56.
7. Galie N, Rubin L, Hoeper M, et al. Treatment of patients with mildly symptomatic pulmonary arterial hypertension with bosentan (EARLY study): a double-blind, randomized controlled trial. Lancet. 2008;371:2093–100.
8. Galie N, Barbera JA, Frost AE, et al. Initial use of ambrisentan plus tadalafil in pulmonary arterial hypertension. N Engl J Med. 2015;373(9):834–44.

Chapter 5
Itch

Nicolas Hunzelmann, Pia Moinzadeh, and Thomas Krieg

Case Vignette

55-year-old male patient with a disease duration of 5 years, a diffuse cutaneous form of SSc (mRSS 20), including GI involvement and stable lung fibrosis, is presenting with dryness of skin and an increased sensation of itch, involving mostly the extremities and parts oft he trunk. Itch is so severe that he gets awakened at night. Use of ointment from a drug store provided no relief. His previous medical history is remarkable for allergic rhino-conjunctivitis due to grass pollen. Furthermore, his only son suffers from atopic eczema.

Background

Itch (pruritus) is a very common problem in the general population with a 12-month incidence of up to 7% [1, 2]. In patients with SSc, itch may be present in up to 60% of cases and a correlation with disease severity has been described

---

N. Hunzelmann (✉) · P. Moinzadeh · T. Krieg
Dept. of Dermatology, University of Cologne, Köln, Germany
e-mail: nico.hunzelmann@uni-koeln.de;
pia.moinzadeh@uk-koeln.de; thomas.krieg@uni-koeln.de

© Springer Nature Switzerland AG 2021
M. Matucci-Cerinic, C. P. Denton (eds.), *Practical Management of Systemic Sclerosis in Clinical Practice*, In Clinical Practice,
https://doi.org/10.1007/978-3-030-53736-4_5

[3–6]. In addition, it has also been shown that the presence of itch correlates independently with the severity of skin hardening and greater GI involvement and remained predominantly stable in the course of the disease [5, 7].

In general, Itch may be directly associated with skin diseases or can be secondary due to internal organ involvement .. The exact causative mechanisms for itch in SSc still have to be elucidated. It is tempting to speculate that several pathophysiological events contribute to the clinical symptom of itch in SSc patients. Inflammatory processes in the dermis, the subsequent loss of skin appendages by the fibrotic process in combination with the loss of the ability to synthesize appropriate amounts of "endogenous lipids and emollients" contributes to skin xerosis are probably major factors [7]. Furthermore, entrapping of sensory nerve fibers can also contribute to the development of pruritus.

Due to comorbidities, itch is often not taken sufficiently into consideration with its effect on well being of the patient, although it may significantly affect quality of life, disturb sleeping and contribute to mood disorders and depression [7]. Therefore adequate symptomatic therapy of itch is an important component of multimodal therapy in SSc patients.

Differential Diagnosis

Differential diagnosis of pruritus encompasses a wide array of dermatological and non-dermatological diseases (see Fig. 5.1). Medical history (including onset, duration, location, quality and severity of itch) and skin examination are the basis of an initial assessment [8].

In chronic pruritus (i.e., persisting longer than 6 weeks) a complete dermatological examination is mandatory to exclude comorbidities and underlying systemic dieseases. It also has to be considered that a number of drugs may induce or maintain chronic pruritus [8].

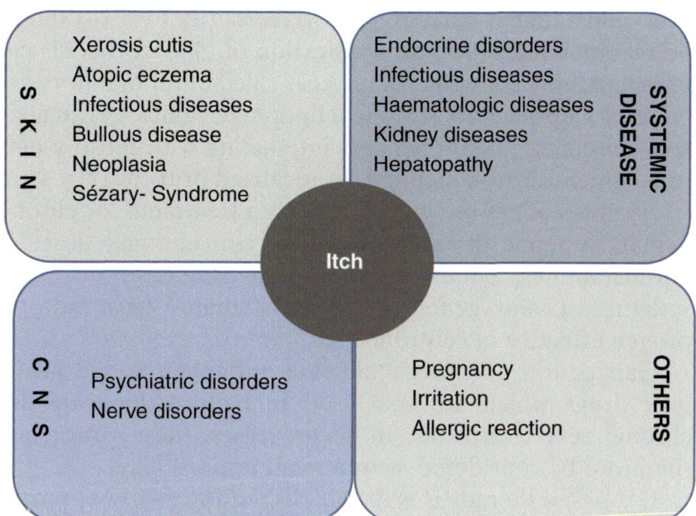

FIGURE 5.1 Differential diagnosis of SSc associated Itch

Therapy

The patient in this vignette suffers from a diffuse cutaneous SSc, but also has a history of atopic disease, indicating an increased risk to have dry skin (xerosis cutis) and develop atopic eczema.

As a first step, the patient should be informed about general pruritus-relieving measures as keeping room temperatures stable and applying moisturizers to improve skin barrier and reduce itching [2]. Although many patients report that hot or cold showers reduce itch, no scientific studies have been performed to confirm this observation and repeated showering leads to drying up of the skin. Avoidance of frequent bathing and showers is strongly recommended.

Topical therapy will be the mainstay of initial treatment. Usually, the patients apply emollients that have a high-water content favoring resorption, but having no effect on the skin texture and reducing itch sensation. Hence, an emollient containing urea (3–10%), lactic acid (1–5%, increasing hydration) and a higher percentage of glycerol (up to 20%) should be recommended. Topical application of glucocorticoids can reduce itching for some time. Also calcineurininhibitors can be used. Capsaicin (0.025% in a lipophilic vehicle), is an alkaloid contained in chili peppers interacting with sensory neurons, which is recommended for localized pruritus [2].

Antihistamines are widely used as a treatment for chronic itch in systemic diseases. However, conventional doses of antihistamines, either sedating first generation or non-sedating second generation antihistamines have not yet proven effective in controlled studies.

Gabapentin and pregabalin are antiepileptic and anxiolytic drugs which are also used in neuropathic pain and chronic severe pruritus. In severe cases, these drugs may therefore be considered as treatment options [2, 9].

UV-based therapy is well established for treating pruritus. UV modalities comprise UVB (290–320 nm) and UVA (320–400 nm). Usually, UV therapy is combined with topical treatment. A number of uncontrolled studies indicate a beneficial effect of UVA1 and photochemotherapy (Psoralen + UVA) on fibrosis in SSc leading to softening of the skin [10, 11] (Morita et al., 1995, 2000). In addition, UV therapy is also reducing the inflammatory response. Therefore, in severe pruritus these options should be considered. Systemic therapy of the underlying disease by mycophenolate mofetil, rituximab or cyclophosphamide in severely affected patients with dsSSc leads to a reduction of the inflammation and can influence the extent of itching.

In conclusion, management of itch in SSc patients comprises proper diagnosis and exclusion of other factors [12]. Treatment consists of topical treatment modalities accompanied by systemic and UV-therapy. In protracted, recalcitrant itch an interdisciplinary approach involving a dermatologist is mandatory.

References

1. Matterne U, Apfelbacher CJ, Vogelgsang L, Loerbroks A, Weisshaar E. Incidence and determinants of chronic pruritus: a population-based cohort study. Acta Derm Venereol. 2013;93(5):532–7.
2. Stander S, Zeidler C, Augustin M, Bayer G, Kremer AE, Legat FJ, et al. S2k guidelines for the diagnosis and treatment of chronic pruritus - update - short version. J Dtsch Dermatol Ges. 2017;15(8):860–72.
3. Haber JS, Valdes-Rodriguez R, Yosipovitch G. Chronic pruritus and connective tissue disorders: review, gaps, and future directions. Am J Clin Dermatol. 2016;17(5):445–9.
4. Razykov I, Thombs BD, Hudson M, Bassel M, Baron M. Canadian Scleroderma Research G. prevalence and clinical correlates of pruritus in patients with systemic sclerosis. Arthritis Rheum. 2009;61(12):1765 70.
5. Razykov I, Levis B, Hudson M, Baron M, Thombs BD, Canadian Scleroderma Research G. Prevalence and clinical correlates of pruritus in patients with systemic sclerosis: an updated analysis of 959 patients. Rheumatology (Oxford). 2013;52(11):2056–61.
6. El-Baalbaki G, Razykov I, Hudson M, Bassel M, Baron M, Thombs BD, et al. Association of pruritus with quality of life and disability in systemic sclerosis. Arthritis Care Res. 2010;62(10):1489–95.
7. Stull CM, Weaver LA, Valdes-Rodriguez R, Naramala S, Lavery MJ, Chan YH, et al. Characteristics of chronic itch in systemic sclerosis: a cross-sectional survey. Acta Derm Venereol. 2018;98(8):793–4.
8. Stander S, Weisshaar E, Mettang T, Szepietowski JC, Carstens E, Ikoma A, et al. Clinical classification of itch: a position paper of the international forum for the study of itch. Acta Derm Venereol. 2007;87(4):291–4.
9. Kaur R, Sinha VR. Antidepressants as antipruritic agents: a review. Eur Neuropsychopharmacol. 2018;28(3):341–52.
10. Breuckmann F, Gambichler T, Altmeyer P, Kreuter A. UVA/UVA1 phototherapy and PUVA photochemotherapy in connective tissue diseases and related disorders: a research based review. BMC Dermatol. 2004;4(1):11.

11. Connolly KL, Griffith JL, McEvoy M, Lim HW. Ultraviolet A1 phototherapy beyond morphea: experience in 83 patients. Photodermatol Photoimmunol Photomed. 2015;31(6):289–95.
12. Pereira MP, Steinke S, Zeidler C, Forner C, Riepe C, Augustin M, et al. European academy of dermatology and venereology European prurigo project: expert consensus on the definition, classification and terminology of chronic prurigo. J Eur Acad Dermatol Venereol. 2018;32(7):1059–65.

Chapter 6
Mood Problems and Depression in Systemic Sclerosis

Alexandra Balbir-Gurman and Yolanda Braun-Moscovici

Introduction

Systemic sclerosis (SSc) is a severe disease with skin and internal organ fibrosis. A progressive course, complications, functional limitations, multiple visits to the clinic, hospitalizations, an uncertain prognosis often lead to mood disorders, such as depression and anxiety. Pain, chronicity, compromised physical health, disfigurement, limited treatment options, and disability negatively affect Health Related Quality of Life (HRQoL) [1]. Mood disorders and depression may overlap with SSc.

Depression is characterized as sad mood, loss of interest or pleasure, feelings of guilt, low self-esteem, poor concentration, disturbed sleep and/or appetite, loss of energy, and psychomotor dysfunction for more than 2 weeks [2]. A diagnosis of depression is based on patient interview, documented use of antidepressants or psychiatric consultation.

A. Balbir-Gurman (✉) · Y. Braun-Moscovici
B. Shine Rheumatology Institute, Rambam Health Care Campus and The Rappaport Faculty of Medicine, Technion, Haifa, Israel
e-mail: a_balbir@rambam.health.gov.il; y_braun@rambam.health.gov.il

© Springer Nature Switzerland AG 2021

M. Matucci-Cerinic, C. P. Denton (eds.), *Practical Management of Systemic Sclerosis in Clinical Practice*, In Clinical Practice,
https://doi.org/10.1007/978-3-030-53736-4_6

The relative risk of depression in SSc patients is 3.3–6.9 [3]; depression comprised 73.2% and anxiety 23.9% of all mood disorders in SSc [4]. About 18.1% of SSc patients hospitalizations were due to depression and about 4.4% to psychosis [5]. SSc patients have a higher incidence of depression than patients with other rheumatic diseases [6–8]. SSc was an independent risk factor for depression [9]. SSc patients may develop adjustment disorders (dysthymia or alexithymia), or a mild, moderate or major depressive disorder (MDD). Mild depression was reported in 36–69%, moderate in 20%, MDD in 5% of patients [10–12]. Lifetime MDD was reported in 22.9%, current MDD (30 days) in 3.8% and 12 months MDD in 10.7% of patients; MDD is associated with low vitality and suicidal ideation [13, 14]. Depression correlated with poor indexes of FACIT-Fatigue score, Health Assessment Questionnaire-Disability Index, and Center for Epidemiologic Studies Depression. Patients with SSc have a reduced capacity to perform previous duties, they are absent from work, lose social position and income [15]. Depression correlated with all case mortality in SSc patients [9]. Depression and psychosis increased the risk of in-hospital mortality among SSc patients [5].

Anxiety is an exaggerated reaction to stress, pain, disability, and uncertainty, presenting with fear, anger, or panic disorder; it often complements depression [16]. The prevalence of anxiety is 35–80% [1, 10, 17, 18]. Patients fear SSc complications, assessments, hospitalization, limited number of specialists specializing in scleroderma, SSc progress, disfigurement, disability and early death [19].

We report on a severe case of MDD. A 42-year-old female school teacher was diagnosed with SSc and myositis 3 years ago. She presented with Raynaud's phenomenon, arthralgia, muscle weakness, dyspepsia, digital ulcers, interstitial lung disease, diffuse skin thickening (DcSSc), severe interstitial cystitis which required self-catheterizations, elevated creatine kinase levels and positive anti-topoisomerase antibodies. The patient was treated with corticosteroids, omeprazole, iloprost, mycophenolate mofetil, elatrol, and intravenous immunoglobulins. She was strongly supported by family members but developed a reduced mood, disturbed sleep and feelings of guilt. Serial psychological interventions, occupational and physical therapy were started; pregabalin was added by a psychiatrist. Later, the patient was admitted for MDD with suicidal ideation; escitalopram and brotizolam were started; pregabalin was changed to duloxetine. Gradually, her condition improved; on her last visit to the clinic, she was physically and mentally stable. *One may learn, that early diagnosis of depression, recruitment of psychologist and psychiatrist, organizing of "supporting circle" could help in stabilization of patient's mental health.*

Contributory Factors Related to Mood Disorders

Pains and pruritus significantly contribute to depression; 75% of patients reported pain; pain impairs sleep, induces fatigue, functional limitation, and disability. *Sleep disorders* aggravate depression, pain, and vice versa [20, 21]; 76% of SSc patients have sleep disturbances [22]. Dyspnea, fatigue, digestive problems, digital ulcers, pruritus, and depression have a major influence on sleep [21,23–25]. *Fatigue* is described as persistent exhaustion, inability to perform, and a need to invest additional effort; 89% of SSc patients reported fatigue [23]. Fatigue is associated with digestive and respiratory problems, pain, depression, impaired coping capacity, and reduced HRQoL [26–28]. Fatigue in SSc patients was significantly worse than in cancer patients in remission, and was compatible with cancer patients on active treatment [29]. The negative effect of fatigue progresses with life-time [30].

Scleroderma-Related Features and Mood Disorders

Hand stiffness, Raynaud's phenomenon, digital ulcers, early SSc, DcSSc, dyspnea, reflux, fecal incontinence, malnutrition, renal crisis, sexual dysfunction, and urinary tract abnormalities are associated with depression and/or anxiety [11, 31–37]. Disfigurement with facial and hand changes and telangiectasia correlated with depression, anxiety, and impaired HRQoL [12, 16, 27, 38–40]. Low Appearance Self-Esteem score in SSc patients correlated with depression, anxiety and disability [19].

Possible Pathogenic Mechanisms of Mood Disorders in SSc

Inability of the immune system may lead to insufficient physical and psychological defense mechanisms; long-lasting psychological and physical distress predisposes to mood disorders. Possible mechanisms for the development of depression were proposed: dysfunction of microvasculature in central nervous system [41], impaired cortisol response to stress [42], dysregulation of serotonin synthesis [43], and excessive production of Interleukin-1, Tumor Necrosis Factor-alpha and Interleukin-6; their levels correlate with active inflammation and fibrosis and induce fatigue and sleep disturbances in patients with inflammatory diseases and correlated with depression.

Patients' Perspectives

A patient's perception of SSc has a major impact on mental scores [44]; patients with "illness identity" had reduced functional capacity and ineffective coping with scleroderma [45]. Patients wish to participate in support groups with emphasis on education, including family members, information on centers specializing in SSc [46]; 78.6% indicated "education" as a major need with an accent on information about SSc, medications, alternative medicine, relaxing strategies and exercise programs, coping with pain, fatigue, stress and changes in appearance, information on social services, disability and prognosis.

Patients' associations are helpful in providing balanced information and sharing coping styles, such as "think positive"; media and the internet can be additional channels to learn about scleroderma [47].

Case 2. A 34-year-old patient has suffered from scleroderma for 4 years; her main problems include skin involvement, digital ulcers, esophageal reflux, and mild interstitial lung disease. The patient was very anxious about her pulmonary condition; in recent months, she arrived at the emergency room several times with severe attacks of cough and dyspnea. Repeated imaging, respiratory function, and oxygen saturation tests showed no worsening of lung condition. In repeated conversations it became clear that the patient had been suffering from esophageal reflux with probable micro-aspirations. She had received a detailed explanation from a rheumatologist, had been evaluated by a gastroenterologist. A detailed explanation of eating arrangements, prevention of food before lying down, lifting of a pillow, conversation with clinical psychologists, and acupuncture treatment resulted in an improvement in respiratory condition. *Symptoms of SSc and anxiety may overlap; patient' education and advices how to manage disease complication may help to both, scleroderma and mood disorder.*

How to Provide Better Health Care to SSc Patients with Mood Disorders

Severe emotional distress in early DcSSc or exhaustion in long-standing disease leads to cognitive impairment, poor compliance with treatment, loss of interest and energy, and progression to MDD; psychosis and delirium are rare in scleroderma. It is crucial to diagnose mood disorders early.

The approach to SSc patients includes proper attention to mood disorders, building a relationship with the patient on the basis of deep empathy and trust, providing available access for help, construction of "supportive circle" with family members and care-providers, and simultaneous treatment of scleroderma symptoms and mood disorders. Physicians should make an effort to understand the patient's feeling to indicate the problem. Detailed anamnesis should include the patient's description of symptoms (pains, pruritus, sleep quality, fatigue, and organ specific problems), family history of autoimmune and mental diseases, smoking, alcohol, and drugs. Compliance with medications and probable adverse events need to be checked. Functional disability, mouth and hand handicap, disfigurement, disability, social aspects (input, role in the family and society, meetings, pleasure) should be appreciated; it is useful to meet family members and informal care-givers. Identification of mood disorder, especially moderate and severe depression, is an indication to assessment by psychologist and psychiatrist and prescription of medications (selective serotonin reuptake inhibitors, selective serotonin and norepinephrine reuptake inhibitors, pregabalin). Treatment of mood disorders should include psychological support, providing the way to "positive" thinking, behavior therapy aimed at restoring a positive attitude, helping in understanding the situation, learning to adapt demands and expectations to new conditions, priorities, and construction problem-solving plans. Patients should be taught how to avoid stressing or challenging situations and how to balance between functioning and disease, how to cope with Raynaud's phenomenon and digital ulcers, how to prevent cough and aspiration caused by reflux, how to keep joint range of movement and muscle strength. Patients need an explanation on the importance of regular blood tests and cardiac and pulmonary assessments, measurement of blood pressure and weight, and treatments options; they need to be sensitive to changes in their body and soul. Providing online support by a nurse, psychologist and the treating rheumatologist with problem-oriented and real-life information is of great importance.

Case 3. A 35-year-old woman developed progressive SSc with joint contractures and digital ucers. She had pain, itching, evere fatigue and could not sleep. Difficulties at work and at home made her sad. We advised her to stop working and adjust activities to her new situation. She was treated with cyclophosphamide, bosentan, and abatacept; there was gradual improvement of skin and joints condition and digital ulcers. In addition, she was putted on multidisciplinary program with contemporary care by nurse, psychologist, occupational therapist and "drama-therapy". Patient' high motivation and "positive attitude", family and care-providers support were fruitful: after 2 years of fighting, she could return to half-time work and some of her regular activities, including social gatherings and trips abroad. During her last visit to the department, she said, "I learned to accept my illness with dignity, to give it a place in my life, I do not like my illness, but I think it changed me and gave me strength to be an another person. I did not realized, how strong I could be!". *It is very important to recruit patient' positive attitude and teach to choose the right priorities and to look for positive side in every situation, be motivated and try to bring life back to normal. Multidisciplinary approach can certainly provide an answer.*

Conclusion

Patients with SSc often have mood disorders; they correlate with more severe skin and joint problems, functional limitation, and disability. SSc is characterized by a variety of organ involvement with a diverse course and severe prognosis; absence of radical treatment makes patients insecure and hopeless. Dyspnea, Raynaud's phenomenon, pain, fatigue, sleep disturbances, gastro-intestinal tract dysmotility and disfigurement induce impaired patients' HRQoL. Mental disorders often run subtle and underdiagnosed; patients with scleroderma receive less or late treatment in this regard. Mood disorders aggravate SSc symptoms, cause poor disease perception and compliance, social isolation and work disability; they have an adverse effect on treatment outcomes and survival of patients with SSc. Building of a multidisciplinary team in centers specializing in the treatment of SSc are of great importance in physicians' and patients' perspectives; they provide advanced support which includes a spectrum of physicians' sub-specialties (rheumatologists, pulmonologists, cardiologists, gastroenterologists, etc.) and health-care providers (nurses, psychologist, occupational therapists, physiotherapists, etc.). Empathic relationships between the patient and treating team, accessebility and personalized care are the best way to achieve patients trust and compliance. Use of various formats for patients' education, such as formal lectures, patients' meetings or support groups; media and on-line facilities will provide better eligibility of information, understanding of SSc features, and treatment modalities. Recruitment of a psychologist and social worker to a multidisciplinary team will contribute to the early recognition of mood disorders and treatment with a positive effect on a feeling of secure, improved compliance, better coping with SSc, and improvement in HRQoL.

References

1. Ostojic P, Zivojinovic S, Reza T, Damjanov N. Symptoms of depression and anxiety in Serbian patients with systemic sclerosis: impact of disease severity and socioeconomic factors. Mod Rheumatol. 2010;20:353–7. https://doi.org/10.1007/s10165-010-0285-7.
2. Kwakkenbos L, Delisle VC, Fox RS, et al. Psychosocial aspects of scleroderma. Rheum Dis Clin N Am. 2015;41:519–28. https://doi.org/10.1016/j.rdc.2015.04.010.
3. Robinson D Jr, Eisenberg D, Nietert PJ, et al. Systemic sclerosis prevalence and comorbidities in systemic sclerosis prevalence and comorbidities in the US 2002-2002. Curr Med Res Opin. 2008;24:1157–66. https://doi.org/10.1185/030079908X280617.
4. Amaral TN, Peres FA, Lapa AT, Marques-Neto JF, Appenzeller S. Neurologic involvement in scleroderma: a systematic review. Semin Arthritis Rheum. 2013;43:335–47. https://doi.org/10.1016/j.semarthrit.2013.05.002.

5. Amoda O, Ravat V, Datta S, Saroha B, Patel RS. Trends in demographics , hospitalization outcomes , comorbidities , and mortality risk among systemic sclerosis patients. Cureus. 2018;10:e2628. https://doi.org/10.7759/cureus.2628.
6. Thombs BD, Taillefer SS, Hudson M, Baron M. Depression in patients with systemic sclerosis: a systematic review of the evidence. Arthritis Rheum. 2007;15(57):1089–97.
7. Malcarne VL, Fox RS, Mills SD. Psychosocial aspects of systemic sclerosis. Curr Opin Rheumatol. 2013;25:707–13. https://doi.org/10.1097/01.bor.0000434666.47397.c2.
8. Hyphantis TN, Tsifetaki N, Siafaka V, et al. The impact of psychological arthritis, functioning upon systemic sclerosis patients' quality of life. Semin Rheum. 2007;37:81–92.
9. Bragazzi NL, Watad A, Gizunterman A, et al. The burden of depression in systemic sclerosis patients: a nationwide population-based study. J Affect Disord. 2019;243:427–31. https://doi.org/10.1016/j.jad.2018.09.075.
10. Leon L, Abasolo L, Redondo M, et al. Negative affect in systemic sclerosis. Rheumatol Int. 2014;34:597–604. https://doi.org/10.1007/s00296-013-2852-7.
11. Faezi ST, Paragomi P, Shahali A, et al. Prevalence and severity of depression and anxiety in patients with systemic sclerosis: an epidemiologic survey and investigation of clinical correlates. J Clin Rheumatol. 2017;23:80–6. https://doi.org/10.1097/RHU.0000000000000428.
12. Tedeschini E, Pingani L, Simoni E, et al. Correlation of articular involvement , skin disfigurement and unemployment with depressive symptoms in patients with systemic sclerosis : a hospital sample. Int J Rheum Dis. 2014;17:186–94. https://doi.org/10.1111/1756-185X.12100.
13. Razykov I, Hudson M, Baron M, Thombs BD. Utility of the patient health Questionnaire-9 to assess suicide risk in patients with systemic sclerosis. 2013;65:753–8. https://doi.org/10.1002/acr.21894.
14. Jewett LR, Razykov I, Hudson M, Baron M, Thombs BD. Prevalence of current , 12-month and lifetime major depressive disorder among patients with systemic sclerosis. Rheumatology (Oxford). 2013;52:669–75. https://doi.org/10.1093/rheumatology/kes347.
15. Singh MK, Clements PJ, Furst DE, Maranian P, Khanna D. Work productivity in scleroderma: analysis from the University of California, Los Angeles, scleroderma quality of life study. 2012;64:176–83. https://doi.org/10.1002/acr.20676.

16. Nguyen C, Ranque B, Baubet T, et al. Clinical, functional and health-related quality of life correlates of clinically significant symptoms of anxiety and depression in patients with systemic sclerosis: a cross-sectional survey. PLoS One. 2014;9:e90484. https://doi.org/10.1371/journal.pone.0090484.
17. Lisitsyna TA, Veltishchev DY, Seravina OF, et al. Comparative analysis of anxiety-depressive spectrum disorders in patients with rheumatic diseases. Ter Arkh. 2018;11(90):30–7. https://doi.org/10.26442/terarkh201890530-37.
18. Baubet T, Ranque B, Taïeb O, et al. Anxiété et dépression chez les patients atteints de sclérodermie systémique. Presse Med. 2011;40:e111–9. https://doi.org/10.1016/j.lpm.2010.09.019.
19. Van Lankveld WGJM, Vonk MC, Teunissen H, van den Hoogen FH. Appearance self-esteem in systemic sclerosis — subjective experience of skin deformity and its relationship with physician-assessed skin involvement , disease status and psychological variables. Rheumatology (Oxford). 2007;46:872–6. https://doi.org/10.1093/rheumatology/kem008.
20. Irwin MR, Miller AH. Depressive disorders and immunity: 20 years of progress and discovery. Brain Behav Immun. 2007;21(4):374–83.
21. Sariyildiz MA, Batmaz I, Budulgan M, et al. Sleep quality in patients with systemic sclerosis: relationship between the clinical variables, depressive symptoms, functional status, and the quality of life. Rheumatol Int. 2013;33:1973–9. https://doi.org/10.1007/s00296-013-2680-9.
22. Bassel M, Hudson M, Taillefer SS, Schieir O, Baron M, Thombs BD. Frequency and impact of symptoms experienced by patients with systemic sclerosis: results from a Canadian National Survey. Rheumatology (Oxford). 2011;50:762–7. https://doi.org/10.1093/rheumatology/keq310.
23. Strickland G, Pauling J, Cavill C, McHugh N. Predictors of health-related quality of life and fatigue in systemic sclerosis: evaluation of the EuroQol-5D and FACIT-F assessment tools. Clin Rheumatol. 2012;31:1215–22. https://doi.org/10.1007/s10067-012-1997-1.
24. Prado GF, Allen RP, Trevisani VM, Toscano VG, Earley CJ. Sleep disruption in systemic sclerosis (scleroderma) patients: clinical and polysomnographic findings. Sleep Med. 2002;3:341–5.
25. Frech T, Hays RD, Maranian P, Clements PJ, Furst DE, Khanna D. Prevalence and correlates of sleep disturbance in systemic sclerosis — results from the UCLA scleroderma quality of

life study. Rheumatology (Oxford). 2011;50:1280–7. https://doi.org/10.1093/rheumatology/ker020.

26. Basta F, Afeltra A, Margiotta DPE. Fatigue in systemic sclerosis: a systematic review. Clin Exp Rheumatol. 2018;36 Suppl 113(4):150–60.
27. Maddali-Bongi S, Del Rosso A, Mikhaylova S, et al. Impact of hand and face disabilities on global disability and quality of life in systemic sclerosis patients. Clin Exp Rheumatol. 2014;32(6 Suppl 86):S-15-20.
28. Frikha F, Masmoudi J, Saidi N, Bahloul Z. Sexual dysfunction in married women with systemic sclerosis. Pan Afr Med J. 2014;17:82. https://doi.org/10.11604/pamj.2014.17.82.3833.
29. Thombs BD, Bassel M, Mcguire L, Smith MT, Hudson M, Haythornthwaite JA. A systematic comparison of fatigue levels in systemic sclerosis with general population , cancer and rheumatic disease samples. Rheumatology. 2008;47:1559–63. https://doi.org/10.1093/rheumatology/ken331.
30. Assassi S, Leyva AL, Mayes MD, Sharif R, Nair DK. Predictors of fatigue severity in early systemic sclerosis: a prospective longitudinal study of the GENISOS cohort. PLoS One. 2011;6:e26061. https://doi.org/10.1371/journal.pone.0026061.
31. Chularojanamontri L, Sethabutra P, Kulthanan K, Manapajon A. Dermatology life quality index in Thai patients with systemic sclerosis: a cross-sectional study. Indian J Dermatol Venereol Leprol. 2011;77:683–7. https://doi.org/10.4103/0378-6323.86481.
32. Khanna D, Ahmed M, Furst DE, et al. Health values of patients with systemic sclerosis. 2007;57:86–93. https://doi.org/10.1002/art.22465.
33. Del Rosso A, Boldrini M, D'Agostino D, et al. Health-related quality of life in systemic sclerosis as measured by the short form 36: relationship with clinical and biologic markers. Arthritis Rheum. 2004;51:475–81. https://doi.org/10.1002/art.20389.
34. Bodukam V, Hays RD, Maranian P, et al. Association of gastrointestinal involvement and depressive symptoms in patients with systemic sclerosis. Rheumatology (Oxford). 2011;50:330–4. https://doi.org/10.1093/rheumatology/keq296.
35. Omair MA, Lee P. Effect of gastrointestinal manifestations on quality of life in 87 consecutive patients with systemic sclerosis. J Rheumatol. 2012;39:992–6. https://doi.org/10.3899/jrheum.110826.
36. Foocharoen C, Tyndall A, Hachulla E, et al. Erectile dysfunction is frequent in systemic sclerosis and associated with severe disease: a study of the EULAR scleroderma trial and research

group. Arthritis Res Ther. 2012;14:R37. https://doi.org/10.1186/ar3748.

37. Sanchez K, Denys P, Giuliano F, et al. Systemic sclerosis: sexual dysfunction and lower urinary tract symptoms in 73 patients. Presse Med. 2016;45(4):e79–89. https://doi.org/10.1016/j.lpm.2015.08.009.
38. Benrud-Larson LM, Haythornthwaite JA, Heinberg LJ, et al. The impact of pain and symptoms of depression in scleroderma. Pain. 2002;95:267–75.
39. Thombs BD, van Lankveld W, Bassel M, et al. Psychological health and Well-being in systemic sclerosis: state of the science and consensus research agenda. Arthritis Care Res. 2010;62:1181–9. https://doi.org/10.1002/acr.20187.
40. Amin K, Sivakumar B, Clarke A, Puri A, Denton C, Butler PE. Hand disease in scleroderma: a clinical correlate for chronic hand transplant rejection. Springerplus. 2013;2:577. https://doi.org/10.1186/2193-1801-2-577.
41. Mohamed RH, Nassef AA. Brain magnetic resonance imaging findings in patients with systemic sclerosis. Int J Rheum Dis. 2010;13:61–7. https://doi.org/10.1111/j.1756-185X.2009.01453.x.
42. Bagnato G, Cordova F, Sciortino D, et al. Association between cortisol levels and pain threshold in systemic sclerosis and major depression. Rheumatol Int. 2018;38:433–41. https://doi.org/10.1007/s00296-017-3866-3.
43. Wipff J, Bonnet P, Ruiz B, et al. Association study of serotonin transporter gene (SLC6A4) in systemic sclerosis in European Caucasian populations. J Rheumatol. 2010;37:1164–7. https://doi.org/10.3899/jrheum.091156.
44. Malcarne VL, Greenbergs HL. Psychological adjustment to systemic sclerosis. Arthritis Care Res. 1996;9:51–9.
45. Arat S, Verschueren P, De Langhe E, et al. The association of illness perceptions with physical and mental health in systemic sclerosis patients: an exploratory study. Musculoskelet Care. 2012;10:18–28. https://doi.org/10.1002/msc.223.
46. Milette K, Thombs BD, Maiorino K, et al. Challenges and strategies for coping with scleroderma: implications for a scleroderma-specific self-management program. Disabil Rehabil. 2018;9:1–10. https://doi.org/10.1080/09638288.2018.1470263.
47. Mura G, Bhat KM, Pisano A, Licci G, Carta M. Psychiatric symptoms and quality of life in systemic sclerosis. Clin Pract Epidemiol Ment Health. 2012;8:30–5. https://doi.org/10.2174/1745017901208010030.

Chapter 7
Raynaud's Phenomenon

John D. Pauling

What Is Raynaud's Phenomenon?

Whereas the majority of medical eponyms describe a constellation of clinical symptoms and signs around a single disease, the term Raynaud's phenomenon (RP) is used to describe a symptom complex that can be present in virtually any form of digital vascular compromise. The existing classification of RP applies the same eponym to both the relatively benign functional vasospasm of primary RP and the more complex (and usually severe) vasospastic, obliterative and vaso-occlusive microangiopathy of systemic sclerosis (SSc). The breadth of pathology associated with the term RP can be traced back to Maurice Raynaud's original treatise which assembled a large number of disparate cases around the common theme of peripheral digital vascular compromise [1]. SSc-RP is generally considered a more severe form of digital vasculopathy than primary RP and can result in impaired dermal nutri-

J. D. Pauling (✉)
Royal National Hospital for Rheumatic Diseases
(at Royal United Hospitals), Bath, UK

Department of Pharmacy and Pharmacology,
University of Bath, Bath, UK
e-mail: JohnPauling@nhs.net

© Springer Nature Switzerland AG 2021
M. Matucci-Cerinic, C. P. Denton (eds.), *Practical Management of Systemic Sclerosis in Clinical Practice*, In Clinical Practice,
https://doi.org/10.1007/978-3-030-53736-4_7

tional flow resulting in tissue injury such as digital ulceration disease and necrosis.

The Clinical Features of Raynaud's Pheneomen

The clinical features of Raynaud's phenomenon are caused by digital ischaemia. Traditional definitions have focussed on the vasospastic component (often precipitated by cold exposure) resulting in discrete 'attacks' manifesting as digital colour changes (white, blue/purple and red) that reflect digital tissue perfusion and oxygenation during vasoactive changes within the digital arteries, arterioles and post-capillary venules. It is sensory symptoms of pain and numbness that result in impaired hand function and reduced quality of life. In SSc-RP, there is a vasospastic component with acute RP 'attacks' (typically precipitated by cold exposure but also the sympathomimetic effects of emotional stress) but also more persistent background digital ischaemic symptoms caused by the obliterative and vaso-occlusive microangiopathy of scleroderma.

The Relevance of Raynaud's Phenomenon in Scleroderma

Endothelial injury is considered an important initiating event in the pathogenesis of systemic sclerosis (SSc) [2]. Evidence of digital vasculopathy is present in virtually all patients at baseline assessment; manifesting as clinical symptoms of digital vascular compromise and confirmed through identification of morphological abnormal capillaries at the nailfold [3, 4]. Indeed, such is the importance of digital vasculopathy, the presence of objective evidence of Raynaud's phenomenon (RP) and nailfold capillaroscopic abnormalities are sufficient to fulfil classification criteria for early SSc [5] and feature, alongside anti-nuclear antibodies and puffy fingers, in the preliminary criteria for very early diagnosis of systemic sclerosis (VEDOSS) [6]. The absence of RP symptoms should prompt clinicians to consider the possibility of a 'SSc mimic' when evaluating a patient with sclerosing skin disease [7].

The Burden of Raynaud's Phenomenon in Systemic Sclerosis

Whilst non-life threatening, SSc-RP is a major cause of disease-related morbidity [8]. Patient survey have ranked RP as the highest disease-specific manifestation of SSc in terms of overall frequency and impact [9]. SSc-RP results in pain, numbness, impaired hand function, emotional distress, impaired health-related quality of life and reduced social participation [10]. The principle goal of treatment is reduce the daily burden of SSc-RP symptoms but it is also hoped that vasoactive medications might modify disease progression. Challenging to demonstrate within the constraints of a clinical trial, observational data from large registries has suggested a lower prevalence of vascular complications of SSc in patients established on calcium channel blockers (CCBs) early in the disease course, offering a tantalising glimpse of the potential disease-modifying potential of such treatments when used over extended periods [11].

Clinical Vignette

Case History

A 72 year old lady presented to the scleroderma clinic in 2014 with an 18-month history of tri-phasic RP and gastro-oesophageal reflux symptoms. Past medical history included hypothyroidism managed with a stable dose of levothyroxine. Clinical examination revealed cool peripheries and grade I sclerodactyly but no other features of SSc. Antinuclear antibody testing revealed an anti-nucleolar stain on indirect immunofluorescence but no SSc-specific autoantibodies were identified using solid phase immunoassays. Nailfold capillaroscopy revealed good preservation of capillary density

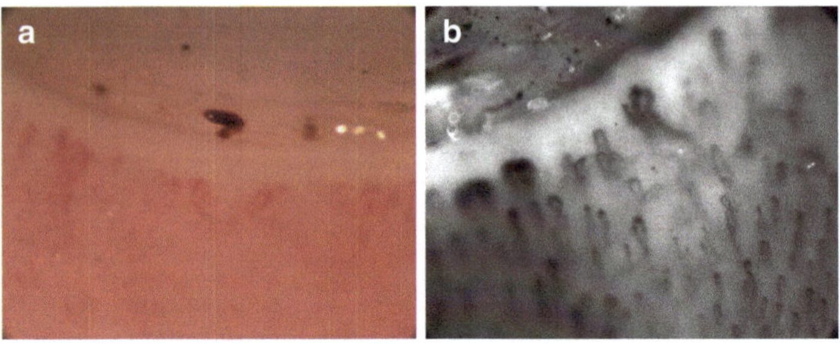

FIGURE 7.1 Nailfold capillary morphology in early systemic sclerosis. (**a**) Left ring finger with evidence of a giant capillary, a few elongated tortuous capillaries and a microhaemorrhage. (**b**) Right ring finger with a few enlarged capillaries. Similar changes were evident in other digits

but there was evidence of SSc changes with the occasional giant capillary, some aberrant neovascularisation and the occasional microhaemorrhage (consistent with 'early' SSc changes using the classification proposed by Cutolo et al.) (Fig. 7.1). A diagnosis of limited cutaneous SSc (lcSSc) was made and low dose nifedpine (5 mg daily) was commenced for Raynaud's symptoms (with a view to dose titration depending on tolerability and efficacy) but not tolerated (vasoactive side effects). Amlodipine 2.5 mg daily was better tolerated and increased to 5 mg daily but stopped after it was concluded it had not helped her RP symptomatically. Her RP remained problematic and treatment was commenced with sildenafil 25 mg daily which was better tolerated and effective at reducing Raynaud's symptoms. In December 2018, she attended a routine clinic review and reported more intrusive Raynaud's symptoms. Clinical examination revealed cool peripheries with patchy blanching and areas of dusky cyanosis affecting several digits (Fig. 7.2). A few small telangiectases were now evident on the palmer aspects of the fingers. There was no overt digital ulceration but minor fissuring of the thumb and index finger of the right hand was noted (Fig. 7.2). Cardiopulmonary screening has remained normal. The sildenafil dose was increased to 50 mg daily, with the opportunity to increase the dose to 50 mg twice daily depending on tolerability and efficacy.

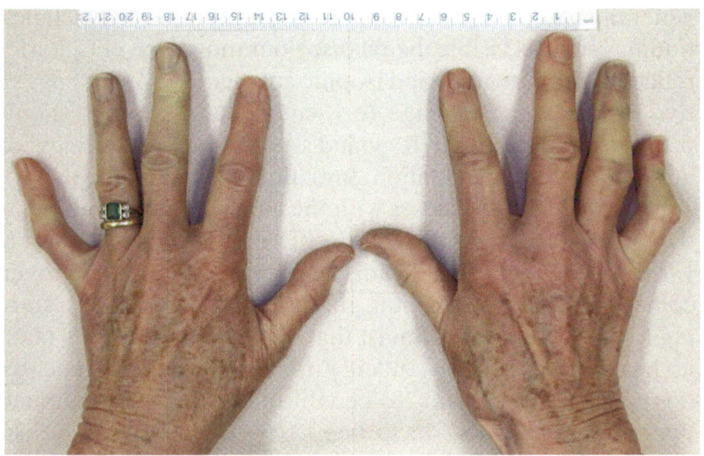

FIGURE 7.2 Appearance of the digits at routine clinic review. Raynaud's is not easily assessed in the clinic setting but the digits may appear cool to touch and there may be visible discolouration of the digits. There is some fissuring of the skin of the right index finger and thumb which reflects impaired digital perfusion

Point for Consideration

The initial presentation included a number of potential 'red flags' to suggest the presence of an underlying autoimmune rheumatic disease including late-onset Raynaud's, gastro-oesophageal reflux symptoms, positive ANA and a history of organ-specific autoimmunity (hypothyroidism). A clinical diagnosis of lcSSc was made based on the distribution of skin involvement and presence of scleroderma-pattern capillaroscopic abnormalities on nailfold microscopy. The patient would have fulfilled classification criteria for early SSc [5] and the preliminary criteria for VEDOSS [6] at presentation. First-line treatment with calcium channel blockers (CCBs) was abandoned due to inefficacy of low-dose therapy and issues around tolerability using higher doses. Despite this, second line treatment with phosphodiesterase V inhibitors (PDEVi) has been better tolerated at low doses and attempts are underway to increase the dose according tolerability and efficacy. The decision to initiate and escalate treatment for SSc-RP is generally based on patient-reported symptom severity. Clinical findings such as visible digital discolouration, cool peripheries, reduced capillary refill and trophic cutaneous changes suggestive of ischaemic damage (e.g. cutaneous fissuring) should prompt enquiry about Raynaud's symptoms and discussion around treatment escalation. Initiation of vasodilator therapy should start with low doses with the aim of escalating the dose depending on tolerability and efficacy. Unwanted transient vasoactive effects (e.g. headaches) can sometimes be overcome with patient education, gradual up-titration from a starting low dose and reassurance that come adverse effects (such as headaches) have a tendency to disappear with repeated dosing; allowing patients to benefit from effective treatments that might otherwise have been stopped prematurely. The preservation of capillary density on nailfold microscopy ('early' changes) was consistent with the early stage of her disease (5 years since first RP symptoms) but may also have accounted for the absence of more overt digital ischaemic lesions such as digital ulcers and normal cardiopulmonary screening. It is possible proactive management of RP symptoms may modify disease progression in SSc.

Assessment and Management of Scleroderma-Related Raynaud's Phenomenon

RP occurs in virtually all patients with SSc and is an important feature of early disease. RP is not life-threatening but is a significant cause of disease-related morbidity and should be treated with the same care as other disease-specific manifestations of SSc. Patient education and advice on important aspects of self-managment (cold avoidance, core temperature control, smoking cessation etc.) are vital, particularly in the early stages of SSc. Patients become adept at cold avoidance and adopting strategies to prevent and/or ameliorate Raynaud's symptoms which can lead to a reduction in the burden of SSc-RP with advancing disease duration; sometimes despite progression of the microangiopathy of SSc [10].

There are a number of available vasodilator therapies that can be used in the management of SSc-RP. Data from large patient registries indicates clinicians do not fully exploit the therapeutic options available (with respect to treatment initiation and optimising dosing) in the management of SSc-RP [12]. Physician attitudes and prescribing practices for SSc-RP management vary considerably. A fifth of SSc experts in one survey considered treatment for RP unnecessary in around half of their SSc patients [13]; surprising given the very high reported burden of RP symptoms reported in surveys capturing the needs of SSc patients [9]. Physician attitudes towards the importance of intervention may be a contributory factor to the significant variation in prescribing practices for SSc-RP [14]. Despite CCBs being recommended for the management of SSc-RP [13, 15], only approximately half of patients have ever received CCB therapy [16, 17]. Variation in clinical practice is even more marked for prostanoid therapy. Despite also being recommended in the management of SSc-RP [13, 15], prostanoid therapy is subject to marked geographic differences in reimbursement policies with higher use at units in Europe compared with North America [16, 17]. The use of PDEVi was not recommended for the management of SSc-RP in the original EULAR recommendations of 2009 [18]. The findings of a subsequent meta-analysis of PDEVi use in SSc-RP (despite indicating only a modest benefit to PDEVi over placebo [19]) have led to PDEVi forming part of the updated 2017 EULAR recommendations [15]. The positioning of PDEVi in the management of SSc-RP is gradually evolving. Previous consensus best practice guidelines proposed PDEVi therapy for SSc-RP in patients for whom prostanoids were ineffective or not tolerated [20]. Clinical experience gained from using PDEVi for SSc-related pulmonary arterial hypertension, the advantages of oral administration and the falling cost of generic preparations have encouraged the earlier use of PDEVi (increasingly in advance of prostanoid therapies) in SSc-RP. A practical approach to the management of SSc-RP and current positioning of the major classes of vasodilator therapy considered useful in SSc-RP is presented in Fig. 7.3.

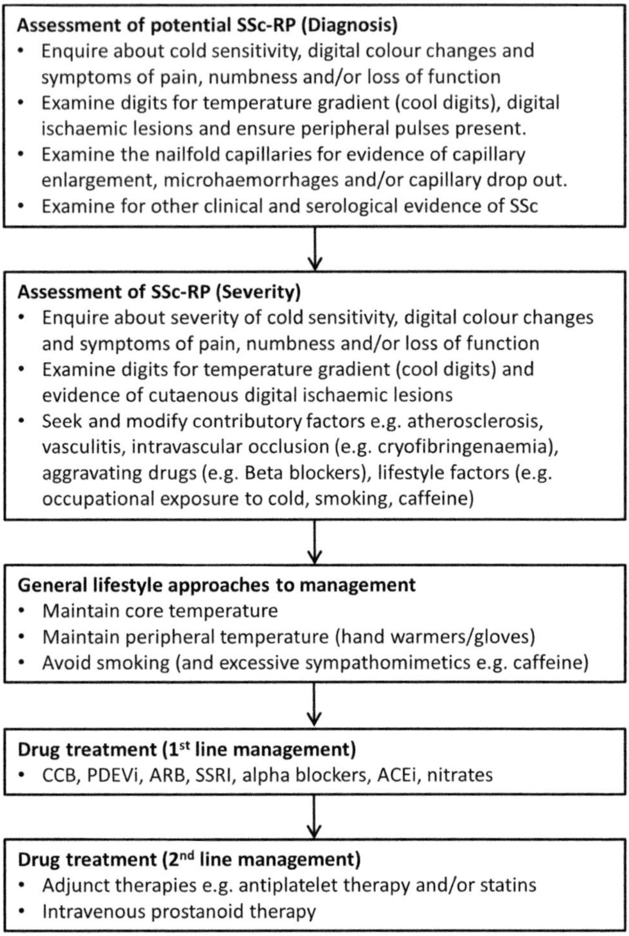

Assessment of potential SSc-RP (Diagnosis)
- Enquire about cold sensitivity, digital colour changes and symptoms of pain, numbness and/or loss of function
- Examine digits for temperature gradient (cool digits), digital ischaemic lesions and ensure peripheral pulses present.
- Examine the nailfold capillaries for evidence of capillary enlargement, microhaemorrhages and/or capillary drop out.
- Examine for other clinical and serological evidence of SSc

↓

Assessment of SSc-RP (Severity)
- Enquire about severity of cold sensitivity, digital colour changes and symptoms of pain, numbness and/or loss of function
- Examine digits for temperature gradient (cool digits) and evidence of cutaenous digital ischaemic lesions
- Seek and modify contributory factors e.g. atherosclerosis, vasculitis, intravascular occlusion (e.g. cryofibringenaemia), aggravating drugs (e.g. Beta blockers), lifestyle factors (e.g. occupational exposure to cold, smoking, caffeine)

↓

General lifestyle approaches to management
- Maintain core temperature
- Maintain peripheral temperature (hand warmers/gloves)
- Avoid smoking (and excessive sympathomimetics e.g. caffeine)

↓

Drug treatment (1st line management)
- CCB, PDEVi, ARB, SSRI, alpha blockers, ACEi, nitrates

↓

Drug treatment (2nd line management)
- Adjunct therapies e.g. antiplatelet therapy and/or statins
- Intravenous prostanoid therapy

FIGURE 7.3 A practical approach to assessment and management of SSc-RP. Adapted from [20]. The assessment and management of SSc-RP starts with careful assessment for contributory factors and patient education. Medication use includes a range of vasoactive medications to improve digital perfusion by either preventing vasoconstriction or encouraging vasodilation. *SSc-RP*, Systemic sclerosis-related Raynaud's phenomenon; *CCB*, calcium channel blockers; *PDEVi*, phosphodiesterase V inhibitors; *ARB*, angiotensin receptor blocker; *SSRI*, selective serotonin receptor inhibitor; *ACEi*, angiotensin converting enzyme inhibitor

Conclusions

Raynaud's phenomenon occurs in virtually all patients with SSc. RP is typically the earliest clinical manifestation of SSc and the identification of digital vasculopathy (clinically manifest as RP and through objective assessment of abnormal capillary morphology) is an important part of SSc diagnosis. RP is not life-threatening but is a major cause of disease-related morbidity. Clinicians should take a proactive approach to RP management, initiating vasodilator therapy and switching to alternative classes of vasodilators where necessary to establish a regime that is effective for the patient. Careful management of SSc-RP can reduce the impact and burden of digital vasculopathy. It may also modify disease progression in SSc.

References

1. Barlow T. On local asphyxia and symmetrical gangrene of the extremities 1862, and new research on the nature and treatment of local asphyxia of the extremities. In: Selected monographs. London: New Sydenham Society; 1874. p. 1888.
2. Herrick AL. Recent advances in the pathogenesis and management of Raynaud's phenomenon and digital ulcers. Curr Opin Rheumatol. 2016;28(6):577–85.
3. Walker UA, Tyndall A, Czirjak L, Denton C, Farge-Bancel D, Kowal-Bielecka O, et al. Clinical risk assessment of organ manifestations in systemic sclerosis: a report from the EULAR scleroderma trials and research group database. Ann Rheum Dis. 2007;66(6):754–63.
4. Koenig M, Joyal F, Fritzler MJ, Roussin A, Abrahamowicz M, Boire G, et al. Autoantibodies and microvascular damage are independent predictive factors for the progression of Raynaud's phenomenon to systemic sclerosis: a twenty-year prospective study of 586 patients, with validation of proposed criteria for early systemic sclerosis. Arthritis Rheum. 2008;58(12):3902–12.
5. LeRoy EC, Medsger TA Jr. Criteria for the classification of early systemic sclerosis. J Rheumatol. 2001;28(7):1573–6.
6. Minier T, Guiducci S, Bellando-Randone S, Bruni C, Lepri G, Czirjak L, et al. Preliminary analysis of the very early diagnosis

of systemic sclerosis (VEDOSS) EUSTAR multicentre study: evidence for puffy fingers as a pivotal sign for suspicion of systemic sclerosis. Ann Rheum Dis. 2014;73(12):2087–93.
7. Morgan ND, Hummers LK. Scleroderma mimickers. Curr Treatm Opt Rheumatol. 2016;2(1):69–84.
8. Pauling JD, Saketkoo LA, Matucci Cerinic M, Ingegnoli F, Khanna D. The patient experience of Raynaud's phenomenon in systemic sclerosis. Rheumatology (Oxford) 2019;58(1):18–26.
9. Bassel M, Hudson M, Taillefer SS, Schieir O, Baron M, Thombs BD. Frequency and impact of symptoms experienced by patients with systemic sclerosis: results from a Canadian National Survey. Rheumatology (Oxford). 2011;50(4):762–7.
10. Pauling JD, Domsic RT, Saketkoo LA, Almeida C, Withey J, Jay H, et al. Multi-national qualitative research study exploring the patient experience of Raynaud's phenomenon in systemic sclerosis. Arthritis Care Res. 2018;70(9):1373–84.
11. Steen V, Medsger TA Jr. Predictors of isolated pulmonary hypertension in patients with systemic sclerosis and limited cutaneous involvement. Arthritis Rheum. 2003;48(2):516–22.
12. Herrgott I, Riemekasten G, Hunzelmann N, Sunderkotter C. Management of cutaneous vascular complications in systemic scleroderma: experience from the German network. Rheumatol Int. 2008;28(10):1023–9.
13. Walker KM, Pope J. Participating members of the scleroderma clinical trials C, Canadian scleroderma research G. treatment of systemic sclerosis complications: what to use when first-line treatment fails--a consensus of systemic sclerosis experts. Semin Arthritis Rheum. 2012;42(1):42–55.
14. Harding S, Khimdas S, Bonner A, Baron M, Pope J. Canadian scleroderma research G. best practices in scleroderma: an analysis of practice variability in SSc centres within the Canadian scleroderma research group (CSRG). Clin Exp Rheumatol. 2012;30(2 Suppl 71):S38–43.
15. Kowal-Bielecka O, Fransen J, Avouac J, Becker M, Kulak A, Allanore Y, et al. Update of EULAR recommendations for the treatment of systemic sclerosis. Ann Rheum Dis. 2017;76(8):1327–39.
16. Pope J, Harding S, Khimdas S, Bonner A, Canadian Scleroderma Research G, Baron M. Agreement with guidelines from a large database for management of systemic sclerosis: results from the Canadian scleroderma research group. J Rheumatol. 2012;39(3):524–31.

17. Moinzadeh P, Riemekasten G, Siegert E, Fierlbeck G, Henes J, Blank N, et al. Vasoactive therapy in systemic sclerosis: real-life therapeutic practice in more than 3000 patients. J Rheumatol. 2016;43(1):66–74.
18. Kowal-Bielecka O, Landewe R, Avouac J, Chwiesko S, Miniati I, Czirjak L, et al. EULAR recommendations for the treatment of systemic sclerosis: a report from the EULAR scleroderma trials and research group (EUSTAR). Ann Rheum Dis. 2009;68(5):620–8.
19. Roustit M, Blaise S, Allanore Y, Carpentier PH, Caglayan E, Cracowski JL. Phosphodiesterase-5 inhibitors for the treatment of secondary Raynaud's phenomenon: systematic review and meta-analysis of randomised trials. Ann Rheum Dis. 2013;72(10):1696–9.
20. Hughes M, Ong VH, Anderson ME, Hall F, Moinzadeh P, Griffiths B, et al. Consensus best practice pathway of the UK Scleroderma Study Group: digital vasculopathy in systemic sclerosis. Rheumatology (Oxford). 2015;54(11):2015–24.

Chapter 8
Critical Ischemia

Jessica G. Huffstuter and Bashar Kahaleh

Critical ischemia is defined as the presence of ischemic symptoms at rest. It identifies patients with high risk of imminent tissue loss. Critical ischemia in SSc results from progressive microvascular insufficiency but occasionally it may result from macrovascular compromise by emboli, thrombosis or vasculitis. Outcome of critical ischemia is contingent on the duration of ischemia, presences of comorbidities, prompt institution of appropriate workup and therapy. Timely and comprehensive therapy is key to prevent loss of threatened tissues.

J. G. Huffstuter · B. Kahaleh (✉)
Division of Rheumatology, Immunology and Allergy, University of Toledo Medical Center, Toledo, OH, USA
e-mail: jessica.huffstutter@utoledo.edu; bashar.kahaleh@utoledo.edu

© Springer Nature Switzerland AG 2021
M. Matucci-Cerinic, C. P. Denton (eds.), *Practical Management of Systemic Sclerosis in Clinical Practice*, In Clinical Practice,
https://doi.org/10.1007/978-3-030-53736-4_8

Case Presentation

The following case presentation will be utilized to illustrate the practical application of the diagnostic and management strategies of critical ischemia.

A 60-year-old female presents to the rheumatology clinic from her primary care provider with a two-week history of worsening digital ulceration on the third and fourth digits of her right hand. Her past medical history includes limited cutaneous systemic sclerosis complicated by significant gastrointestinal involvement, and subcutaneous calcinosis. She is known to be anticentromere positive. Despite her efforts at primary prevention of ulceration (wearing protective clothing, warming her hands, limiting time outside, and taking her prescribed medications including CCB), she developed the digital ulcerations. Her primary care physician started her on a course of steroids, and when she did not improve, he sent a referral to rheumatology for the next available appointment.

Upon arrival to the rheumatology office 2 weeks later, the patient was in distress and her ulcerations had progressed despite the patient's strict adherence to her prescribed steroids. Her clinical exam was benign aside from digital gangrene (Fig. 8.1).

She was admitted to the hospital, and despite administration of prostacyclin analog and other therapy, she did not regain perfusion to any portion of the effected digits. Unfortunately, she lost one half of her third digit and the tip of her fourth by means of autoamputation.

Cases with this outcome prompt investigation into root cause as well as appropriate quality care measures. There is always the question of what could be done differently, and could this outcome have been avoided. This chapter aims to further prepare clinicians for similar clinical scenario.

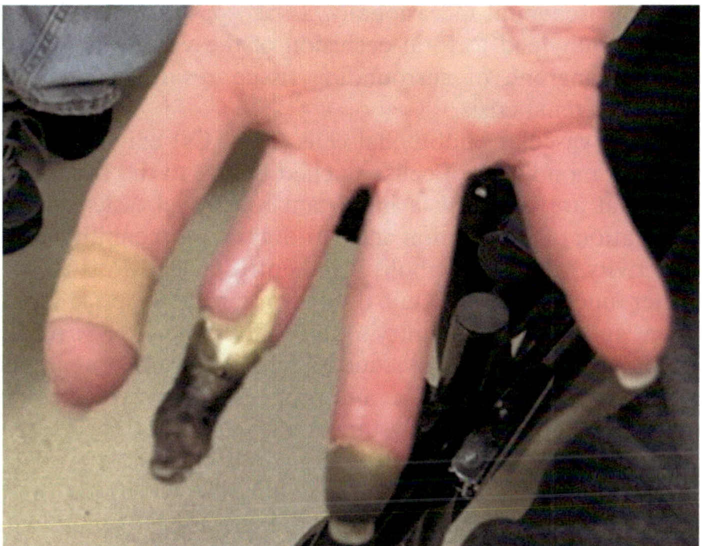

FIGURE 8.1 Digital gangrene in patient with limited cutaneous systemic sclerosis

Definitions and Pathogenetic Pathways

Vascular features dominate the clinical presentation of systemic sclerosis (SSc). Raynaud's phenomenon (RP) is the most characteristic early and persistent vascular symptom [1]. A Raynaud-like vasoconstriction associated with decrease blood flow has been also described in the cardiac, pulmonary and renal circulations. A fibroproliferative remodeling of the vascular wall at the arteriolar level leads to fixed narrowing of lumina, and the subsequent rigidity of the vascular wall leading to vascular stiffness [2]. Ischemia of tissues eventually ensues and progressively intensifies leading to ischemic symptoms when blood supply does not meet tissue demand. Further progression of imbalanced supply and demand lead to ischemic symptoms at rest. This state is best described as 'critical ischemia'. Occasionally, a vasospastic attack in this setting may lead to total occlusion of the vessel and subsequent gangrene of surrounding tissue resulting in digital ulcers or renal crisis.

Microvascular endothelial cells (MVECs) exist as a continuous monolayer of cells attached tightly to the basal lamina, that are involved in important functional tasks such as regulation of coagulation and fibrinolysis, permeability, vasoreactivity, cellular metabolism and nutrition [3]. MVECs have other functions that include fluid filtration, neutrophil recruitment and trafficking. Injury to the endothelium in SSc results in profound MVECs dysfunction that is prominent in the early stages of the disease and progressively worsens as the disease progresses. This dysfunction is manifested by increase vascular permeability and dysregulated control of vascular tone that is clinically best illustrated by the puffy hand stage and by RP. An imbalance in endothelial vascular signals with increased endothelin production and impaired nitric oxide as well as prostacyclin release mediates the vasospasm and contributes to the intimal proliferation, vascular fibrosis and stiffness of the vessel wall. Platelet activation and enhanced coagulation with reduced fibrinolysis may contribute to fibrin deposits and the evolution of the intimal fibroproliferative lesion resulting in luminal narrowing. Enhanced MVECs apoptosis and injury is proposed as a crucial initiating event leading to capillary breakdown, vascular remodeling, and ultimately to blood vessel occlusion. Attacks of RP leads to ischemia-reperfusion injury to the vessel wall and the activation of the NF-kB pathways leading to the generation of oxidative stress that add further insult to the endothelium. Immune activation and generation of autoantibodies and defective angio/vasculogenesis lead to impaired regeneration of blood vessels and restoration of adequate blood supply to affected tissues [4].

A distinct events and pathways are involved in the initiation and evolution of the critical ischemia that are inferred from the pathogenetic observations are listed (Table 8.1). The

Table 8.1 Potential targets for therapy

• Endothelial apoptosis
• Immune activation and the generation of anti-endothelial antibodies and harmful cytokines
• Oxidative injury
• Adhesion molecule expression and endothelial activation
• Enhanced cellular proliferation
• Platelet activation
• Hypercoagulation
• Defective fibrinolysis
• Impaired production of endothelial nitric oxide and prostacyclin
• Enhanced endothelin production
• Defective angiogenesis and vasculogenesis
• Tissue hypoxia

observed pathways act consecutively or simultaneously and represent attractive targets for the prevention and treatment of critical ischemia.

Not all critical ischemia in SSc are entirely related microvascular disease. Macrovascular occlusion by thrombosis, emboli or vasculitis can occur and need to be promptly investigated. The key point is that digital ischemia and ulceration in SSc patient may be due to large vessel as well as to small vessel disease. The association of vasculitis and scleroderma is unusual but well documented in the literature. The most commonly observed vasculitis is anti-neutrophil cytoplasmic antibody (ANCA)-associated vasculitis [5]. The presence of ANCA in in the setting of SSc critical ischemia should raise the possibility of an associated vasculitis. Digital ischemia, similar to ones seen in SSc, is reported in patients with granulomatosis with polyangiitis (formerly termed Wegener's) [6].

Risk Factors for Developing Critical Ischemia

Risk factors associated with poor outcome and development of gangrenous lesions were proposed by analysis of the Digital Ulcer Outcomes (DUO) Registry (Table 8.2). This European prospective multicenter observational cohort enrolled 4944 patients with past or current DUs from April 2008 to November 2014 [7]. The data demonstrated that gangrene is a common event that occurred in 18% of patients with DUs. The data also can help to risk stratify patients with SSc-DUs and to assess preventive and management strategies. Anticentromere antibody positivity has been previously linked with the severity of vascular disease [8]. Thus, SSc patients with positive anticentromere antibody had increased risk of major peripheral vascular occlusive disease. Ischemia and digital loss were also reported in non-SSc patients with anti-centromere antibody, suggesting that the antibody may play a causal role in vascular damage [9].

Therapeutic Approaches

Approximately 11% of patients with systemic sclerosis will develop critical limb ischemia during the course of their disease, and 18% of all SSc patients have DUs [10]. Therapeutic

Table 8.2 Risk factors for developing gangrene

• Smoking status
• Previous gangrene
• Previous autoamputation
• Previous soft tissue infection requiring systemic antibiotics
• Previous osteomyelitis
• Previous hospitalization(s) for DUs (at least 1 day)
• Upper limb sympathectomy

interventions must be initiated quickly and imperatively. Rheumatologists experienced in the management of SSc complication should be responsible for initiating the diagnostic workup and for coordinating patient's care. Primary care physicians are not prepared to act fast or to choose the appropriate therapy as illustrated by the presented case. The treatment of critical ischemia should be individualized and must utilize a multidisciplinary approach. The stage, location, and comorbidities of the patient must be considered to achieve optimal outcome.

Interdisciplinary Team Care

Critical Ischemia in SSc requires a multidisciplinary management, since pharmacological therapy is indicated for some cases and complementary surgical management is better for others. A team of professionals representing different disciplines to assist in the evaluation and management of the patient with critical ischemia is essential for rational and timely care. The team typically include individuals who are skilled in in the management of critical ischemia (Table 8.3).

Table 8.3 Interdisciplinary team

• Vascular and orthopedic surgeons
• Infectious disease specialists
• Radiology and vascular imaging specialists
• Physical medicine and rehabilitation clinicians
• Physical and occupational therapists
• Pain management specialists
• Nutrition and dieticians

Table 8.4 Initial laboratory workup

• ANA titer and staining pattern
• SSc specific autoantibodies: Centromere, Scl-70, and RNP polymerase III antibodies
• Phospholipid antibodies and lupus anticoagulant
• Cytoplasmic neutrophil cytoplasmic antibody ANCA,
• Lupus serology: DNA, Smith, RNP antibodies.
• Circulating immune complex levels, cryoglobulins, complement levels
• Urinalysis, renal and hepatic function
• Hepatitis serology
• ESR and CRP

Initial approach—Hospital admission should be initiated immediately, patient should be stabilized and a central line need to be established. Pain management is important first step to reduce reflux vasospasm associated with pain. Laboratory workup including serologic testing of possible associated or overlapping disorders should be obtained (Table 8.4). Next, vascular imaging to detected possible large vessel disease should be completed as soon as feasible.

Pain management—Intense pain is associated with critical ischemia and can be quite punishing and exhausting. Pain management experts should be involved early after hospital admission to plan an individualized approach to achieve safe and effective analgesia by utilizing short and long acting analgesic agents. Opioids remain the principal agents, however, they should be used at the lowest effective doses to avoid short and long-term complications.

Vascular imaging—Duplex ultrasound, and non-invasive angiography with computerized tomography (CTA) or magnetic resonance (MRA), can demonstrate arterial obstruction. CTA requires iodinated contrast that may compromise kidney function. Non-contrast MRA is prone to artifact and concerns for nephrogenic systemic fibrosis from gadolinium contrast limit the use of contrast MRA in patients with kidney disease. CTA and MRA can help localize disease targets and help plan the mode and approach to revascularization. Still, invasive angiography is often used to clarify the potential for revascularization and should be considered prior to any surgical intervention.

Wound care—The wound should be assessed for infection. Broad-spectrum systemic antibiotics should be instituted if infection is suspected. Carful debridement may be required if necrotic tissue develops, but should be done with extreme caution given the underlying vascular compromise that extends beyond the area of necrosis.

Detailed Treatment Approach

Treatment options with the most crucial therapies will be discussed first. While there are a number of surgical approaches and techniques, the overall focus will be on medical therapy both in this urgent setting as well as adjunctive therapies. The first step in therapy is to determine if the ischemia is related to macrovascular or microvascular disease since the two require distinct treatment strategies.

Macrovascular Ischemia

Critical ischemia secondary to larger vessel occlusion should be fully evaluated on initial presentation to search for reversible process like vasculitis, embolic, or thrombotic events. Arteriography is indicated in critical ischemia when macrovascular cause is suspected and the option of surgery is considered. There are obvious differences in the treatment of macro- and microvascular disease. From a macrovascular perspective, the American Heart Association guidelines for treatment of peripheral vascular disease dictate that inflow disease be treated first. This is either addressed by surgery or percutaneous intervention. At that point outflow disease would then be addressed [11]. The decision on whether to pursue a bypass surgery rather than an angioplasty first approach depends on the complexity and location of the lesion. The gold standard for revascularization remains surgical bypass, but the endovascular first approach may be appropriate in those patients with significant comorbidities as a 2013 meta-analysis points out [12]. AHA guidelines also state that angioplasty should be offered first to patients with significant comorbidities who are not expected to live more than 2 years [13]. Upper extremity interventions for critical ischemia are generally successful with the rare need for immediate amputations [14]. However, despite efforts for limb salvaging surgery, approximately 25% of patients with chronic ischemia undergo amputation within 1 year. Those who are at higher risk of needing an amputation are those with pain in the limb at rest, septic complications, flexion contractures, and those who have necrosis of weight baring parts of the feet [9, 11]. Recovering from any of the aforementioned procedures is complemented with aggressive wound care and physical therapy. Surveillance of bypass typically involves evaluation by a vascular specialist at least twice yearly for the first 2 years, ultrasound of the bypass, and measurements of ankle-brachial index when applicable (11). After surgery, the American College of Chest Physician's (ACCP) states that aspirin therapy should begin perioperatively and continue indefinitely. Clopidogrel can be used in those patients who cannot tolerate aspirin [15].

Microvascular Ischemia—The Acute Setting

Upon suspicion of microvascular critical ischemia, medical approaches in conjunction with surgical opinion are utilized for managing the microvascular insult. In the case of a critical digital ischemic event, patients will present with intense pain and debility which must be promptly and aggressively managed to preserve functionality. After confirming the diagnosis and mapping out vascular targets, the initial pain caused by vasospasm can be mitigated by local injection of lidocaine or bupivacaine at the base of the digit [15, 16]. Once the initial pain had been managed, prompt administration of vasodilating agents should be provided. Short acting calcium channel blockers may be used, but in the case of rapidly progressing ischemia, IV prostacyclin analogs are the treatment of choice [15, 16]. Thrombotic events would prompt inhibition of platelet aggregation and evaluation for angioplasty or digital sympathectomy [16].

Sympathectomy—Clinical experience support sympathectomy early in course of critical ischemia. Chemical sympathectomy can be achieved by digital or regional administration of lidocaine or bupivacaine. Temporary cervical or lumbar sympathectomy may help for short period of time.

Digital sympathectomies/adventitial stripping are salvage procedures that should be considered only when more conservative therapies have been tried and failed or when there is a particular digit that appears to be imminently at risk for tissue loss. The procedure may improve blood flow in the digital arteries by interrupting the sympathetic vasoconstrictor supply to the superficial palmar arch, the common and main digital arteries of the fingers and stripping the periadventitial fibrotic tissues from around the arteries. The effect on blood flow can be immediate and long lasting. One study reported a mean follow-up period of 46 months with continues improvement in blood flow, healing of ulcers and rare recurrences of ulcers [17]. while, another study reported up to 26% of digits required surgical amputation on follow-up [18].

Pharmacologic therapy—Therapy is aimed at reliving symptoms and preventing further injury. Medications preferred for their vasodilatory effect include calcium channel blockers, cyclic guanosine monophosphate (cGMP) specific phosphodiesterase type 5 inhibitors, prostacyclin analogs, and alpha-1 blockers. Other therapies include, statins, botulinum toxin, and antioxidants.

Prostacyclin (PGI2)—Prostacyclin is an arachidonic acid derivative that is generated by the vascular endothelium. PGI2 is a potent vasodilator, it inhibits platelet aggregation and adhesion, and is a strong inhibitor of smooth muscle cells proliferation. These biologic effects propose PGI2 as a potent inhibitor of the fibroproliferative vasculopathy [15, 19, 20]. Furthermore, and relevant to SSc pathogenesis, PGI2 is shown to facilitate angiogenesis and repair of injured endothelium [19]. PGI2 effects are analogous to the effects of nitric oxide and it may offset the loss of NO in certain pathologic states. Accordingly, PGI2 can maintain endothelial function when NO signaling is deficient [20]. Epoprostenol and iloprost are analogs of PGI2 that are used clinically for the management of variety of vascular disorder and should be considered as first line therapy in SSc of critical ischemia. Both analogs are administered parenterally as a continuous intravenous infusion via a central venous catheter. Doses are escalated gradually to the maximal effective or tolerable dose. Duration of infusion is 72 hours in hospitalized patients and 6 hours per day in the outpatient setting that can be repeated 5 days in a row. Common side effects include flushing, cough, nausea, vomiting, jaw pain, insomnia, palpitations, muscle pain and headaches that increase transiently with dose escalation. Uncommon, but potentially severe adverse events include pulmonary edema, hypotension, syncope and hemoptysis [15, 16].

Epoprostenol was approved for use in the United States in 1995, the typical dose is 2 ng per kg body weight per minute. The dose can be increased every 15–30 min in increments of 1 to 2 ng/kg/min, up to 8 ng/kg/min based on clinical response and tolerance. Limited evidence supports the use of epoprostenol in SSc critical ischemia. The largest study reported acceptable safety and efficacy in the treatment of digital ischemia [21]. In that study, 29 out of 46 epoprostenol infusions had documented improvement in pain, increased perfusion of digits and reduction in the number and size of DUs.

Iloprost is a more stable and has a longer half-life than epoprostenol and is fourfold more potent. The starting dose is 0.5 ng/kg/min that is increased to a maximum of 2 ng/kg/min. A landmark study that popularized the use of Iloprost in therapy of SSc critical ischemia reported good efficacy and safety [22]. In this study 126 SSc patients completed 6-hour intravenous infusions of iloprost (0.5 to 2.0 ng/kg per min) or placebo. Significant improvement in the number of Raynaud attacks, global Raynaud severity score and healing of DUs were all noted.

Calcium channel blockers are the most common first line treatment for RP. Primary RP is considered to be a self-limiting and benign pathology which is generally not associated with gangrene and digital ulcerations [23]. Calcium channel blockers are the first line medical treatment when conservative rewarming and protective measures are not adequate [15]. They act on vascular smooth muscle to cause arterial dilatation via action on L-type calcium channels thereby dampening vasoconstrictive response [15, 16]. Members of the dihydropyridine class (nifedipine and amlodipine) are the most commonly used agents. Dosing ranges for these medications are from 30-180 mg daily for nifedipine and 5-20 mg daily for amlodipine [16]. Other members of the calcium channel blocker class may be used, but there is no proven added benefit [16]. A 2017 Cochran review demonstrated that the dihydropyridine calcium channel blockers may be useful in reducing the frequency, duration, severity of attacks, and pain with an overall 1.72 fewer attacks per week (95% CI, 0.06–2.84) [24]. Side effects are generally mild and included headache, dizziness, nausea, palpitations, and ankle edema [15, 24].

Phosphodiesterase type 5 inhibitors are indicated should calcium channel blockers not be effective. Agents like sildenafil, tadalafil, vardenafil, pentoxifylline, and cilostazol have been used since 2003 when the first successful use of nightly sildenafil produced remarkable relief from RP in ten patients [15, 16, 25]. These medications act by inhibition of PDE-5 activity which allows cGMP to accumulate within the endothelial cells. This accumulation changes the cellular response to prostacyclin and nitric oxide whereby resulting in vascular smooth muscle relaxation resulting in increase perfusion to distal tissues [15, 16, 26]. These medications received a class A recommendation by the European League Against Rheumatism (EULAR), and a 2017 literature review noted that PDE-5 inhibitors improve healing of digital ulcers in patients with systemic sclerosis, and that they may prevent the development of new digital ulcerations [27]. Current dosing regiments include sildenafil 20 mg three times daily, tadalafil 5 mg–20 mg daily, and vardenafil 10 mg twice daily [15]. Common side effects of these medications include flushing, headache, and dizziness. Hypotension, arrhythmia, vision changes, and stroke have been observed but are less frequent [16].

Adjunctive Therapies

A lesser reviewed class of effective medication are the **alpha-adrenergic blockers**. These medications play a significant role in thermoregulation [16]. The most notable member of this class is prazosin the effects of which were studied in the 2000 Cochrane Review [28]. Here the 3 mg daily and the 4 mg daily regimens were studied, the data showed that it was more effective than placebo in the treatment of Raynaud's secondary to scleroderma, but there are no recommendations for it's use in acute critical ischemia (28).

Glyceryl triturate (GTN) has been studied using an intravenous approach but the effect was transient. GTN patches (0.2 mg/h) were also investigated however, the side effects, and in particular headaches, were intolerable. Unlike phosphodiesterase inhibitors which increase the availability of endogenous nitric oxide in smooth muscle, **topical nitroglycerin** preparations have been used for decades as a more direct way of inducing vasodilatation [29, 30]. There are several preparations of nitrates, and while the first preparation of IV nitrates was discontinued due to intolerable headaches, the process is more refined and suitable for treating ischemia [15, 29, 30]. This diversity of the modes of administration has made it more difficult to study all preperations in a standardized setting, and many of the patients evaluated were treated with MQX-503 which is a gel not currently approved by the FDA [29, 30]. The currently available forms have more systemic side effects, but when used in conjunction with calcium channel blockers, they are effective in restoring perfusion [30, 31]. Dosing amounts and intervals will depend on the type of preparation used, but overall the side effect profile is the same. Headaches are the most common side effect, and larger doses are generally not well tolerated [15, 29–31]. Other side effects include hypotension, flushing, dizziness, tachycardia, and GERD. These agents should be used with caution or not at all in those with heart failure, use of a PDE inhibitor, or in dehydrated patients [30, 31].

Hyperbaric oxygen therapy has been used as an adjunctive treatment in critical ischemia for decades [32]. It is often utilized when CCB, vasodilators, and prostanoids fail, and for patients who need to avoid invasive treatments. The main mechanism is fairly straight forward and acts by increasing the amount of dissolved oxygen in the arterial supply whereby relieving the hypoxia of the skin and surrounding tissues [33]. This increased oxygen will also stimulate endothelial cell growth and promote neovascularization.

Botulinum toxin A has increasingly been investigated as a method to reduce pain from RP. When applied to supplying blood vessels, it improves surgical flap survival via oxygen delivery [34]. The toxin's main mechanism is inhibition of presynaptic acetylcholine release, but it may also block sympathetic vasoconstriction of the smooth muscle by inhibition of the norepinephrine vesicle release [35]. A pilot study demonstrated increase digital pulp temperature that persisted for up to 6 weeks after injection into the palmar arch [36]. A randomized double-blind placebo controlled clinical study of 40 patients was conducted wherein investigators injected one randomly chosen hand with botulinum toxin (50 units in 2.5 mL) and the contralateral hand with normal saline. The primary outcome was change in blood flow measured by laser Doppler imaging, but no significant benefits were noted at 4 months. However, clinical measures including cold sensitivity score, and pain on a visual analog scale improved briefly in the botulinum toxin treated hands [37]. Overall, this agent will benefit from further investigation especially in acute digital ischemia cases.

Angiotensin converting enzyme inhibitors (ACEi) and angiotensin receptor blockers (ARBs) have been suggested as therapies in ischemic events. Initial investigations of captopril in 1987 demonstrated improvement in cutaneous blood flow, but there was no difference in frequency or severity of ischemic attacks [16, 38]. Subsequent studies involving other agents from both of these classes has likewise yielded mixed results. The overall consensus is that these drugs are not recommended as first line or monotherapy for digital ischemia [15, 16].

Fluoxetine is a member of the selective serotonin reuptake inhibitor class (SSRI), and at a dose of 20 mg daily it was shown to reduce the severity and frequency of the attacks of RP in a prospective pilot study [39]. The effects of serotonin on vascular tone are complex, and both vasodilatation and vasoconstriction are mediated through separate serotonin channels [40]. There is limited available data, and the initial pilot study as well as recent criticisms have brought up the need for a randomized double-blind trial [39, 40]. SSRIs have found their niche in those patients in whom CCBs cannot be titrated upwards due to hypotension [16].

Statins have demonstrated efficacy in digital ulcer healing, but the data on their use in critical ischemia is lacking [16, 41, 42]. They are known to be vasoprotective as they decrease LDL and increase HDL. This change in turn decreased free radicals and coagulation [16]. Overall, they are generally added when everything else failed.

N-acetylcysteine (NAC) is the precursor of a major antioxidant, glutathione that may have beneficial effects in SSc ischemia due to its vasodilating properties and impact on platelet aggregation. A pilot study of intravenous NAC in 20 patients with SSc-DUs showed that more than half of the DUs present at baseline healed after 5-day infusion [43]. A prospective observational study of intravenous NAC dosed at 15 mg/kg/h for 5 hours every 14 days was recently reported [44]. The median treatment was 3 years, and the mean of ulcers/patient/year decreased significantly from 4.5 to 0.81 with minimal reported side effects. Although promising, this agent should be evaluated in a prospective, placebo controlled, randomized trials.

Revisiting the Case

At the beginning of the chapter, the case report discussed an unfortunate incidence of late diagnosis of critical ischemia. A long-term scleroderma patient with positive centromere presented to her PCP with digital ulcerations. At that point, initiating further workup including hospitalization and the chain of events illustrated in Fig. 8.2 would have been appropriate to do. Administering steroids in the absence of further diagnostic evaluation is not standard of care, and in this case led to delay in her care resulted in digital loss.

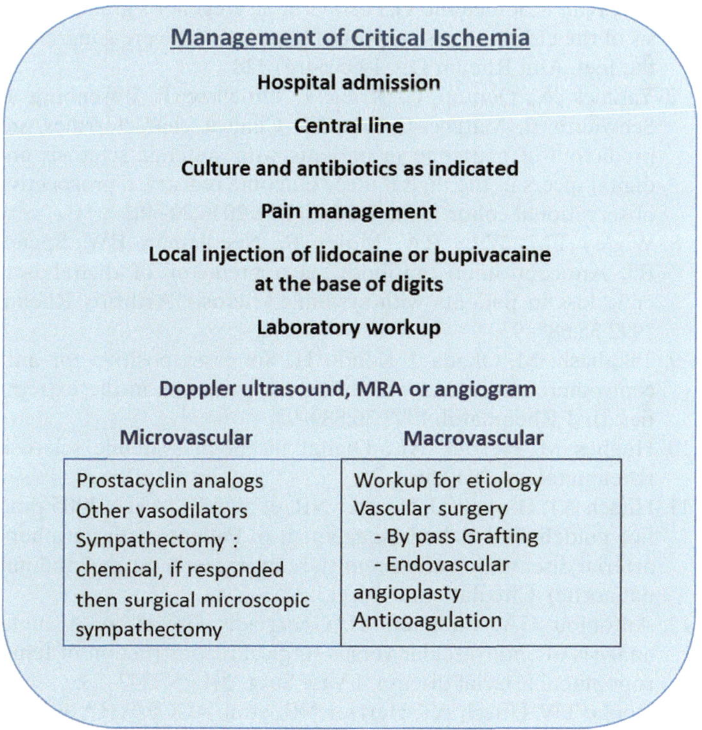

Figure 8.2 Evaluation and management algorithm for scleroderma patients with critical ischemia

References

1. Abraham DJ, Varga J. Scleroderma: from cell and molecular mechanisms to disease models. Trends Immunol. 2005;26(11):587–95.
2. Rajendran P, et al. The vascular endothelium and human diseases. Int J Biol Sci. 2013;9(10):1057–69.
3. Kahaleh B. The microvascular endothelium in scleroderma. Rheumatology (Oxford). 2008;47(5):14–5.
4. Distler JH, Gay S, Distler O. Angiogenesis and vasculogenesis in systemic sclerosis. Rheumatology (Oxford). 2008;47(2):234–5.
5. Rho YH, Choi SJ, Lee YH, Ji JD, Song GG. Scleroderma associated with ANCA associated vasculitis. Rheumatol Int. 2006;26(5):369–75.
6. La Civita L, Jeracitano G, Ferri C, et al. Wegener's granulomatosis of the elderly: a case report of uncommon severe gangrene of the feet. Ann Rheum Dis. 1995;54(4):328.
7. Yannick A, Denton C, Krieg T, Ornelisse P, Rosenberg D, Schwierin B, Matucci-Cerinic M. Clinical characteristics and predictors of gangrene in patients with systemic sclerosis and digital ulcers in the digital ulcer outcome registry: a prospective, observational cohort. Ann Rheum Dis. 2016;209481
8. Wigley FM, Wise RA, Miller R, Needleman BW, Spence RJ. Anticentromere antibody as a predictor of digital ischemic loss in patients with systemic sclerosis. Arthritis Rheum. 1992;35:688–93.
9. Takahashi M, Okada J, Kondo H. Six cases positive for anticentromere antibodies with ulcer and gangrene in the extremities. Br J Rheumatol. 1997;36:889–93.
10. Hughes M, Herrick AL. Digital ulcers in systemic sclerosis. Rheumatology. 2017;56:4–25.
11. Hirsch AT, Haskal ZJ, Hertzer NR, et al. ACC/AHA 2005 practice guidelines for the Management of Patients with peripheral arterial disease (lower extremity, renal, mesenteric, and abdominal aortic). Circulation. 2006;113:e463–654.
12. Antoniou GA, Chalmers N, Georgiadis GS, et al. A meta-analysis of endovascular versus surgical reconstruction of femoropopliteal arterial disease. J Vasc Surg. 2013;57:242–53.
13. Rooke TW, Hirsch AT, Hertzer NR, et al. ACCF/AHA focused update of the guideline for the Management of Patients with peripheral artery disease (updating the 2005 guideline) a report of the American College of Cardiology Foundation/American

Heart Association task force on practice guidelines. Circulation. 2011;124(18):2020–4529.

14. Cheun T, Jayakumar L, Sheehan M, et al. Outcomes of upper extremity interventions for chronic critical ischemia. J Vasc Surg. 2019;69(1):120–8. e2
15. Stringer T, Femia AN. Raynaud's phenomenon: current concepts. Clin Dermatol. 2018;36(4):498–507.
16. McMahan ZH, Wigley FM. Raynaud's phenomenon and digital ischemia: a practical approach to risk stratification, diagnosis and management. Int J Clin Rheumtol. 2010;5(3):355–70.
17. Ruch DS, Holden M, Smith B, Koman A. Periarterial sympathectomy in scleroderma patients: intermediate-term follow-up. J Hand Surg. 2002;27A:258–64.
18. Tristain L, Hartzell E, Makhni C, Sampson C. Long-term results of Periarterial Sympathectomy. J Hand Surg Am. 2009;34(8):1454–60.
19. Visalli E, Amato G, Di Gangi M, et al. Treatment with intravenous iloprost in patients with systemic sclerosis: a short review. J Rare Dis Res Treat. 2017;2(4):6–13.
20. Fati R, Visalli E, Amato G, et al. Long-term clinical stabilization of scleroderma patients treated with a chronic and intensive IV iloprost regimen. Rheumatol Int. 2017;37:245–9.
21. Law S, Simms RW, Farber HW. Use of intravenous Epoprostenol as a treatment for the digital vasculopathy associated with the scleroderma Spectrum of diseases [abstract]. Arthritis Rheumatol. 2016;68(suppl 10)
22. Wigley FM, Wise RA, Seibold JR, et al. Intravenous iloprost infusion in patients with Raynaud phenomenon secondary to systemic sclerosis. A multicenter, placebo-controlled, double-blind study. Ann Intern Med. 1994;120(3):199–206.
23. Rodriguez-Franco K, Miranda-Diaz A, Hoyes-Restrepo J, Melendez G. Systemic scleroderma: an approach from plastic surgery. Rev Fac Med. 2018;66(2):237–45.
24. Rirash F, Tingey PC, Harding SE, Maxwell LJ, et al. Calcium channel blockers for primary and secondary Raynaud's phenomenon. Cochrane Database Syst Rev. 2017;(12):CD000467.
25. Fries R, Shariat K, Wilmowsky H, Böhm M. Sildenafil in the treatment of Raynaud's phenomenon resistant to vasodilatory therapy. Circulation. 2005;112:2980–5.
26. Andrigueti F, Ebbing P, Arismendi M, Kayser C. Evaluation of the effect of sildenafil on the microvascular blood flow in

patients with systemic sclerosis: a randomized, double-blind, placebo- controlled study. Clin Exp Rheumatol. 2017;35:151–8.
27. Kowal-Bielecka O, Fransen J, Eustar AJ, et al. Update of EULAR recommendations for the treatment of systemic sclerosis. Ann Rheum Dis. 2017;76:1327–39.
28. Harding SE, Tingey PC, Pope J, et al. Prazosin for Raynaud's phenomenon in progressive systemic sclerosis. Cochrane Database Syst Rev. 1998;(2):CD000956.
29. Qiu O, Chan T, Luen M, et al. Use of nitroglycerin ointment to treat primary and secondary Raynaud's phenomenon: a systemic literature review. Rheumatol Int. 2018;38:2209–16.
30. Chung L, Shapiro L, Fiorentino D, Baron M, et al. MQX-503, a novel formulation of nitroglycerin, improves the severity of Raynaud's phenomenon: a randomized, controlled trial. Arthritis Rheum. 2009;60:870–7.
31. Khanna PP, Maranian P, Gregory J, et al. The minimally important difference and patient acceptable symptom state for the Raynaud's condition score in patients with Raynaud's phenomenon in a large randomized controlled clinical trial. Ann Rheum Dis. 2010;69:588–91.
32. Dowling GB, Copeman PW, Ashfield R. Raynaud's phenomenon in scleroderma treated with hyperbaric oxygen. Proc R Soc Med. 1967;60(12):1268–9.
33. Sato T, Arai K, Ichioka S. Hyperbaric oxygen therapy for digital ulcers due to Raynaud's disease. Case Reports Plast Surg Hand Surg. 2018;5(1):72–4.
34. Schweizer D, Schweizer R, Zhang S, et al. Botulinum toxin a and B raise blood flow and increase survival of critically ischemic skin flaps. J Surg Res. 2013;184:1205–13.
35. Berk-Krauss J, Christman MP, Franks A, Sicco KL, Liebman TN. Botulinum toxin for treatment of Raynaud phenomenon in CREST syndrome. Dermatol Online J. 2018;24(12)
36. Jenkins S, Neyman K, Veledar E, et al. A pilot study evaluating the efficacy of botulinum toxin a in the treatment of Raynaud phenomenon. J Am Acad Dermatol. 2013;69:834–5.
37. Bello R, Cooney C, Melamed E, et al. The therapeutic efficacy of botulinum toxin in treating scleroderma-associated Raynaud's phenomenon: a randomized, double-blind, placebo-controlled clinical trial. Arthritis Rheumatol. 2017;69:1661–9.
38. Tosi S, Marchesoni A, Messina K, et al. Treatment of Raynaud's phenomenon with captopril. Drugs Exp Clin Res. 1987;13(1):37–42.

39. Coleiro B, Marshall SE, Denton CP, Howell K, Blann A, Welsh KI, et al. Treatment of Raynaud's phenomenon with the selective serotonin reuptake inhibitor fluoxetine. Rheumatology. 2001;40(9):1038–43.
40. Khouri C, Gailland T, Lepelley M, Roustit M, Cracowski JL. Fluoxetine and Raynaud's phenomenon: friend or foe? Br J Clin Pharmacol. 2017;83(10):2307–9.
41. Kuwana M, Okazaki Y, Kaburaki J. Long-term beneficial effects of statins on vascular manifestations in patients with systemic sclerosis. Mod Rheumatol. 2009;19:530–5.
42. Abou-Raya A, Abou-Raya S, Helmii M. Statins: potentially useful in therapy of systemic sclerosis-related Raynaud's phenomenon and digital ulcers. J Rheumatol. 2008;35:1801–8.
43. Sambo P, Amico D, Giacomelli R, et al. Intravenous N-acetylcysteine for treatment of Raynaud's phenomenon secondary to systemic sclerosis: a pilot study. J Rheumatol. 2001;28:2257–62.
44. Rosato E, Borghese F, Pisarri S, Salsano F. The treatment with N-acetylcysteine of Raynaud's phenomenon and ischemic ulcers therapy in sclerodermic patients: a prospective observational study of 50 patients. Clin Rheumatol. 2009;28:1379–84.

Chapter 9
Increase in Pulmonary Artery Pressures

Nkemamaka Okonkwo and J. Gerry Coghlan

Patient 1: Routine Follow-Up Patient

A 58-year-old female with a 10 year history of anti-centromere antibody (ACA) positive limited SSc and telangiectasias is seen for annual review. She does not volunteer a change in effort tolerance and has no new symptoms related to her SSc. Her echocardiogram report reveals an estimated pulmonary artery systolic pressure (estPASP) of 35 mmHg, the ECG shows ST depression and T-wave inversion in right precordial leads and on lung function testing she has a DLCO (diffusion capacity of carbon monoxide) of 38%. How would you manage this patient?

This is clearly a patient at risk of pulmonary arterial hypertension (PAH), while all patients with SSc are at increased risk of developing pulmonary hypertension PH, PAH domi-

N. Okonkwo
Dept of Pulmonary Hypertension, Royal Free NHS Trust Hospital, London, UK
e-mail: nkemamka.okonkwo@nhs.net

J. G. Coghlan (✉)
Department of Cardiology, Royal Free NHS Trust Hospital, London, UK
e-mail: gerry.coghlan@nhs.net

© Springer Nature Switzerland AG 2021
M. Matucci-Cerinic, C. P. Denton (eds.), *Practical Management of Systemic Sclerosis in Clinical Practice*, In Clinical Practice,
https://doi.org/10.1007/978-3-030-53736-4_9

nates in limited SSc especially those that are ACA positive. In diffuse SSc PAH, post capillary PH and lung associated PH are all common [1].

This patient has been seen routinely, and we are not told of any exercise limitation. To date all trials of therapy have been in patients with at least some breathlessness on effort [2]. We have no reason to believe that the treatments are ineffective in the absence of symptoms. Most patients with SSc have some exercise limitation, but being tolerant of this simply do not exercise to the point of breathlessness [3]. Focused questioning will often reveal breathlessness and an exercise test (such as a 6-min walking test) can also be helpful. Even in the absence of symptoms, PAH is a relentless progressive disorder so unless co-morbidity is a reason one would not treat PAH, investigation should be undertaken [4] [5],.

The echocardiogram data provided seems relatively reassuring. But we are provided with minimal data. If correct a PASP of 35 mmHg would be associated with a mean pulmonary artery pressure of around 20 mmHg [6]—below the diagnostic threshold in current guidelines. However, we also know that the accuracy of estPASP is ± 40 mmHg—so pressures may be entirely normal or very elevated [7]. Cardiac involvement in SSc is common, we are not told about the size of the left atrium (LA) or diastolic or systolic parameters—so left heart issues remains on the cards.

The DLCO is very low, but no other lung function data has been provided. While low gas transfer is associated with PAH in the setting of SSc, this is also seen in lung fibrosis and emphysema—so if pressures are elevated this could be due to lung disease [8]. A low DLCO is also associated with pulmonary veno-occlusive disease [9]—which is common in SSc and rapidly lethal unless transplantation is an option.

There is therefore insufficient information to provide reassurance to this patient. Further information is required to determine the pre-test probability that the echo data supports or excludes PAH. From the ECG whether right axis deviation is present. We also need the urate and N terminal probrain natriuretic peptide (NT-proBNP) levels and FVC (forced vital capacity), only then can we use the DETECT algorithm [10] to determine the pre-test probability of PAH for any given echocardiographic findings.

From the echocardiogram we need to know the right atrial area (the probability of PAH increases as right atrial area increases), and the triscuspid velocity (TV—estPASP includes an inaccurate estimate of right atrial pressure that increases the error significantly): above 2.3 m/s, or 22mmmHg the probability of PAH increases [10], above 3.4 m/s or est PAPS of 50 mmHg PH is highly probable irrespective of other findings [11]. It is important to also look at the left heart—reduced left ventricular ejection fraction (LVEF), left ventricular hypertrophy, valve disorders, left atrial enlargement or abnormal diastolic function all increase the likelihood that a left heart abnormality is present.

A flow-chart of how to screen and subsequently investigate for SSc PH is presented below (Fig. 9.1), an outline of management options is shown in Fig. 9.2.

Patient 2: Elevated Pulmonary Pressures with Breathlessness

A 55-year-old male with a 6 month history of diffuse Systemic Sclerosis, anti-Scl-70 positive and overlap myositis (CK 630iu) presents with breathlessness on modest exertion and palpitations. He denies any syncopal or presyncopal events. He is noted to have a persistent positive Troponin between 62 and 70 ng/L, an echocardiogram has reported LVEF of 55%, and estimated PASP of 55 mmHg. How should one proceed?

This patient may have a triscuspid velocity of 3.5 m/s and thus almost certain PH if the RA was estimated to be 5 mmHg, or <3.4 m/s if the RA is estimated as ≥10 mmHg, in which case supportive evidence of right heart abnormalities is recommended as detailed in Fig. 9.1 [2]. If PH is present, this may be due to PAH but there are pointers suggesting that postcapillary PH is more likely.

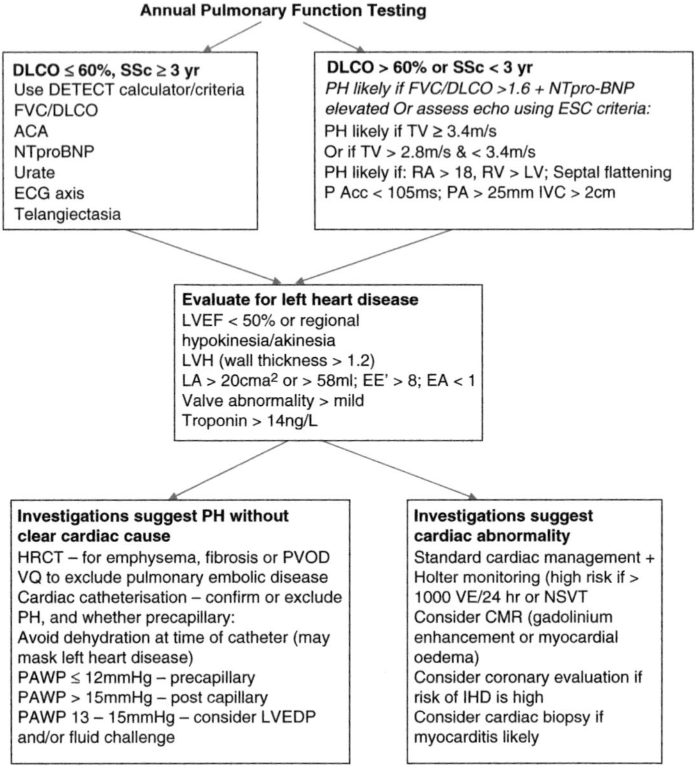

Legend. Flow chart illustrating the issues arising during screening. Patients may or may not meet criteria for DETECT, if not there is only consensus guidance on how to screen. Once echo is done as part of screening one may incidentally find cardiac abnormalities, that cannot be ignored.
ACA – anticentromere antibody status; LVEF left ventricular ejection fraction; LVH left ventricular hypertrophy; HRCT high resolution CT scanning; VQ – ventilation perfusion scan, PAWP – pulmonary artery wedge pressure; VE ventriculr ectopy; CMR cardiac magnetic resonance

Figure 9.1 Annual Pulmonary Function Testing

Patients with early DSSc and myositis are reported to be at higher risk of severe cardiac involvement, though it can occur in all SSc patients and at any time during the disease course [12]. Cardiac involvement is usually subclinical with minor ECG abnormalities (such as intraventricular conduction defects or loss of R wave in septal leads) [13], mild to

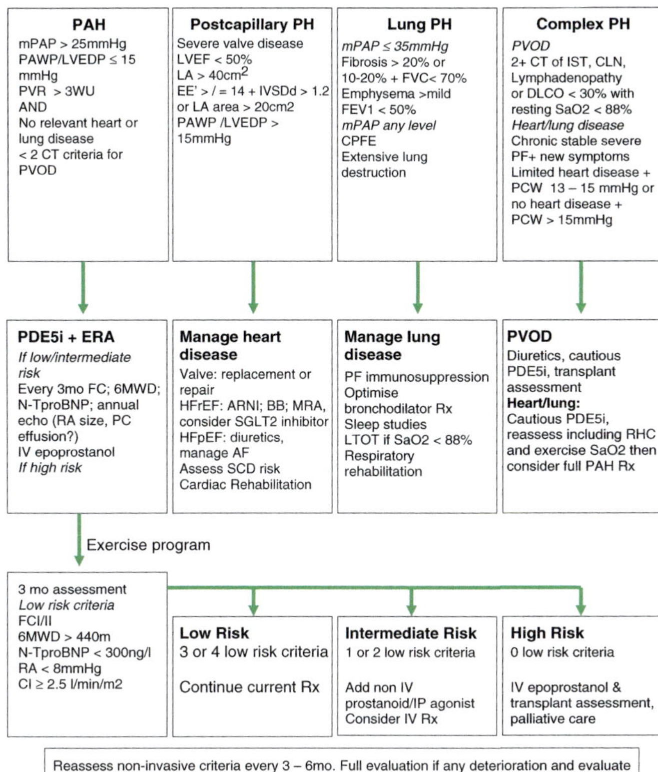

Legend: LVEDP - left ventricular end diastolic pressure; PVR – pulmonary vascular resistance; PAWP – pulmonary artery wedge pressure; IVSDd – interventricular septal diameter in diastole; CT computerised tomography; IST interlobular septal thickening; CLN – centrilobular nodules; PDE5i – phosphodiesterase type 5 inhibitor; ERA endothelin receptor antagonist; FC – functional class; RA – right atrium; 6MWD – six minute walking distance; ACEi – angiotensin converting enzyme inhibitors; BB – betablockers; CRT(D) – cardiac resynchronisation therapy (defibrillator); SCD – sudden cardiac death; PC – pericardial; AF – atrial fibrillation; LTOT – longterm oxygen therapy; ARNI - angiotensin receptor neprilysin inhibitor; MRA - mineralocorticoid receptor antagonist

FIGURE 9.2 Overview of SSc PH management

moderate diastolic impairment on echo [13], and cardiac magnetic resonance (CMR) scanning with wall thickness abnormalities or regional late gadolinium enhancement [14].

HFpEF (heart failure with preserved ejection fraction) is the most common form of symptomatic cardiac disease in SSc [12]. Previously this was called diastolic heart failure. In breathless patients the EE' is high (often >\=14), there is left atrial dilation (usually >24 cm^2 or 69 mL) and atrial fibrillation is common [15]. Pulmonary hypertension is common and may be severe. NT-proBNP is usually elevated and often quite high (>1000 ng/L). Breathless occurs on effort and may progress to overt heart failure. Because systolic function is preserved and pulmonary hypertension develops gradually, the echo appearances can be almost indistinguishable from PAH—with a dilated poorly functioning right heart and even septal flattening in advanced HFpEF associated PH (mPAP >40 mmHg) [15]. In such cases LA enlargement usually provides the clue that the problem is left sided. Differentiating incidental left atrial dilation and PAH from HFpEF in patients with SSc is an art rather than a science and best done in expert centres. The only therapy that is established in HFpEF is diuretics [15].

Arrhythmias may or may not cause symptoms, in the setting of PH atrial arrhythmias worsen breathlessness and prognosis. Atrial fibrillation is strongly associated with HFpEF [15], in PAH atrial flutter is the more common atrial arrhythmia [16]. Sudden cardiac death due to ventricular tachyarrhythmias are strongly associated with high ventricular ectopic burden (>1000/24 h), NSVT and impaired systolic function with regional myocardial fibrosis [17]. In high risk cases an ICD is required [13], where the risk is uncertain, implantable monitors should be considered.

Coronary disease is believed to be more common in SSc than in the general population [18], though the data are inconsistent [19]. IHD should be considered where risk factors are identified or there is exertional chest discomfort. The presence of coronary disease complicates the management of PH.

HFrEF (heart failure with reduced ejection fraction) is relatively uncommon but important [12], PH is relatively less common in HFrEF but can occur. It is associated with male sex, older age, overlap myositis, and lung involvement [20], it may be driven by an inflammatory myocarditis with persistently elevated troponin. Once the diagnosis is established immunosuppressive therapy is recommended in addition to all standard therapies for systolic heart failure [13]. In this population betablocker treatment is required despite the presence of Raynaud's, carvedilol is often well tolerated as a vasodilating betablocker. In patients that progress to end stage heart failure despite standard treatment cardiac transplantion is an option.

In this case we see high risk features (DSSc, overlap myositis, persistent Troponin elevation) but preserved ejection fraction. The elevated estPASP is a concern and cardiac catheterisation would be required to determine if PH is present. If postcapillary PH is confirmed, diuretics are required as stated above [15]. Confirmatory catheterisation is not required where PH is clearly postcapillary, for example the LA area is >40 cm^2 and there is no septal flattening [15]. A CMR and rhythm monitoring are essential in this case, if there is evidence of myocardial inflammation, then immunosuppression should be considered. If this is necessary from a non-cardiac perspective then one should simply proceed and monitor the Troponin and LVEF. If there is no non-cardiac indication, then we advise monitoring the Troponin and LVEF on a 6 monthly basis [13]. If the troponin escalates or the EF falls then immunosuppression should be considered, cardiac biopsy to exclude viral infection and confirm inflammatory cell infiltration and ideally chemokine drivers may help guide choice of therapy.

References

1. Nihtyanova SI, Schreiber BE, Ong VH, Rosenberg D, Moinzadeh P, Coghlan JG, Wells AU, Denton CP. Prediction of pulmonary complications and long-term survival in systemic sclerosis. Arthritis Rheumatol. 2014;66(6):1625–35.
2. Galiè N, et al. 2015 ESC/ERS Guidelines for the diagnosis and treatment of pulmonary hypertension. The Joint Task Force for the Diagnosis and Treatment of Pulmonary Hypertension of the European Society of Cardiology (ESC) and the European Respiratory Society (ERS). Eur Heart J. 2016;37:67–119.

3. Rizzi M, Sarzi-Puttini P, Airoldi A, Antivalle M, Battellino M, Atzeni F. Performance capacity evaluated using the 6-minute walk test: 5-year results in patients with diffuse systemic sclerosis and initial interstitial lung disease. Clin Exp Rheumatol. 2015;33(4 Suppl 91):S142–7.
4. Condliffe R, Kiely DG, Peacock AJ, Corris PA, Gibbs JS, Vrapi F, Das C, Elliot CA, Johnson M, DeSoyza J, Torpy C, Goldsmith K, Hodgkins D, Hughes RJ, Pepke-Zaba J, Coghlan JG. Connective tissue disease-associated pulmonary arterial hypertension in the modern treatment era. Am J Respir Crit Care Med. 2009;179:151–7.
5. Humbert M, Sitbon O, Yaïci A, et al. Survival in incident and prevalent cohorts of patients with pulmonary arterial hypertension. Eur Respir J. 2010;36:549–55.
6. Aduen JF, et al. Accuracy and precision of three echocardiographic methods for estimating mean pulmonary artery pressure. Chest. 2011;139(2):347–52.
7. Fisher MR, Forfia PR, Chamera E, et al. Accuracy of Doppler echocardiography in the hemodynamic assessment of pulmonary hypertension. Am J Respir Crit Care Med. 2009;179:615–21.
8. Antoniou KM, et al. Combined pulmonary fibrosis and emphysema in scleroderma-related lung disease has a major confounding effect on lung physiology and screening for pulmonary hypertension. Arthritis Rheumatol. 2016;68(4):1004–12.
9. Connolly MJ, Abdullah S, Ridout DA, Schreiber BE, Haddock JA, Coghlan JG. Prognostic significance of computed tomography criteria for pulmonary veno-occlusive disease in systemic sclerosis-pulmonary arterial hypertension. Rheumatology (Oxford). 2017;56(12):2197–203.
10. Coghlan JG, Denton CP, Grünig E, Bonderman D, Distler O, Khanna D, Müller-Ladner U, Pope JE, Vonk MC, Doelberg M, Chadha-Boreham H, Heinzl H, Rosenberg DM, McLaughlin VV, Seibold JR, DETECT study group. Evidence-based detection of pulmonary arterial hypertension in systemic sclerosis: the DETECT study. Ann Rheum Dis. 2014;73(7):1340–9.
11. Mukerjee D, St George D, Knight C, et al. Echocardiography and pulmonary function as screening tests for pulmonary arterial hypertension in systemic sclerosis. Rheumatology (Oxford). 2004;43:461–6.
12. Bissell LA, Md Yusof MY, Buch MH. Primary myocardial disease in scleroderma-a comprehensive review of the literature to

inform the UK systemic sclerosis study group cardiac working group. Rheumatology (Oxford). 2017;56(6):882–95.

13. Bissell LA, Anderson M, Burgess M, Chakravarty K, Coghlan G, Dumitru RB, Graham L, Ong V, Pauling JD, Plein S, Schlosshan D, Woolfson P, Buch MH. Consensus best practice pathway of the UK systemic sclerosis study group: management of cardiac disease in systemic sclerosis. Rheumatology (Oxford). 2017;56(6):912–21.
14. Hachulla AL, Launay D, Gaxotte V, et al. Cardiac magnetic resonance imaging in systemic sclerosis: a cross-sectional observational study of 52 patients. Ann Rheum Dis. 2009;68(12):1878–84.
15. Vachiéry JL, Tedford RJ, Rosenkranz S, et al. Pulmonary hypertension due to left heart disease. Eur Respir J. 2018. pii: 1801897;53:1801897. https://doi.org/10.1183/13993003.01897-2018.
16. Mercurio V, Peloquin G, Bourji KI, Diab N, Sato T, Enobun B, Housten-Harris T, Damico R, Kolb TM, Mathai SC, Tedford RJ, Tocchetti CG, Hassoun PM. Pulmonary arterial hypertension and atrial arrhythmias: incidence, risk factors, and clinical impact. Pulm Circ. 2018;8(2):2045894018769874. https://doi.org/10.1177/2045894018769874.
17. De Luca G, Bosello SL, Gabrielli FA, et al. Prognostic role of ventricular ectopic beats in systemic sclerosis: a prospective cohort study shows ECG indexes predicting the worse outcome. PLoS One. 2016;11(4):e0153012. https://doi.org/10.1371/journal.pone.0153012. eCollection 2016
18. Ungprasert P, Charoenpong P, Ratanasrimetha P, Thongprayoon C, Cheungpasitporn W, Suksaranjit P. Risk of coronary artery disease in patients with systemic sclerosis: a systematic review and meta-analysis. Clin Rheumatol. 2014;33(8):1099–104.
19. Colaci M, Giuggioli D, Spinella A, Vacchi C, Lumetti F, Mattioli AV, Coppi F, Aiello V, Perticone M, Malatino L, Ferri C. Established coronary artery disease in systemic sclerosis compared to type 2 diabetic female patients: a cross-sectional study. Clin Rheumatol. 2019;38:1637–42. https://doi.org/10.1007/s10067-019-04427-2.
20. Allanore Y, Meune C, Vonk MC, et al. Prevalence and factors associated with left ventricular dysfunction in the EULAR Scleroderma Trial and Research group (EUSTAR) database of patients with systemic sclerosis. Ann Rheum Dis. 2010;69(1):218–21.

Chapter 10
Digital Ulcers

Michael Hughes and Cosimo Bruni

Introduction

Digital ulcers (DU) are common (Fig. 10.1) in patients with SSc and are a major non-lethal complication associated with the disease. Around half of patients report a history of DUs [1, 2]. Common sites for DUs include the fingertips and over the dorsal aspect of the fingers [2]. They can also occur on the lower limbs/toes [3]. Fingertip DUs are ischaemic and driven by the progressive vasculopathy observed in SSc. Whereas, dorsal aspect DUs are driven by the progressive thinning of the skin/contractures and recurrent trauma to these exposed surfaces. DUs can also develop from existing digital pitting scars and in relation to underlying calcinosis [2]. They can also occur on the lateral aspects of the digits and at the base of the nail (Fig. 10.1).

M. Hughes (✉)
Department of Rheumatology, Royal Hallamshire Hospital, Sheffield Teaching Hospitals NHS Foundation Trust, Sheffield, UK
e-mail: Michael.hughes-6@postgrad.manchester.ac.uk

C. Bruni
Department of Experimental and Clinical Medicine, Division of Rheumatology, University of Florence, Florence, Italy

© Springer Nature Switzerland AG 2021

M. Matucci-Cerinic, C. P. Denton (eds.), *Practical Management of Systemic Sclerosis in Clinical Practice*, In Clinical Practice,
https://doi.org/10.1007/978-3-030-53736-4_10

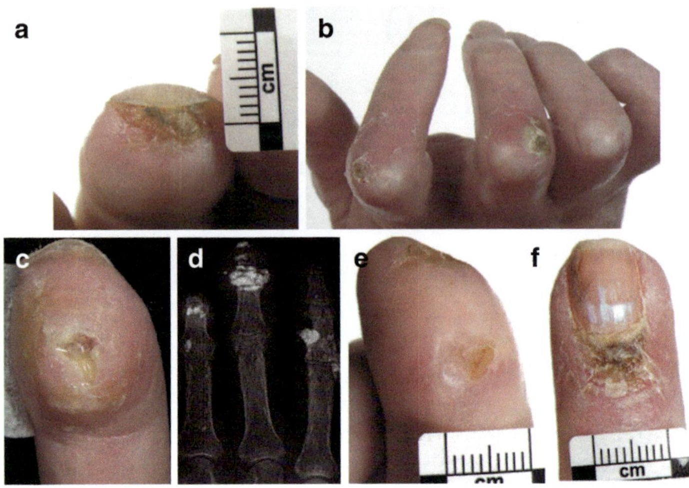

FIGURE 10.1 SSc-DUs. Fingertip (**a**), extensor (**b**), overlying subcutaneous calcinosis as seen on a plain radiograph (**c** and **d**, respectively), and on the lateral aspect (**e**) and the nailbed of the fingers (**f**). Reproduced with permission [10]

Microvascular and Microvascular Assessment

Both microvascular and macrovascular involvement are implicated in SSc-DUs. The progressive microangiopathy (e.g. enlarged capillaries with areas of avascularity) which characterises the SSc disease process is easily appreciated by nailfold capillaroscopy. Although videocapillaroscopy (magnification ×200–600) is considered the 'gold standard', capillaroscopy can also be performed using a number of other lower-magnification techniques such as the dermatoscope [4] or USB-microscope. A number of authors [5–7] have reported that nailfold capillaroscopic abnormalities are highly predictive of the development of future DU (and in their absence are reassuring to the clinician). Thermography which measures surface temperature can differentiate between patients with primary and secondary Raynaud's phenomenon (RP) [8], however, at present its use is limited to a number of specialist centres. A key point is the need to distinguish between primary ('idiopathic) and secondary RP (i.e. due to an underlying medical condition such as SSc) because patients with PRP do not develop ischaemic tissue damage such as DUs. Macrovascular involvement is a very important feature that must not be neglected including abnormalities of the digital and ulnar arteries. An increased risk of cardiovascular disease has also been reported in patients with SSc [9]. The peripheral pulses should be assessed in all patients with digital ischaemia. Arterial Doppler scanning should be performed early if there is any clinical suspicion of proximal (large) vessel disease and confirmed by large vessel imaging [10]. Large vessel disease should be identified early as this potentially could be amenable to successful therapeutic intervention.

Pain Evaluation and its Management

SSc-DUs can be exceptionally painful and disabling, and therefore the evaluation of pain is mandatory. A simple method to evaluate pain is to perform a visual analogue scale using a 10 cm long line in which the patient indicates their level of pain (the left being the lowest possible and the right representing the highest). Such an approach can be used to track DU progression/healing and to inform changes in pain management. Patients not uncommonly require strong (i.e. opioid-based) analgesia. Nocturnal pain can be very disabling and can significantly disturb sleep. A key approach is to consider and identify DU infection early and to treat with appropriate anti-microbial therapy, as this may contribute to the patient's pain generation. Severe pain and tenderness are a potential indication for surgical intervention which can suggest the collection of pus and/or necrotic material [11]. This should be suspected where palpation of the DU is associated with significant pain [11].

Disability and Functionality Assessment and its Management

As previously described, DUs are associated with significant disability including all of the activities of daily living and occupation. In routine practice it is very important for the clinician to actively ask about function including the activities of daily living/occupation during their consultation. The impact of SSc-DU on personal relations including emotional health, sexual relationships and social participation should also be examined. There is no disease-specific patient reported outcome instrument to assess the severity and impact of SSc-DUs. In general, there is a reliance of legacy instruments to assess the patient experience of SSc-DUs [12]. Patients should be managed as part of a dedicated multidisciplinary team including (but not limited to) physicians, nurses and physiotherapists who understand the challenges of caring for patients with SSc [13]. The goal is to identify any associated disability and functional impairment early so that patients can receive prompt intervention. For example, specialist input from colleagues in physiotherapy and occupational therapy for issues relating to physical function and the activities of daily living.

Complications and Their Management

Infections are a frequent complication of SSc-DUs, and are often caused by *Staphylococcus aureus*, *Pseudomonas aeruginosa* or faecal pathogens. As previously discussed, infection can cause significant pain and is associated with the presence of the signs of inflammation [14].

Although rare, fistula can develop from infection, representing a communication between the DU and a deeper layer of the skin (in particularly in calcinosis induced DU) [15]. Fistulae can be suspected in the case of the appearance of a second satellite lesion, depression of wound edges or, when aboundant exudate is present [15].

Infections can spread to the surrounding soft tissues, causing cellulitis, or to the bone, resulting in ostomyelitis. While elevated acute phase reactants and/or an increase in the neutrophil count may raise the suspicion of presence of infection, radiographs and MRI are considered the first line and confirmatory tests for osteomyelitis, respectively. Osteopenia and periosteal reactions on radiography guide the clinician to request a MRI scan, showing the presence of bone oedema if there is bone Infection [14].

Gangrene represents the most severe DU complication. This should be suspected when a line of demarcation appears, representing the inflammatory reaction dividing dead and living tissues [16]. Gangrene can present as a dry, dark coloured area, evolving into dehydration and rarely mummification, otherwise as wet, when bacterial infecion determine purulent liquefaction [16]. The latter is frequently associated with soft tissue oedema, maceration and a characteristic odor. In the case of gangrene, it is mandatory to evaluate macrovascular blood flow, in order to exclude vascular stenosis/large vessel disease (.e.g. by performing Allen's test and Doppler ultrasound) [16].

Local Treatment: Wound Bed Preparation

The principles of local treatment of DUs are derived from the "Wound bed preparation" algorithm from diabetic ulcer care, which includes all the possible intereventions which favour lesion healing. All these concepts are included in the acronym "TIME" [17]: "T" for tissue management, which includes a deep agitation to remove dirt, necrotic tissue and remnants of previous dressings, and allows tissue evaluation [18]. This is followed by evaluation of "I", including both inflammation/infection, which should be suspected in the case of redness and swelling of surrounding skin and in case of exudate/purulent slough in the wound bed [18]. Once washed, DU should undergo debridement to remove all necrotic tissues which may prevent the lesion from promoting self-healing. Debridement requires adequate anesthesia to be perfomed physically with a scalpel [19, 20], otherwise this can be done chemically, using autolytic dressings, such as alginate for exudating wounds or hydrogels and hydrocolloids for dry or poorly exudating wounds. The general status of "M", the moisture balance of the wound, is of pivotal importance: as both excessive dryness or exudation are not efficient in promoting wound healing, and an appropriate dressing choice should help in restoring a correct hydration status [21]. Finally, DU edges ("E") evaluation is important, as it reflects the attempt and the evolution of healing, from periphery to centres and from bottom to top: hyper-proliferation or undermining of the edges should always be checked and locally treated [18].

Systemic Treatment: Healing and Prevention

Systemic medical treatment (Fig. 10.2) is of pivotal importance and aims at both preventing and healing DUs [22]. Prevention includes education of the patient in cold exposure and trauma avoidance and pharmacological treatment of Raynaud's phenomenon, which commonly includes calcium-channel blockers. DU vasodilating and vasoactive treatments targets the three main pathways of SSc vasculopathy: prostanoids, in particular intravenous Iloprost over 3–5 days, which compensates for prostacyclin deficiency, and have proven efficacy in DU healing and preventing DU recurrency when administered chronically [23, 24]. Similarly, phosphodiesterase 5 inhibitors restore the lack of nitric oxide. The SEDUCE trial showed a trend for higher DU healing rate, in particular when used in combination with Bosentan [25]. Endothelin 1 receptor antagonists, i.e. Bosentan, have a vasoactive effect, promoting vasodilation and vascular-remodelling. Both the RAPIDS-1 and RAPIDS-2 studies showed beneficial effect in DU prevention, and this was more significant in those patients with more than 3 DUs [26, 27].

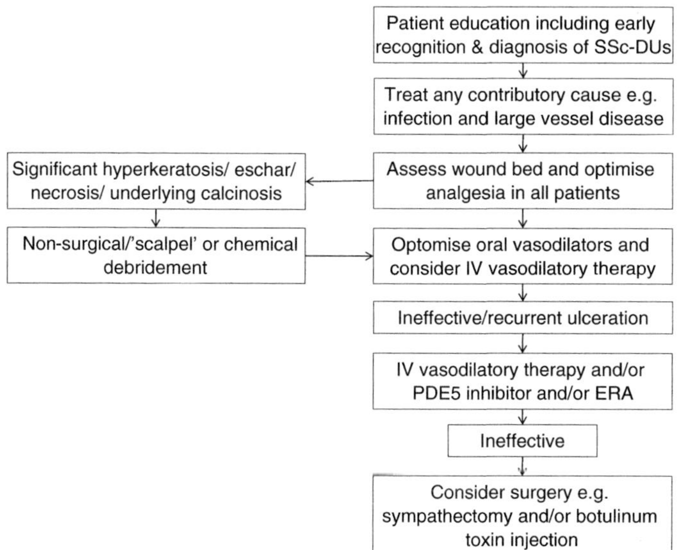

FIGURE 10.2 The management of SSc-DUs. Adapted from the UK Scleroderma Study Group Best Practice Recommendations on the management of DUs in patients with SSc [10]. ERA: Endothelin receptor antagonist. IV: Intravenous. PDE5: Phosphodiesterase type-5

In the case of non-resolving local infection when treated with topical anti-septic dressings or systemic infection, then systemic antibiotic treatment is of pivotal importance. This can include empirical treatment with broad-spectrum drugs, obtaining a swab sample with microbiologic isolation, and then targeted antibiotic therapy (Fig. 10.3). Hospitalisation for intravenous treatment is indicated for cases of septic/ osteomyelitis evolution [28].

In the case of medical treatment failure, then surgical options should be considered. Botulinum A toxin injection is a mini-invasive procedure, promoting local arterial vasodilation [29]. The same effect can also be obtained with a deep-surgical peripheral sympathectomy [11]. As a promising rescue treatment, a single injection of autologous fat tissue derived stem cells has proven to be effective in DU healing [30].

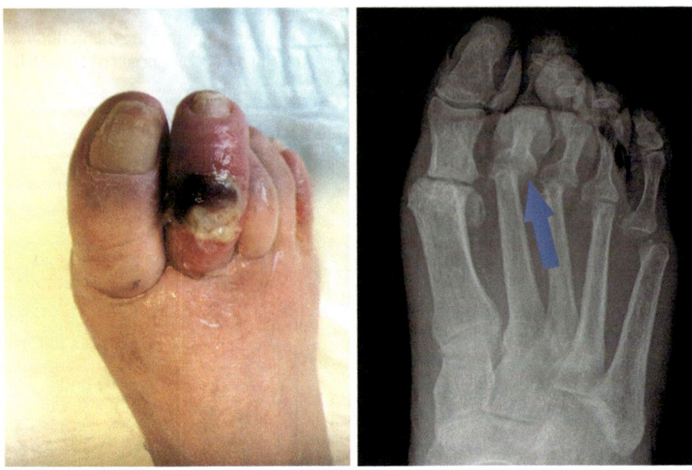

FIGURE 10.3 Management of SSc-DU. A 55 years old female patient with limited SSc and overlap with anti-phospholipid syndrome presented with a painful ulcer on the second toe of the right foot. Despite common vasodilating and vasoactive treatments, combined with wound bed-preparation and local dressings, the ulcer remained very painful and did not tend to improve. When radiography was performed, an area of bone reabsorption was seen at the basis of the proximal phalanx of the second toe (blue arrow), and was later confirmed by MRI as compatible with ostomyelitis. Treatment with Ciprofloxacine and Trimetoprim-Sulphametoxazole was used in association with the above mentioned treatment, with final ulcer healing

Conclusion

DUs are common and represent a serious complication of SSc. Different types of DU exist based upon the underlying pathophysiology. Microvascular and macrovascular assesment is needed. Both medical and surgical options are avaliable to treat SSc-DUs. Careful attention must be paid to wound bed management and the treatment of complications (e.g. infection). Associated pain and disability/impairment of function must be identified and managed appropriately.

Through prompt assessment and the initiation of targeted treatment for DUs, clinicians can preserve patients hand function and prevent the development of devastating ischaemic tissue loss.

References

1. Tiev KP, Diot E, Clerson P, Dupuis-Simeon F, Hachulla E, Hatron PY, et al. Clinical features of scleroderma patients with or without prior or current ischemic digital ulcers: post-hoc analysis of a nationwide multicenter cohort (ItinerAIR-Sclerodermie). J Rheumatol. 2009;36(7):1470–6. https://doi.org/10.3899/jrheum.081044.
2. Hughes M, Herrick AL. Digital ulcers in systemic sclerosis. Rheumatology (Oxford). 2017;56(1):14–25. https://doi.org/10.1093/rheumatology/kew047.
3. Blagojevic J, Piemonte G, Benelli L, Braschi F, Fiori G, Bartoli F, et al. Assessment, definition, and classification of lower limb ulcers in systemic sclerosis: a challenge for the rheumatologist. J Rheumatol. 2016;43(3):592–8. https://doi.org/10.3899/jrheum.150035.
4. Hughes M, Moore T, O'Leary N, Tracey A, Ennis H, Dinsdale G, et al. A study comparing videocapillaroscopy and dermoscopy in the assessment of nailfold capillaries in patients with systemic sclerosis-spectrum disorders. Rheumatology (Oxford). 2015;54(8):1435–42. https://doi.org/10.1093/rheumatology/keu533.
5. Sebastiani M, Manfredi A, Vukatana G, Moscatelli S, Riato L, Bocci M, et al. Predictive role of capillaroscopic skin ulcer risk index in systemic sclerosis: a multicentre validation study. Ann Rheum Dis. 2012;71(1):67–70. https://doi.org/10.1136/annrheumdis-2011-200022.
6. Manfredi A, Sebastiani M, Carraro V, Iudici M, Bocci M, Vukatana G, et al. Prediction risk chart for scleroderma digital ulcers: a composite predictive model based on capillaroscopic, demographic and clinico-serological parameters. Clin Hemorheol Microcirc. 2015;59(2):133–43. https://doi.org/10.3233/CH-141809.

7. Cutolo M, Herrick AL, Distler O, Becker MO, Beltran E, Carpentier P, et al. Nailfold Videocapillaroscopic features and other clinical risk factors for digital ulcers in systemic sclerosis: a multicenter, Prospective Cohort Study. Arthritis Rheumatol. 2016;68(10):2527–39. https://doi.org/10.1002/art.39718.
8. Anderson ME, Moore TL, Lunt M, Herrick AL. The 'distal-dorsal difference': a thermographic parameter by which to differentiate between primary and secondary Raynaud's phenomenon. Rheumatology (Oxford). 2007;46(3):533–8. https://doi.org/10.1093/rheumatology/kel330.
9. Man A, Zhu Y, Zhang Y, Dubreuil M, Rho YH, Peloquin C, et al. The risk of cardiovascular disease in systemic sclerosis: a population-based cohort study. Ann Rheum Dis. 2013;72(7):1188–93. https://doi.org/10.1136/annrheumdis-2012-202007.
10. Hughes M, Ong VH, Anderson ME, Hall F, Moinzadeh P, Griffiths B, et al. Consensus best practice pathway of the UK scleroderma study group: digital vasculopathy in systemic sclerosis. Rheumatology (Oxford). 2015;54(11):2015–24. https://doi.org/10.1093/rheumatology/kev201.
11. Muir J, AL H. Surgical approaches including sympathectomy. In: Matucci Cerinic M, Denton CP, editors. Atlas of ulcers in systemic sclerosis. Berlin: Springer; 2019. p. 173–82.
12. Hughes M, Pauling JD. Exploring the patient experience of digital ulcers in systemic sclerosis. Semin Arthritis Rheum. 2019; [Epub ahead of print];48:888–94. https://doi.org/10.1016/j.semarthrit.2018.08.001.
13. Bruni C, Pucci T, Rasero L, Denton CP. The team and the assessment. In: Matucci Cerinic M, Denton CP, editors. Atlas of ulcers in systemic sclerosis. Berlin: Springer; 2019.
14. Bellando-Randone S, Lepri G. Infections, cellulitis and osteomyelitis. In: Matucci Cerinic M, Denton CP, editors. Atlas of ulcers in systemic sclerosis. Berlin: Springer; 2019. p. 95–8.
15. Piemonte G, Braschi F, Fistulas RL. In: Matucci Cerinic M, Denton CP, editors. Atlas of ulcers in systemic sclerosis. Berlin: Springer; 2019. p. 89–94.
16. Blagojevic J. Digital loss (gangrene, amputation, autoamputation). In: Matucci Cerinic M, Denton CP, editors. Atlas of ulcers in systemic sclerosis. Berlin: Springer; 2019. p. 99–104.
17. Schultz GS, Sibbald RG, Falanga V, Ayello EA, Dowsett C, Harding K, et al. Wound bed preparation: a systematic approach to wound management. Wound Repair Regen. 2003;11(Suppl 1):S1–28.

18. Piemonte G, Benelli L, Braschi F, Rasero L. The local treatment: methodology, debridement and wound bed preparation. In: Matucci Cerinic M, Denton CP, editors. Atlas of ulcers in systemic sclerosis. Berlin: Springer; 2019. p. 145–60.
19. Braschi F, Bartoli F, Bruni C, Fiori G, Fantauzzo C, Paganelli L, et al. Lidocaine controls pain and allows safe wound bed preparation and debridement of digital ulcers in systemic sclerosis: a retrospective study. Clin Rheumatol. 2017;36(1):209–12. https://doi.org/10.1007/s10067-016-3414-7.
20. Giuggioli D, Manfredi A, Vacchi C, Sebastiani M, Spinella A, Ferri C. Procedural pain management in the treatment of scleroderma digital ulcers. Clin Exp Rheumatol. 2015;33(1):5–10.
21. Lebedoff N, Frech TM, Shanmugam VK, Fischer A, Erhardt D, Kolfenbach J, et al. Review of local wound management for scleroderma-associated digital ulcers. J Scleroderma Rel Disord. 2018;3(1):66–70. https://doi.org/10.5301/jsrd.5000268.
22. Bruni C, Bellando-Randone S, Denton CP, Matucci Cerinic M. Ulcer healing and prevention in systemic sclerosis. In: Matucci Cerinic M, Denton CP, editors. Atlas of ulcers in systemic sclerosis. Berlin: Springer; 2019. p. 167–71.
23. Zachariae H, Halkier-Sorensen L, Bjerring P, Heickendorff L. Treatment of ischaemic digital ulcers and prevention of gangrene with intravenous iloprost in systemic sclerosis. Acta Derm Venereol. 1996;76(3):236–8. https://doi.org/10.2340/0001555576236238.
24. Wigley FM, Seibold JR, Wise RA, McCloskey DA, Dole WP. Intravenous iloprost treatment of Raynaud's phenomenon and ischemic ulcers secondary to systemic sclerosis. J Rheumatol. 1992;19(9):1407–14.
25. Hachulla E, Hatron PY, Carpentier P, Agard C, Chatelus E, Jego P, et al. Efficacy of sildenafil on ischaemic digital ulcer healing in systemic sclerosis: the placebo-controlled SEDUCE study. Ann Rheum Dis. 2016;75(6):1009–15. https://doi.org/10.1136/annrheumdis-2014-207001.
26. Korn JH, Mayes M, Matucci Cerinic M, Rainisio M, Pope J, Hachulla E, et al. Digital ulcers in systemic sclerosis: prevention by treatment with bosentan, an oral endothelin receptor antagonist. Arthritis Rheum. 2004;50(12):3985–93. https://doi.org/10.1002/art.20676.
27. Matucci-Cerinic M, Denton CP, Furst DE, Mayes MD, Hsu VM, Carpentier P, et al. Bosentan treatment of digital ulcers related to systemic sclerosis: results from the RAPIDS-2 ran-

domised, double-blind, placebo-controlled trial. Ann Rheum Dis. 2011;70(1):32–8. https://doi.org/10.1136/ard.2010.130658.
28. Raja J, Ong VH. Antibiotic treatment. In: Matucci Cerinic M, Denton CP, editors. Atlas of ulcers in systemic sclerosis. Berlin: Springer; 2019. p. 183–92.
29. George N, Kanzara T, Chakravarty K. Alternative therapeutic approaches in skin ulcers due to systemic sclerosis. In: Matucci Cerinic M, Denton CP, editors. Atlas of ulcers in systemic sclerosis. Berlin: Springer; 2019. p. 193–208.
30. Del Papa N, Di Luca G, Andracco R, Zaccara E, Maglione W, Pignataro F, et al. Regional grafting of autologous adipose tissue is effective in inducing prompt healing of indolent digital ulcers in patients with systemic sclerosis: results of a monocentric randomized controlled study. Arthritis Res Ther. 2019;21(1):7. https://doi.org/10.1186/s13075-018-1792-8.

Chapter 11
Lower Limb Ulcers

Jelena Blagojevic and Silvia Bellando-Randone

Background

Prevalence of lower limb ulcers in SSc has not been investigated, but our unpublished data suggest that around 10% of patients develop leg ulcers. It seems that patients with long-lasting limited cutaneous form of SSc are at highest risk.

Their etiopathogenesis is often multifactorial. Microangiopathy is one of the disease hallmarks [1] and may be the primary cause of leg ulcers. Concomitant arterial and/or venous macrovascular disease can overlap. Lymphedema may contribute to fluid stasis and facilitate ulcer formation. In addition, cutaneous traction over the bone prominences and repetitive trauma, calcinosis, hyperkeratosis, often related to articular deformities, loss of the fat pad and altered posture, may be involved [2].

Clinical case: You are called to evaluate a patient with SSc and lower limb ulcers referred to the Wound Clinic.

J. Blagojevic (✉) · S. Bellando-Randone
Department of Experimental and Clinical Medicine, University of Florence, Florence, Italy

Department of Geriatric Medicine, Division of Rheumatology and Scleroderma Unit, AOUC, Florence, Italy
e-mail: blagojevicj@aou-careggi.toscana.it

© Springer Nature Switzerland AG 2021

M. Matucci-Cerinic, C. P. Denton (eds.), *Practical Management of Systemic Sclerosis in Clinical Practice*, In Clinical Practice,
https://doi.org/10.1007/978-3-030-53736-4_11

70-years old female with limited cutaneous form of systemic sclerosis diagnosed 30 years before was referred to the Wound Clinic for lower limb ulcers evaluation. She has a long-standing history of recurrent digital ulcers and hand calcinosis. Current medications: calcium channel blockers, proton pomp inhibitors, cholecalciferol. On clinical examination there are sclerodactyly and digital pitting scars on the fingertips. There are two leg cutaneous lesions: right pretibial ulcer and left perimalleolar medial ulcer. There is hard whitish material in the bed of the pretibial lesion and perilesional skin is very inflamed. She has leg edema, more evident on the left, varicose veins on both legs and there is cutaneous dyschromia in the gaiter region of the left leg.

1. **Describe clinical assessment of these lesions?**
2. **How would you classify the limb ulcers described above?**
3. **How should these ulcers be managed?**

Clinical Assessment of the Lower Limb Lesions

Diagnostic work-up of leg ulcers should always include:

- *Clinical history*: Thorough clinical history including medications must be collected. History of hand DU, ulcers in other sites and calcinosis should be investigated.
- *The elements suggestive of macrovascular arterial involvement* are intermittent claudication, pain that worsens following leg elevation, cardiovascular risk factors, previous cardiovascular events
- *The elements suggestive of venous disease* are previous venous thrombo-embolism, varicose veins or their treatment, multiple pregnancies, obesity, occupation that require prolonged standing or sitting. The ulcer-related pain is usually relieved by elevation of the leg and is more intense in the evening.
- *Clinical examination*: In addition to general examination, assessment of peripheral pulses and auscultation of the bruits, evaluation of venous insufficiency, search of calci-

nosis, hyperkeratosis and foot deformities should be performed. Asymmetrical/abolished pulses and arterial bruits are suggestive of macrovascular arterial peripheral diseases. Oedema, varicosities, skin hyperpigmentation and/or discoloration, inverted “champagne bottle” aspect of the leg, atrophie blanche and lipodermatosclerosis are indicative of venous pathology.

- *Ulcer assessment*: The following characteristics should be registered: localization, dimensions, borders, features of the bed of the lesion and of the perilesional skin, depth of the ulcer. Ulcer related pain should be registered, using VAS scale. Signs of infection ought to be searched.
- *Examinations*: All patients with lower limb ulcers should perform arterial and venous colour Doppler ultrasound (US) examination and ABI (ankle-brachial index) assessment. Patients with hemodynamically significant peripheral arterial disease on arterial colour Doppler US, with distribution consistent with the ulcer site, should undergo digital subtraction angiography (arteriography), if endovascular intervention is feasible and planned. Not-invasive CT/MR angiography should be performed if conventional angiography is contraindicated or in selected cases in order to assess localization and severity of arterial lesions and guide interventional strategies. The advantages of MR over CT angiography are no exposure to radiation and iodine contrast and higher soft tissue resolution [3]. However, it has higher motion artefacts and underestimates arterial calcifications [3]. Clinical utility of complementary exams, such as toe systolic blood pressure, toe-brachial index and transcutaneous oxygen pressure measurement, that may be useful in patients with medial calcinosis and incompressible arteries in other clinical setting [3, 4] has not been investigated in SSc.
- In patients with arterial macrovasular disease, the involvement of upper limb arteries ought to be assess. Carotid and coronary vessel disease should be also investigated especially in patients with traditional cardio-vascular risk factors.

- Supplementary investigations of the venous circulation, such as intravenous ultrasound and venography may be indicated in the selected cases. Angiologist/vascular surgeon must be actively involved in the decision making about the invasive procedures.
- Podiatric evaluation should be performed in patients with altered posture and foot deformities.
- If infection is suspected wound swab has to performed and if there is a suspicion of osteomyelitis, bone X-ray and subsequently MRI and CT ought to be done.
- If clinically indicated, additional examination (as Echocardiogram, Holter electrocardiogram, etc) should be performed for differential diagnosis with distal embolization, hematological disorders and overlap syndromes. Concurrent diabetes mellitus should be ruled out.
- All patients with lower limb ulcer ought to have the reassessment of disease activity and of internal organ involvement.

How Would you Classify the Limb Ulcers Described Above?

In SSc, the lower limb ulcers can be classified according to their origin and clinical features into:

1. **Ulcers associated with hyperkeratosis** (Fig. 11.1): Hyperkeratosis is represented by hypertrophy of the stratum corneum (eg callus and corn), located mainly in areas submitted to increased friction or pressure and fostered by foot deformities, loss of the fat pad, altered posture and microtrauma [2]. Hyperkeratosis promote an ulcer formation by pressing underneath tissues and causing their maceration, haematoma and autolysis, as occur in diabetic foot [5]. Ulcers associated with hyperkeratosis are usually hidden below the hyperkeratotic tissue and may be suspected when there is inflammation and oedema of perilesional skin. The final diagnosis can be made only after debridement, which is also mandatory for ulcer heling [2].

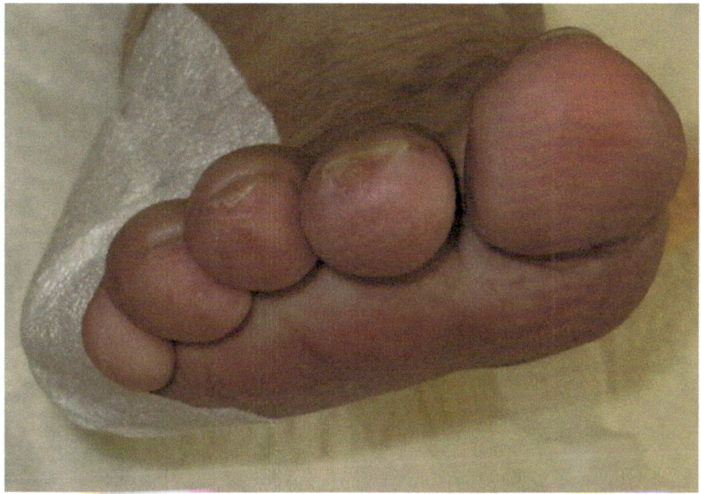

FIGURE 11.1 Ulcer associated with hyperkeratosis (reprinted with permission from Springer Nature)

2. **Ulcers secondary to calcinosis** (Fig. 11.2): These ulcers are directly caused by a mechanical action of calcinosis erupting through the skin. They are localised most frequently on pretibial area, have irregular borders and inflamed perilesional skin and calcinotic material erupting through the skin is often visible [2].
3. **Pure ulcers:** They can be defined as loss of epidermal covering with a break in the basement membrane not occurring in association with hyperkeratosis or with calcinosis. These lesions may be additionally classified into arterial, venous, mixed arterial-venous and pure microvascular ulcers, according to their origin.

    (a) **Venous ulcers** (Fig. 11.3)**:** Venous insufficiency seems to be the most frequent cause of lower limb ulcers in SSc. It has been estimated that 35–50% of ulcers have venous aetiology [2, 6]. Risk factors for venous disease have not been investigated is SSc, but traditional risk factors as previous thrombo-embolic events, vari-

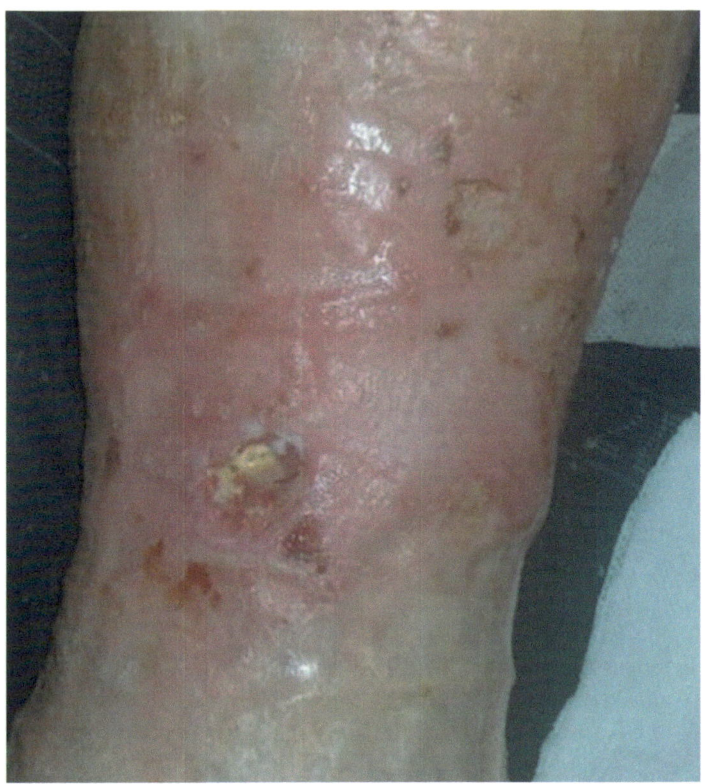

FIGURE 11.2 Ulcers secondary to calcinosis (reprinted with permission from Springer Nature)

cosities, pregnancies and obesity are probably involved. Venous ulcers are usually localized around the gaiter region, in SSc patients most frequently in the perimalleolar medial area [2]. They are typically shallow, have irregular shape, bed of the lesions is often covered by granulation tissue [4, 7, 8] and surrounding skin presents signs of venous insufficiency as described above [7, 8, 9].

(b) **Arterial ulcers** (Fig. 11.4): In the lower limbs, arterial disease may be the result of SSc-related macrovascular involvement and/or accelerated atherosclerosis [10–

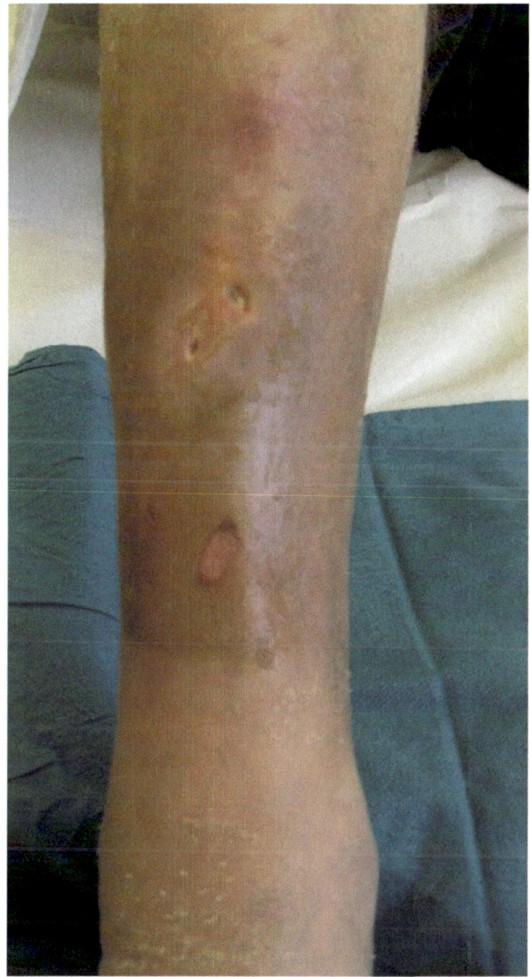

FIGURE 11.3 Venous ulcer (reprinted with permission from Springer Nature)

14]. Severe arterial involvement leading to lower limb ulcers has been described in 10–15% of SSc patients [2, 6]. Importantly, not all patients with significant arterial macrovascular involvement present leg ulcers. It seems that arterial involvement is more frequent in long

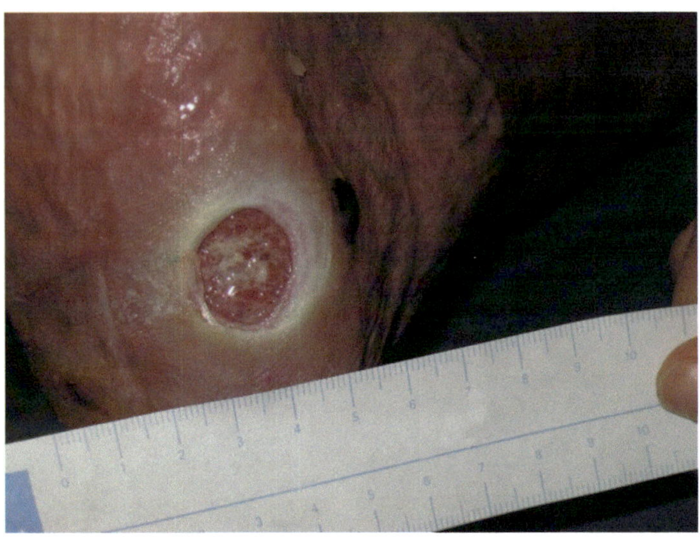

FIGURE 11.4 Arterial ulcer (reprinted with permission from Springer Nature)

standing limited cutaneous form of disease (**10,** personal observation), but risk factors/predictors for macrovascular arterial involvement in SSc has still to be determined.

Arterial ulcers have distinct borders, punched out appearance and cold surrounding skin [4, 7–9]. In SSc patients, they are localized more frequently on toes and heels and are the more painful than other types of leg ulcers [2].

(c) **Mixed arterial-venous ulcers:** Arterial macrovascular involvement and venous disease may overlap and contribute to the ulcer formation, as described in other clinical settings [4]. They have characteristics of both arterial and venous lesions, most frequently features of a venous ulcer in combination with signs of arterial impairment, such as absent or abolished pulses [7, 8].

(d) **Pure microvascular ulcers** (Fig. 11.5): These ischemic lesions are a consequence of SSc-related microangi-

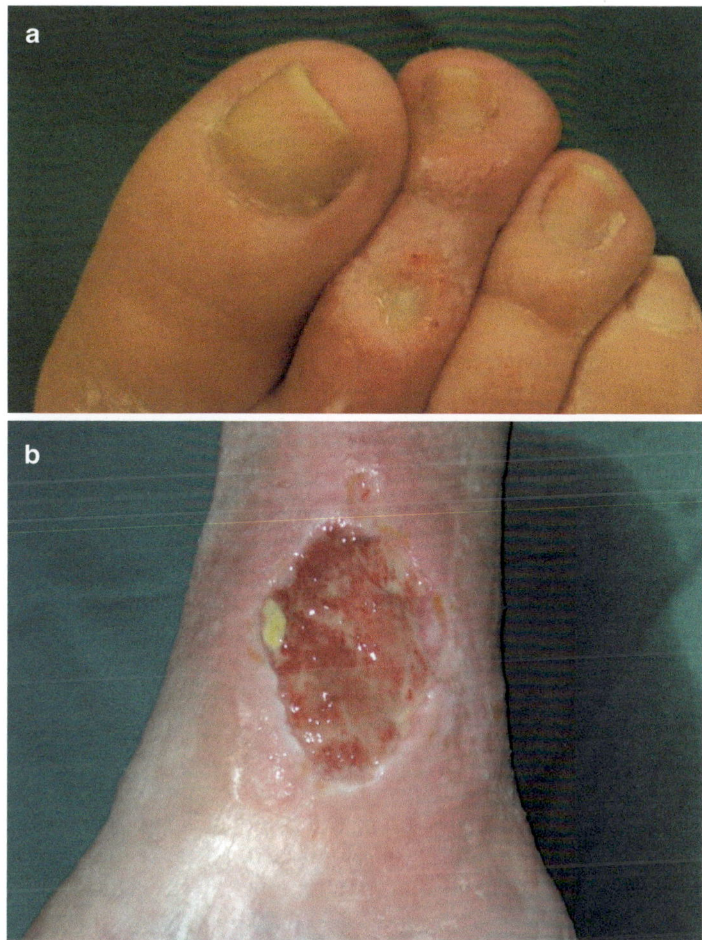

FIGURE 11.5 Pure microvascular ulcers (**a**) digital ulcer. (**b**) medial malleolus ulcer (reprinted with permission from Springer Nature)

opathy as digital ulcers in the upper limbs, although factors as tight skin and traction over the bony prominences (e.g malleolus) may contribute to the ulcer formation. Our personal observations suggest that longstanding limited cutaneous form of SSc, history of digital ulcers and ulcers in other locations may represent risk factors for these lesions. Pure microvascular ulcers have morphological characteristics of arterial ulcers in the absence of signs of macrovascular impairment (such as absent or diminished peripheral pulses) and are most frequently found on toes and on perimalleolar lateral area [2].

How Should These Ulcers Be Managed?

The general management of the lower limb ulcers is based on few fundamental steps:

1. *Removing/avoiding factors that may contribute to the ulcer formation*: adequate footwear, insoles and foot orthotics when indicated, avoiding trauma, smoking cessation, treatment of cardiovascular risk factors, elastic compression for venous insufficiency and lymphedema, lymph drainage for lymphedema
2. *Supportive measures*: prompt analgesia, maintenance of adequate nutritional status
3. *Local treatment based on wound care principles*. To ensure ulcer healing, lesions must be vascularized, free of necrotic and nonviable tissue, without infection, and kept moist. One of the pivotal steps of the local treatment is debridement which consists in removal of necrotic, nonviable and infected tissue and is fundamental for the healing. Sharp debridement is the main treatment for ulcers associated with hyperkeratosis and ulcers secondary to calcinosis. Simple hyperkeratosis should be promptly debrided in order to prevent ulcer formation.
4. *Pharmacological treatment*: optimization of vasodilating/vasoactive treatment, consideration/increase of immunosuppression/immunomodulation, treatment of cardiovascular risk factors. Statins and anti-platelet medications may be useful, especially in patients with macrovascular arterial disease
5. *Additional treatments*: topical vitamin E, hyperbaric oxygen for severe and persistent ulcers [15].

Patients with critical arterial macrovascular disease with distribution consistent with the ulcer site and lesions suitable for endovascular treatment should be referred for digital subtraction angiography and endovascular procedures. The role of surgical revascularisation for SSc-related leg ulcers have not been established, but limited data suggest that its long-term outcome is significantly worse than those in non-scleroderma patients [16, 17]. For arterial ulcers intravenous prostanoids, statins and anti-platelet agents should be prescribed. Cardiovascular risk factors should be treated aggressively.

Treatment *pure microvascular ulcers* is based on optimizing vasodilating/vasoactive treatment and increasing of immunosuppression/immunomodulation, taking into account other disease manifestations. Anti-platelet agents and statins should be considered.

Treatment of *venous ulcers* is based on elastic compression (at least 18–24-mmHg pressure) [9]. Medications that that may aggravate peripheral oedema, as calcium channel blockers, should be avoided if possible. Role of endovascular venous ablation and/or radiofrequency ablation or laser therapy have not been established in SSc but might be discussed in selected cases.

Mixed arterial-venous ulcers should be managed closely with angiologist/vascular surgeon. Venous insufficiency should be treated with compression therapy and in selected cases superficial venous ablation may be considered. Indication for arterial revascularization in mixed ulcers is based on clinical presentation and ABI (generally <0, 7) [4].

Regarding compressive therapy for venous and mixed arterial-venous ulcers, there is a potential concern that the excessive compression might worsen arterial insufficiency; therefore, reduced compression is usually advised. However, it has been reported that even anelastic compression up to 40 mmHg does not obstruct arterial perfusion in patients with mixed arterial-venous ulcers with ABI >0, 5 and ankle pressure >60 mmHg [18].

Wound swab should be performed, and antibiotic treatment should be started if clinical signs of infection are present (purulent exudate, inflammation of perilesional skin).

Diagnostic and treatment algorithm is shown in Fig. 11.6.

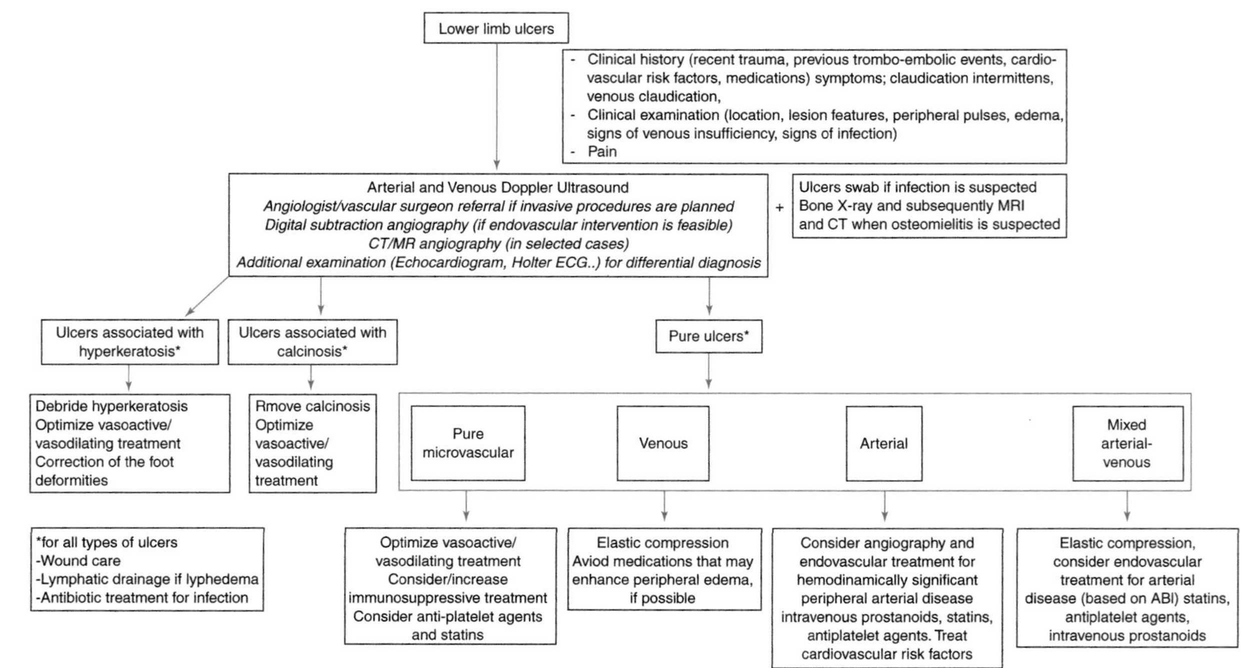

FIGURE 11.6 Leg ulcers: diagnostic and therapetic algorythm

Comments to the Questions Regarding Clinical Case

Left ulcer is likely of venous origin. Varicose veins, peripheral oedema and dyschromia in the gaiter region of the left leg are indicative of venous insufficiency. However, significant macrovascular arterial involvement should be always ruled out. The treatment is based on wound care and elastic compression. Topical vitamin E may be helpful. Substitution of calcium channel blockers with other vasoactive/vasodilating that cause les peripheral oedema should be considered.

Right ulcer is probably secondary to calcinosis (hard whitish material in the bed of the lesion is suggestive for stone calcinosis). The treatment is based on calcinosis removal and wound care. For calcinosis a number of different treatments, such as vasoactive/vasodilating drugs, bisphosphonates, colchicine, minocycline, warfarin, intravenous immunoglobulins and Rituximab have been proposed, with unsatisfactory results [19].

Take home points. Lower limb ulcers are often multifactorial in SSc and more than one type of ulcer may occur in the same patient. Macrovascular arterial and/or venous involvement must be always investigated. Local factors that may predispose to the ulcer formation should be removed. Topical wound management and optimising pharmacological therapy are mandatory for ulcer healing. Elastic compression is the main therapy for venous ulcers. Endovascular treatment should be considered for arterial macrovascular ulcers.

References

1. Varga J, Trojanowska M, Kuwana M. Pathogenesis of systemic sclerosis: recent insights of molecular and cellular mechanisms and therapeutic opportunities. J Scleroderma Relat Disord. 2017;2:137–52.
2. Blagojevic J, Piemonte G, Benelli L, Braschi F, Fiori G, Bartoli F, et al. Assessment, definition and classification of lower limb ulcers in systemic sclerosis: a challenge for the rheumatologist. J Rheumatol. 2016;43(3):592–8.

3. Aboyans V, Ricco JB, Bartelink MEL, Björck M, Brodmann M, Cohnert T, Collet JP, Czerny M, De Carlo M, Debus S, Espinola-Klein C, Kahan T, Kownator S, Mazzolai L, Naylor AR, Roffi M, Röther J, Sprynger M, Tendera M, Tepe G, Venermo M, Vlachopoulos C, Desormais I, ESC Scientific Document Group. 2017 ESC guidelines on the diagnosis and treatment of peripheral arterial diseases, in collaboration with the European Society for Vascular Surgery (ESVS): document covering atherosclerotic disease of extracranial carotid and vertebral, mesenteric, renal, upper and lower extremity arteries endorsed by: the European stroke organization (ESO)the task force for the diagnosis and treatment of peripheral arterial diseases of the European Society of Cardiology (ESC) and of the European Society for Vascular Surgery (ESVS). Eur Heart J. 2018;39(9):763–816.
4. Hedayati N, Carson JG, Chi YW, Link D. Management of mixed arterial venous lower extremity ulceration: a review. Vasc Med. 2015;20(5):479–86.
5. Edmonds ME, Foster AV. Diabetic foot ulcers. BMJ. 2006;18(332):407–10.
6. Bohelay G, Blaise S, Levy P, Claeys A, Baudot N, Cuny JF, et al. Lower-limb ulcers in systemic sclerosis: a multicentre retrospective case-control study. Acta Derm Venereol. 2018;98(7):677–82.
7. Mekkes JR, Loots MA, Van Der Wal AC, Bos JD. Causes, investigation and treatment of leg ulceration. Br J Dermatol. 2003;148:388–401.
8. Wound and Skin Care Clinical Guidelines 2007, VIHA.www.viha.ca
9. Grey JE, Harding KG, Enoch S. Venous and arterial leg ulcers. BMJ. 2006;332:347–50.
10. Youssef P, Brama T, Englert H, Bertouch J. Limited scleroderma is associated with increased prevalence of macrovascular disease. J Rheumatol. 1995;22:469–72.
11. Ho M, Veale D, Eastmond C, Nuki G, Belch J. Macrovascular disease and systemic sclerosis. Ann Rheum Dis. 2000;59:39–43.
12. Blagojevic J, Matucci CM. Macrovascular involvement in systemic sclerosis: comorbidity or accelerated atherosclerosis? Curr Rheumatol Rep. 2007;9(3):181–2.
13. Hettema ME. Bootsma H, Kallenberg CG macrovascular disease and atherosclerosis in SSc. Rheumatology (Oxford). 2008;47:578–83.
14. Nordin A, Jensen-Urstad K, Björnådal L, Pettersson S, Larsson A, Svenungsson E. Ischemic arterial events and atherosclerosis

in patients with systemic sclerosis: a population-based case-control study. Arthritis Res Ther. 2013;15(4):R87. https://doi.org/10.1186/ar4267.

15. Mirasoglu B, Bagli BS, Aktas S. Hyperbaric oxygen therapy for chronic ulcers in systemic sclerosis - case series. Int J Dermatol. 2017;56(6):636–40.
16. Deguchi J, Shigematsu K, Ota S, Kimura H, Fukayama M, Miyata T. Surgical result of critical limb ischemia due to tibial arterial occlusion in patients with systemic scleroderma. J Vasc Surg. 2009;49:918–23.
17. Arhuidese I, Malas M, Obeid T, Massada K, Khaled A, Alzahrani A, Samaha G, Reifsnyder T. Outcomes after open infrainguinal bypass in patients with scleroderma. J Vasc Surg. 2016;64(1):117–23.
18. Valenzuela A, Chung L. Calcinosis: pathophysiology and management. Curr Opin Rheumatol. 2015;27(6):542–8.
19. Mosti G, Iabichella ML, Partsch H. Compression therapy in mixed ulcers increases venous output and arterial perfusion. J Vasc Surg. 2012;55:122–8.

Chapter 12
Interpretation of PFTs and Decline in PFTs

Eric S. White, Pier Valerio Mari, and Dinesh Khanna

Spirometry is a non-invasive, semi-objective physiological test that assesses basic lung function by evaluating measures of lung volume, expiratory time, and airflow rates. Despite being an easily administered and reproducible test, clinicians should be aware that spirometry does not provide an etiological diagnosis. Rather, spirometry may best be used to detect the presence of lung disease and monitor the effect of therapy or environmental/occupational exposures on lung function. The objective of this chapter is to guide rheumatologists in the basic knowledge of spirometry testing and its interpretation in the clinical setting according to the latest respiratory society guidelines.

E. S. White
Divison of Pulmonary and Critical Medicine Interstitial Lung Disease Program, Ann Arbor, MI, USA
e-mail: docew@umich.edu

P. V. Mari
Agostino Gemelli University Hospital, Rome, Italy

D. Khanna (✉)
Division of Rheumatology/Dept. of Internal Medicine, University of Michigan Scleroderma Program, University of Michigan, Ann Arbor, MI, USA
e-mail: khannad@med.umich.edu

© Springer Nature Switzerland AG 2021
M. Matucci-Cerinic, C. P. Denton (eds.), *Practical Management of Systemic Sclerosis in Clinical Practice*, In Clinical Practice,
https://doi.org/10.1007/978-3-030-53736-4_12

Although beyond the scope of this article, clinicians should be aware of some important aspects of pulmonary function testing. Machine calibration is necessary for reproducible, interpretable results and must be performed daily prior to testing [1]. Accurate recordings of patient height, weight, sex, ethnicity, and age are crucial since they are necessary to calculate predicted values. Co-morbid conditions, such as scoliosis, recent thoracic surgery or trauma with associated pain, and pneumothorax among others may also impact interpretation of studies and must be considered. Finally, patient understanding of instructions is important in order to obtain accurate and interpretable results per International Guidelines [2].

Spirometry is physically and technically demanding [3], requiring the patient to inhale fully and to exhale as forcibly as possible, continuing the expiratory maneuver until reaching at least one of three end-of-test criteria: 1) Smooth curvilinear rise of volume-time tracing followed by a plateau of at least 1 second duration; 2) If there is not a plateau, then a forced expiratory time of at least 6 s must be reached; and/or 3) Patients unable to continue forced expiration.

Figure 12.1 is an example of testing sessions showing the flow-volume and volume-time curves with the American Thoracic Society (ATS) / European Respiratory Society (ERS) Criteria for acceptable spirometry [4]:

The term “spirometry” refers to the mechanics of air movement and includes (among other values):

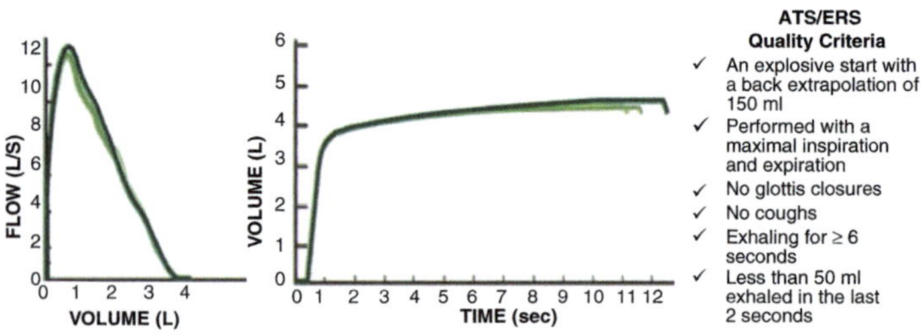

FIGURE 12.1 Flow-volume and volume-time spirometric curves with ATS/ERS Quality Criteria

- **FVC**: Forced Vital Capacity. The maximal total volume of air exhaled with a forced effort from a maximal inspiration.
- **FEV1**: Forced Expiratory Volume in 1 second. FEV_1 is the volume of air exhaled in the very first second of a forced expiration from a full inspiration position.
- **FEV1/FVC Ratio**: This ratio, also called the Tiffeneau-Pinelli index, represents the proportion of vital capacity that is exhaled in the first second of a forced expiration. A value less than 0.70 is diagnostic of an obstructive ventilatory defect. A value >0.8 *may* indicate a restrictive ventilatory defect, which must be confirmed with a total lung capacity (TLC) measurement (see below).

In the presence of a possible restrictive ventilatory defect, lung volume determination provides useful information in order to confirm the clinical suspicion of restrictive disease. This can be accomplished using **helium gas dilution, nitrogen wash-out, or whole-body plethysmography.** By using these techniques, the physician can obtain measures of the following lung volumes and may confirm or disprove the suspected restrictive pattern:

- **RV**: Residual Volume. The volume of air in the lungs after a maximal exhalation.
- **TLC**: Total Lung Capacity. This value represents the total volume in the lungs at maximal inspiration. By definition, restrictive lung diseases must have a TLC lower than the lower limit of normal predicted values.
- **RV/TLC Ratio**: This ratio, if more than 35%, may suggest air trapping with obstructive lung disease and hyperinflation.

While pulmonary volumes or flow rates may be assessed using the described methods, a different technique is necessary to measure the lung's ability to transfer gases across the alveolar basement membrane, called the diffusing capacity of the lung for carbon monoxide (DL_{CO}) [5]. DL_{CO} is a useful early marker for interstitial lung diseases (including those associated with systemic sclerosis and other connective tissue disorders), chronic pulmonary vascular disease (i.e. thromboembolic disease and pulmonary arterial hypertension), or diseases associated with chronic hypoxia. DL_{CO} is tested by having patients inhale a known quantity of carbon monoxide (CO), hold their breath for 10 s and then forcefully and completely exhaling. The difference between inhaled and exhaled CO concentrations allows for the DL_{CO} calculation.

Interpretation of pulmonary function studies requires comparison against predicted values for populations of individuals with similar ethnicity, age, gender, height, and weight (see Fig. 12.2 for a quick guide to PFT interpretation). Based on a normal standard deviation of about 10%, the normal range of spirometric values which encompass about 95% of the population is set between the LLN of 80% predicted and an Upper Limit of Normal (ULN) of 120% predicted. Clinicians should be aware that ratios have different normal ranges:

- FEV_1/FVC: Normal if ≥70% or 0.70. Obstructive pattern is diagnosed when the ratio is ≤70% or 0.70

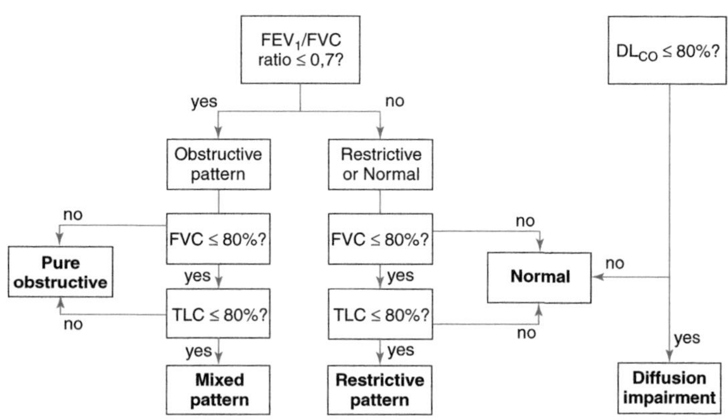

FIGURE 12.2 Fast Interpretation of Pulmonary Function Test (PFT)

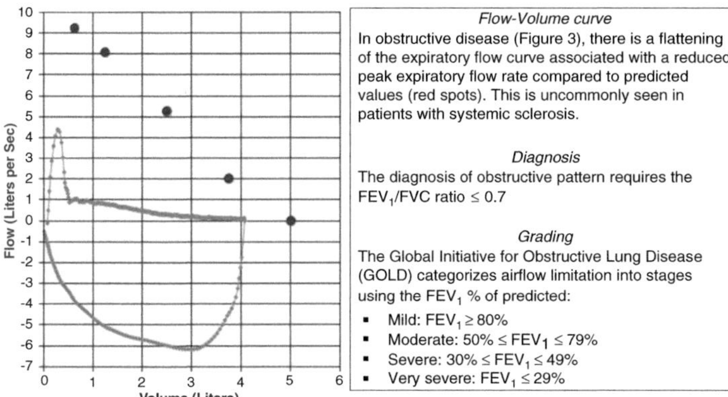

FIGURE 12.3 Obstructive pattern. Deidentified flow-volume curve provided by Eric S. White, MD, MS.

- RV/TLC: Hyperinflation when ≥35% or normal value if ≤35%

Good quality spirometry can lead the clinician to identify underlying respiratory abnormalities; it is worthwhile to summarize them showing flow-volume curve features, diagnostic criteria and disease grading [6]:

- **Obstructive pattern** (Fig. 12.3)

When obstruction is identified, reversibility testing with an inhaled bronchodilator may be performed to determine degree of airflow reversibility. International guidelines state there should be at least a 12% increase from baseline and 200 mL improvement in FEV_1 in order to diagnose reversibility, a hallmark of asthma.

- **Restrictive Pattern** (Fig. 12.4)
- **Combined obstructive and restrictive pattern** (Fig. 12.5)
- **Diffusion Impairment** (Fig. 12.6)

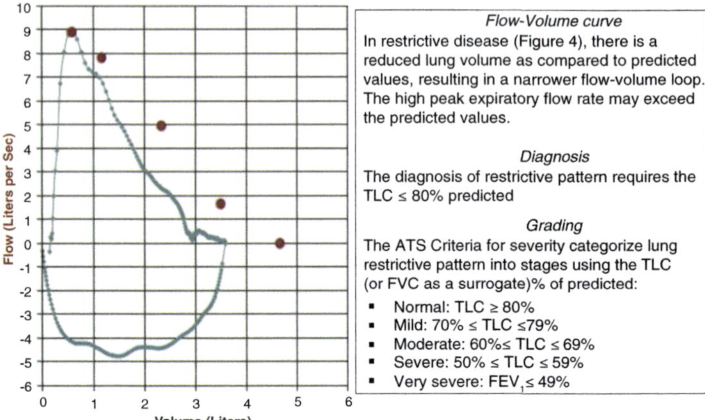

Figure 12.4 Restrictive pattern. Deidentified flow-volume curve provided by Eric S. White, MD, MS

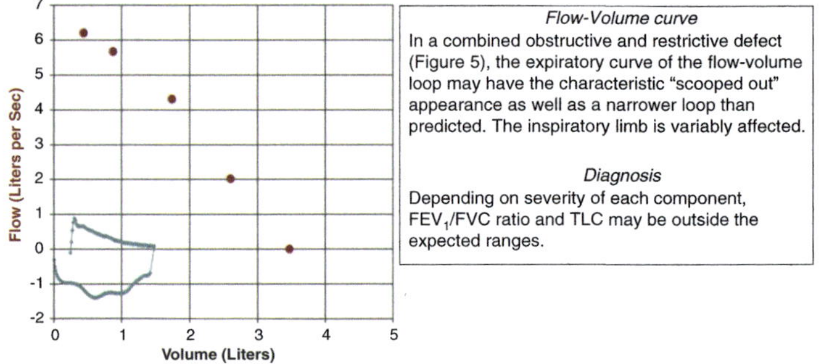

Figure 12.5 Mixed pattern. Deidentified flow-volume curve provided by Eric S. White, MD, MS

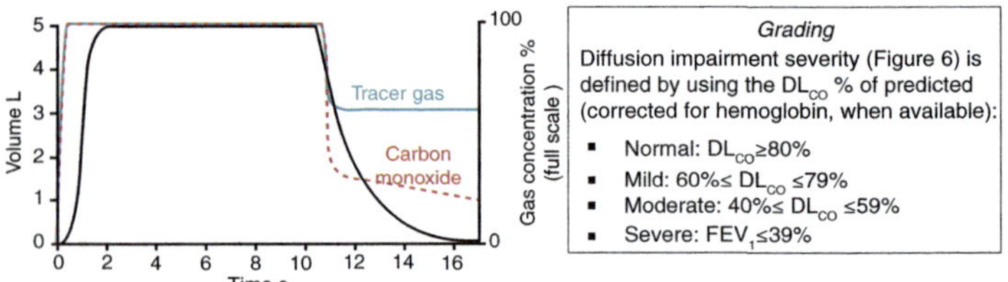

Figure 12.6 Measurement of DL_{CO}

Patient Examples

Patient AB is a 40-year-old female who presented to the Michigan Medicine Scleroderma Clinic with 18-month history of Raynaud's phenomenon, progressive skin thickening, and progressive dyspnea on exertion. Examination showed diffuse cutaneous systemic sclerosis, presence of bilateral crackles at lung bases, presence of small and large joint contractures, and Raynaud's phenomenon. PFTs showed no evidence of obstructive disease, low FVC and a proportionate decline in DLCO% predicted (Fig. 12.7). HRCT showed a non-specific interstitial pneumonitis (NSIP) pattern (the most commonly observed HRCT pattern in scleroderma patients). The PFT pattern is diagnostic of a restrictive lung disease associated with SSc-ILD because TLC < 80% predicted and there is proportionate decline in the DLCO%. FVC% can be incorporated as a physiological measure to assess for stabilization vs. worsening of underlying ILD [7]. A decline in FVC of >10% or a decline in FVC of 5–9% and in DLCO >15% is considered to be clinically meaningful, although a smaller change with worsening symptoms or changes in the HRCT may represent worsening of ILD [8].

Patient CD is a 61-year-old female who presented with 24 months' history of Raynaud's phenomenon, progressive skin thickening, and progressive dyspnea on exertion. Examination showed diffuse cutaneous systemic sclerosis, digital pitting scars, and small joint contractures of fingers. Complete PFT showed no evidence of obstructive disease, normal FVC and TLC and a disproportionate decline in DLCO% predicted (FVC%/ DLCO% ratio of 2.7) (Fig. 12.8). HRCT showed mild NSIP pattern. Her transthoracic echocardiogram showed tricuspid regurgitation of 2.8 m/sec and increased right ventricular load. The right heart catheterization showed mean pulmonary artery pressure of 36 mmHg, a pulmonary wedge pressure of 12 mmHg and a normal cardiac output, consistent with pulmonary arterial hypertension. A disproportionate decline in DLCO or an FVC%/ DLCO% ratio > 1.8 is suggestive of pulmonary hypertension [9].

	Baseline		
SPIROMETRY:	Actual	Pred	%Pred
FVC liters	2.30	3.66	63%
FEV1 liters	2.17	2.85	76%
FEV1/FVC %	94%	78%	121%
FEV6 liters	2.30	3.74	61%
FET sec	6.43		
FEFMAX l/sec	5.78	6.36	91%
FEF25-75 l/sec	3.64	3.25	112%
FIVC liters	2.10	3.66	57%
FIFMAX l/sec	3.33	6.36	52%
FIF50 l/sec	2.00	4.53	44%
FEF50/FIF50 %	236%	100%	236%
MVV l/min	94	107	88%

	Baseline		
LUNG VOLUMES:	Actual	Pred	%Pred
VC liters	2.30	3.66	63%
IC liters	1.44	2.27	63%
ERV liters	0.86	1.39	62%
FRC pleth liters	2.24	2.87	78%
RV pleth liters	1.38	1.48	93%
TLC pleth liters	3.68	5.14	72%
RV/TLC pleth %	38%	29%	130%
Raw cm H20/l/s	0.92	<2.00	
Sgaw s/cmH2O*l^2	0.42	>0.21	

	Baseline		
DIFFUSION:	Actual	Pred	%Pred
DLCO ml/min/mmHg	13.42	24.24	55%
IVC liters	2.02	2.30*	88%
VA liters	3.17	5.14	62%
DL/VA ml/m/Hg/l	4.23	4.71	90%

FIGURE 12.7 Patient AB, complete pulmonary function study

	Baseline		
SPIROMETRY:	Actual	Pred	%Pred
FVC liters	2.74	3.31	83%
FEV1 liters	2.03	2.45	83%
FEV1/FVC %	74%	74%	100%
FEV6 liters	2.73	3.42	80%
FET sec	6.98		
FEFMAX l/sec	4.38	6.10	72%
FEF25-75 l/sec	1.53	2.72	56%
FIVC liters	2.66	3.31	80%
FIFMAX l/sec	4.05	6.10	66%
FIF50 l/sec	3.90	4.13	94%
FEF50/FIF50 %	53%	100%	53%
MVV l/min	91	95	95%

	Baseline		
LUNG VOLUMES:	Actual	Pred	%Pred
VC liters	2.74	3.31	83%
IC liters	1.72	2.02	85%
ERV liters	1.02	1.29	79%
FRC pleth liters	2.49	2.93	85%
RV pleth liters	1.47	1.64	89%
TLC pleth liters	4.21	4.95	85%
RV/TLC pleth %	35%	33%	105%
Raw cm H20/l/s	1.46	<2.00	
Sgaw s/cmH2O*l^2	0.24	>0.21	

	Baseline		
DIFFUSION:	Actual	Pred	%Pred
DLCO ml/min/mmHg	6.66	22.47	30%
IVC liters	2.60	2.74*	95%
VA liters	3.92	4.95	79%
DL/VA ml/m/Hg/l	1.70	4.54	37%
Hgb mg/dl	9.10	13.40	68%
DLCOcorrH ml/m/Hg	7.96	22.47	35%

FIGURE 12.8 Patient CD, complete pulmonary function

Take Home Messages

1. Standardization of PFTs and accurate recordings of patient height, weight, sex, ethnicity, and age are crucial for correct interpretation of pulmonary physiology.
2. A low FVC% or TLC% is not diagnostic for ILD in patients with systemic sclerosis—HRCT is required to show the parenchymal changes consistent with an ILD.
3. Ratio of FEV1%/FVC% of ≤ 0.70 is suggestive of obstructive lung disease, or that obstructive lung disease is more severe than a concomitant restrictive lung defect.
4. In a scleroderma patient with established ILD, declining FVC% along with a proportionate decline in DLCO% is suggestive of progressive ILD.
5. In a scleroderma patient with established ILD, declining FVC% along with a disproportionate decline in DLCO% may suggest pulmonary vascular disease, if DLCO% has been performed properly and there is no significant decline in the red blood cells. Suggestive of progressive ILD.

References

1. Miller MR, Crapo R, Hankinson J, Brusasco V, Burgos F, Casaburi R, Coates A, Enright P, van der Grinten CP, Gustafsson P, Jensen R, Johnson DC, MacIntyre N, McKay R, Navajas D, Pedersen OF, Pellegrino R, Viegi G, Wanger J, Force AET. General considerations for lung function testing. Eur Respir J. 2005;26(1):153–61. https://doi.org/10.1183/09031936.05.00034505.
2. Miller MR, Hankinson J, Brusasco V, Burgos F, Casaburi R, Coates A, Crapo R, Enright P, van der Grinten CP, Gustafsson P, Jensen R, Johnson DC, MacIntyre N, McKay R, Navajas D, Pedersen OF, Pellegrino R, Viegi G, Wanger J, Force AET. Standardisation of spirometry. Eur Respir J. 2005;26(2):319–38. https://doi.org/10.1183/09031936.05.00034805.
3. Moore VC. Spirometry: step by step. Breathe. 2012;8(3):232–40. https://doi.org/10.1183/20734735.0021711.

4. Culver BH, Graham BL, Coates AL, Wanger J, Berry CE, Clarke PK, Hallstrand TS, Hankinson JL, Kaminsky DA, MacIntyre NR, McCormack MC, Rosenfeld M, Stanojevic S, Weiner DJ. Laboratories ATSCoPSfPF. Recommendations for a standardized pulmonary function report. An official American Thoracic Society technical statement. Am J Respir Crit Care Med. 2017;196(11):1463–72. https://doi.org/10.1164/rccm.201710-1981ST.
5. Graham BL, Brusasco V, Burgos F, Cooper BG, Jensen R, Kendrick A, MacIntyre NR, Bruce R. 2017 ERS/ATS standards for single-breath carbon monoxide uptake in the lung. Thompson and Jack Wanger. Eur Respir J. 2017;49:1600016. The European respiratory journal. 2018;52(5). https://doi.org/10.1183/13993003.50016-2016.
6. Pellegrino R, Viegi G, Brusasco V, Crapo RO, Burgos F, Casaburi R, Coates A, van der Grinten CP, Gustafsson P, Hankinson J, Jensen R, Johnson DC, MacIntyre N, McKay R, Miller MR, Navajas D, Pedersen OF, Wanger J. Interpretative strategies for lung function tests. Eur Respir J. 2005;26(5):948–68. https://doi.org/10.1183/09031936.05.00035205.
7. Kafaja S, Clements P, Wilhalme H, Furst D, Tseng CH, Hyun K, Goldin J, Volkmann E, Roth M, Tashkin D, Khanna D. Reliability and Minimal Clinically Important Differences (MCID) of Forced Vital Capacity: Post-Hoc Analyses from the Scleroderma Lung Studies (SLS-I and II). The American College of Rheumatology Annual Meeting in Washington, DC (November 2016), (Oral Presentation, Abstract 971).
8. Khanna D, Mittoo S, Aggarwal R, Proudman SM, Dalbeth N, Matteson EL, Brown K, Flaherty K, Wells AU, Seibold JR, Strand V. Connective tissue disease-associated interstitial lung diseases (CTD-ILD) - report from OMERACT CTD-ILD working group. J Rheumatol. 2015;42(11):2168–71. https://doi.org/10.3899/jrheum.141182.
9. Coghlan JG, Denton CP, Grunig E, Bonderman D, Distler O, Khanna D, Muller-Ladner U, Pope JE, Vonk MC, Doelberg M, Chadha-Boreham H, Heinzl H, Rosenberg DM, McLaughlin VV, Seibold JR, Group Ds. Evidence-based detection of pulmonary arterial hypertension in systemic sclerosis: the DETECT study. Ann Rheum Dis. 2014;73(7):1340–9. https://doi.org/10.1136/annrheumdis-2013-203301.

Chapter 13 Arrhythmias

Yannick Allanore and Christophe Meune

Definitions

Arrhythmias are categorized according to rate, origin, regularity.

Bradycardia is defined as a resting heart rate of fewer than 60 beats per minute. Injury or scarring near the sinus node may slow down or block the electrical impulses. A block can happen anywhere along the heart's electrical pathways.

Tachycardia is defined as a resting heart rate of more than 100 beats per minute. **Supraventricular tachycardia** (SVT) origins above the ventricle, it can be chronic or transient. Atrial fibrillation is the most frequent SVT. **Ventricular tachycardia** (VT) is a life-threatening arrhythmia, is increased by the existence of heart failure and/or myocardial ischemia

Y. Allanore (✉)
Rheumatology Department, Cochin Hospital, APHP, Paris Descartes University, Paris, France
e-mail: yannick.allanore@aphp.fr

C. Meune
Cardiology Department, Avicenne Hospital, APHP, Paris 13 University, Bobigny, France
e-mail: christophe.meune@aphp.fr

© Springer Nature Switzerland AG 2021
M. Matucci-Cerinic, C. P. Denton (eds.), *Practical Management of Systemic Sclerosis in Clinical Practice*, In Clinical Practice,
https://doi.org/10.1007/978-3-030-53736-4_13

(microvascular or as a consequence of coronary artery stenosis/occlusion). Ventricular fibrillation (VF) is the most severe arrhythmia and corresponds to cardiac arrest.

Clinical Cases

1/ A 67-year old SSc woman was referred to our institution for palpitations and being breathless. She suffered from the diffuse cutaneous subset of the disease from >15 years. Organ involvements include severe esophageal and gastrointestinal dysmotility, mild lung fibrosis (<20%) and past atrial fibrillation (AF). Latest cardiac examination performed 1 year ago showed normal ventricle surface and volumes, normal LVEF of 55%, normal pulmonary arterial pressure and no pericardial effusion.

She has been treated with clopidogrel (mistakenly ordered for AF) verapamil and flecainide. On examination, heart rate was 70/min, blood pressure was 150/70 mmHg, heart sounds were irregular with premature beats, and she presented with signs of mild left and right heart failure. ECG showed normal sinus rhythm with ventricular premature beats.

Blood tests were unremarquable excepted NT-proBNP that averaged 1200 ng/L and high-sensitivity troponin that was 45 ng/L (N < 14 ng/L) at presentation and 3 h later. On echocardiography, LV volume and LVEF were unchanged, there was evidence of diastolic dysfunction with mild elevated LV filling pressure, elevated systolic pulmonary arterial pressure (sPAP) of 45 mmHg. A 24-h holter ECG was ordered and showed frequent ventricular beats, but without ventricular tachycardia.

Second-line test included a coronary angiogram that showed normal coronary arteries, and cardiac MRI that showed no myocardial fibrosis; echo was re-performed after successful treatment of heart failure with diuretic and systolic sPAP was 25 mmHg.

Flecaidine, verapamil and clopidogrel were withdrawn, a treatment with oral anticoagulation, metoprolol, amlodipine and low-dosage loop diuretic was introduced. Follow-up remained uneventful, a 24 h holter ECG showed only rare and isolated ventricular premature beats, exercise testing showed no arrhythmias.

2/ A 50 year old woman was referred for systematic cardiac screening. She suffered from Raynaud phenomenon and arthralgia for >5 year, more recently from dyspepsia. A diagnosis of systemic sclerosis, of the diffuse cutaneous subset, was affirmed 3 years ago with positivity of anti-topoisomerase antibodies. She was still treated with low-dose prednisone and methotrexate, and her routine follow-up included visits in a department of rheumatology every 6 months.

She was referred to our institution for a complete re-assessment of the disease. She complained of no cardiac symptoms but has very limited physical activity. On examination, heart rate was 95/min, blood pressure was 120/60 mmHg and cardiac examination revealed a pericardial friction rub; there was no sign of heart failure. First-line tests included routine blood test, C-reactive protein, NT-proBNP and high-sensitivity Troponin measurements, resting ECG, echocardiography and 24 h holter monitoring.

The results were as follow: C-reactive protein of 15 mg/L, NTproBNP of 325 ng/L (N < 125 ng/L), normal troponin concentration, ECG showed incomplete left bundle branch block (Fig. 13.1), 24 h holter monitoring showed frequent

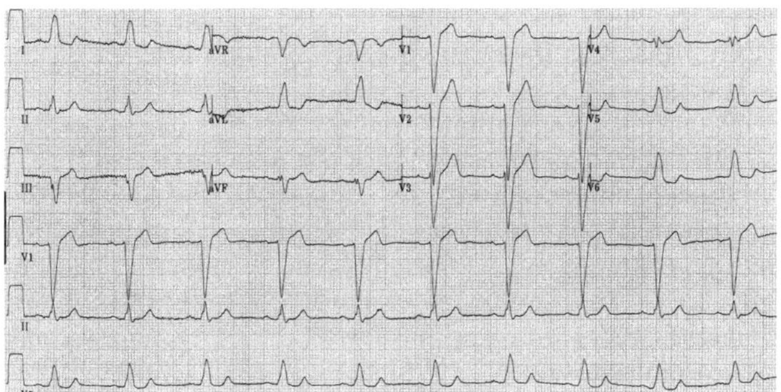

FIGURE 13.1 Electrocardiogram with left bundle branch block

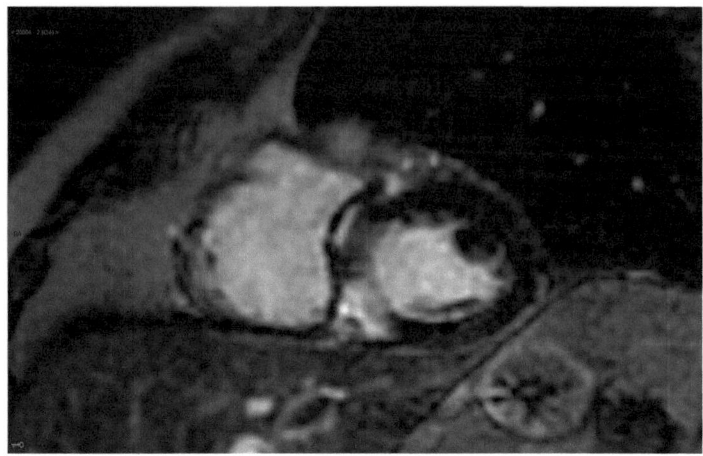

FIGURE 13.2 Late gadolinium enhancement on cardiac MRI

ventricular and atrial premature beats and the presence of 3 episodes on non-sustained ventricular tachycardia and echocardiography showed normal left and right ventricle dimensions, LVEF of 50%, normal LV filling pressure, no valvular stenosis/regurgitation, normal systolic PAP of 25 mmHg, normal RV contractility (Tricuspid AnteroPosterior Excursion), minimal pericardial effusion.

Second line tests included cardiac MRI that showed pericardial thickening and minimal pericardial effusion, LVEF was 45%, and there was linear late gadolinium enhancement (LGE) that was inconsistent with coronary artery distribution (Fig. 13.2).

A coronary angiography was nevertheless performed and showed normal coronary arteries. She was treated with ACE inhibitor and metoprolol, in addition to the switch from methotrexate to mycophenolate mofetil as immunosuppressant. At 6 months she remained asymptomatic, ECG was unchanged, NTproBNP concentration was 250 ng/L, echocardiography showed the persistence of mild pericardial effusion, LVEF of 55%, normal LV filling pressure, normal RV function, normal pulmonary arterial pressure; 24 h holter monitoring showed the persistence of isolated and are (<5%) ventricular premature beats. Catheter-ablation of VT and internal cardioverter implantation were initially discussed and there was a consensus that they were not indicated. Tight follow-up with 24 h Holter every 6 months was planned.

Discussion

Although cardiac involvement is often clinically occult, myocardial involvement is common in SSc [1]. When sensitive tools are used it has been estimated to occur in up to 100% of SSc patients. Once cardiac involvement is clinically evident, it is recognized as a poor prognostic factor [2, 3].

Studies looking at resting ECG show abnormal features in 30–50% of the patients but when 24-hour Holter ECG monitoring is performed, it shows disturbances even more commonly [4]. However, there might be a patient selection bias in such studies and findings are very heterogeneous and sometimes non-specific (high sensitivity and low specificity of Holter-ECG). Commonly, the prevalence and severity of ventricular arrhythmias did not correlate with clinical variants or with other symptoms and signs of the disease. It is generally acknowledged that the presence of abnormal ventricular arrhythmias or even frequent ventricular ectopic beats identify patients at high risk of life-threatening arrhythmic complications, particularly when multiform and/or repetitive ventricular premature beats are observed. These abnormalities have even a poorer prognostic value when associated with altered myocardial function as showed by echocardiography. Despite the very frequent occurrence of ventricular arrhythmias, sudden cardiac death is not very common in SSc. The worst prognosis due to severe cardiac arrhythmias is significantly more frequent in patients with concomitant skeletal and cardiac muscle involvement [4].

With regards to conduction abnormalities, although being frequent in SSc patients with myocardial disease, specific conduction system disease is almost never the cause of death in SSc patients. In fact, the conduction system appeared to be relatively spared from the myocardial changes of SSc, and the high incidence of conduction disturbances may be a consequence, rather than a specific damage to the proximal portion of the specialized conduction tissue. The most common alterations are left bundle branch block, followed by first-degree atrioventricular block, whilst second- and third-degree atrioventricular block are very infrequent [5, 6].

Cardiac involvement is the result of microvascular lesions, collagen deposit, complex immune system dysregulation and autonomic dysfunction. A variable combination of the above mechanisms promotes ischemic, fibrotic and inflammatory lesions involving all the cardiac structures, included the electrical system. Histologic examinations reveal the presence of patchy myocardial fibrosis that can involve the conduction system in SSc [7]. However, the demonstration of fibrosis as being the only responsible for the pathophysiology of these conduction defects is not so far achieved.

Diagnostic Work-Up

Standard 12-lead ECG should be performed routinely to all SSc patients such as Doppler echocardiography, even if the patient is asymptomatic. Moreover, if the patient complains of palpitations, syncope or dizziness the next steps must include 24-hour Holter monitoring and also exercise testing and upright tilt-table testing. Although not endorsed by any guideline, some teams recommend that 24-hour Holter monitoring should be considered on a yearly basis even if the patient remains asymptomatic.

The patient should be investigated about the presence of systemic illness that may promote arrhythmias such as chronic obstructive pulmonary disease, thyrotoxicosis, pericarditis, or congestive heart failure. Invasive electrophysiologic studies are required in patients who have atrioventricular block, intraventricular conduction disturbance, sinus node dysfunction, tachycardia, and unexplained syncope or palpitations [8].

When significant changes are detected with regards to conduction and rhythm systems, careful investigations for heart disease must be performed (see above cases). Firstly, classic cardiovascular risk factors should be analyzed together with signs or symptoms of ischemic heart disease. If scleroderma related heart disease is suspected, echocardiography should be performed implemented, when possible, by pulsed Doppler Imaging and/or strain rate imaging. In addition, cardiac MRI may be discussed case by case to evaluate tissue damages particularly in case of any signs of myositis in order to rule out myocarditis which demands specific management [8].

Treatment

First of all, some drugs may induce conduction abnormalities and arrhythmias: corticosteroids at high intravenous dose are associated with tachyarrhythmias, methotrexate may exceptionally induce right bundle branch block and ventricular arrhythmias, hydroxychloroquine is safer than chloroquine in terms of heart conduction disorders.

Personalized medicine should be applied in the context of SSc heart disease and the choice of treatment must be adapted to the individual patient. As no randomized controlled trials have been conducted to assess the proper management in SSc, the therapy should be similar to that of patients without SSc, but physicians should consider:

1. Raynaud's phenomenon, with adverse effects of β-blockers whereas calcium channel blockers offer beneficial effects as well as their possible preventive effect on left ventricular ejection fraction deterioration. Thus, verapamil-like calcium channel blockers might be recommended in the treatment of atrial or intra-nodal tachycardia, although their efficacy is somewhat limited. In case β-blockers are truly advocated, metoprolol has proven not to worsen RP

if associated with CCB. Also not studied, nebivolol might be safe thanks to its NO liberation.

2. the prevalence of myocardial ischaemia and, as a consequence, the possible detrimental effect of class I antiarrhythmic drugs (see case report 1); They are contra-indicated in patients with reduced EF.
3. In patients with heart failure with reduced ejection fraction, non-dihydropyridines CCB are detrimental. Dihydropyridines CCB are neutral. Patients' treatment should be based on the guidelines on the management of heart failure primarily with ACE inhibitors (or sacubitril/valsartan), β-blockers, MRA and possibly loop diuretics to avoid congestion (see case report 2).
4. Amiodarone is the most effective antiarrhythmic drug. Side effects include immuno-allergic pneumonia than can be a concern in SSc; there is no evidence that pre-existing pulmonary fibrosis increases the risk of immuno-allergic pneumonia but it will worsen its consequences.
5. Implantable cardioverter defibrillator (ICD), which monitors the cardiac rhythm and can deliver competing pacing stimuli and low- and high-energy shocks, has been used effectively in selected patients to prevent malignant ventricular arrhythmias. Thus, they are indicated in secondary prevention of ventricular fibrillation (tachycardia) or in patients with very low EF (<35%). Catheter ablation of a unique and localized source of ventricular tachycardia should be considered, in patients already implanted with ICD or not. (in cases 1 and 2, ICD was not indicated in the absence of malignant arrhythmias, because EF was >35%, and medical treatment was effective in the relief of arrhythmias).
6. Catheter ablation is also indicated for recurrent reentrant tachycardia and/or atrial flutter/fibrillation.
7. Pacemaker implantation is the treatment of choice for complete heart block and other serious brady-arrhythmias.

References

1. Allanore Y, Meune C. Primary myocardial involvement in systemic sclerosis: evidence for a microvascular origin. Clin Exp Rheumatol. 2010;28(5 Suppl 62):S48–53.
2. Elhai M, Meune C, Boubaya M, Avouac J, Hachulla E, Balbir-Gurman A, et al. Mapping and predicting mortality from systemic sclerosis. Ann Rheum Dis. 2017;76(11):1897–905.
3. Assassi S, Del Junco D, Sutter K, McNearney TA, Reveille JD, Karnavas A, Gourh P, Estrada-Y-Martin RM, Fischbach M, Arnett FC, Mayes MD. Clinical and genetic factors predictive of mortality in early systemic sclerosis. Arthritis Rheum. 2009;61(10):1403–11.
4. Vacca A, Meune C, Gordon J, Chung L, Proudman S, Assassi S, Nikpour M, Rodriguez-Reyna TS, Khanna D, Lafyatis R, Matucci-Cerinic M, Distler O, Allanore Y, Scleroderma Clinical Trial Consortium Cardiac Subcommittee. Cardiac arrhythmias and conduction defects in systemic sclerosis. Rheumatology (Oxford). 2014;53(7):1172–7.
5. Draeger HT, Assassi S, Sharif R, Gonzalez EB, Harper BE, Arnett FC, Manzoor A, Lange RA, Mayes MD. Right bundle branch block: a predictor of mortality in early systemic sclerosis. PLoS One. 2013;8(10):e78808.
6. De Luca G, Bosello SL, Gabrielli FA, Berardi G, Parisi F, Rucco M, Canestrari G, Loperfido F, Galiuto L, Crea F, Ferraccioli G. Prognostic role of ventricular ectopic beats in systemic sclerosis: a prospective cohort study shows ECG indexes predicting the worse outcome. PLoS One. 2016;11(4):e0153012.
7. Muresan L, Oancea I, Mada RO, Petcu A, Pamfil C, Muresan C, Rinzis M, Pop D, Zdrenghea D, Rednic S. Relationship between ventricular arrhythmias, conduction disorders, and myocardial fibrosis in patients with systemic sclerosis. J Clin Rheumatol. 2018;24(1):25–33.
8. Bissell LA, Anderson M, Burgess M, Chakravarty K, Coghlan G, Dumitru RB, Graham L, Ong V, Pauling JD, Plein S, Schlosshan D, Woolfson P, Buch MH. Consensus best practice pathway of the UK systemic sclerosis study group: management of cardiac disease in systemic sclerosis. Rheumatology (Oxford). 2017;56(6):912–21.

Chapter 14
Pericardial and Pleural Complications in Systemic Sclerosis

Shannon Alyssa Sylvie Meilleur and Murray Baron

Background

Pericardial Disease: Pericardial involvement in systemic sclerosis (SSc) is relatively common based on autopsy studies, but less apparent clinically. Cardiac involvement is more commonly diagnosed in SSc and is represented by heart block and/or myocardial fibrosis [1]. Autopsy studies, however, show that 33–72% of people with SSc have pericardial involvement at autopsy, while 15–43% have detectable pericardial involvement on echocardiography [2]. Only about 5–10% of patients will have clinically symptomatic disease [3]. Pericardial involvement consists of fibrinous pericarditis, pericardial adhesions, and acute or chronic pericarditis with or without effusion [2]. The pathophysiology of pericardial disease is not well understood; on pericardial biopsy, the most

S. Alyssa Sylvie Meilleur
Division of Rheumatology, McGill University, Montreal, QC, Canada
e-mail: smeilleur@qmed.ca

M. Baron (✉)
Chief Division of Rheumatology, Jewish General Hospital, McGill University, Montreal, QC, Canada
e-mail: mbaron@jgh.mcgill.ca

© Springer Nature Switzerland AG 2021
M. Matucci-Cerinic, C. P. Denton (eds.), *Practical Management of Systemic Sclerosis in Clinical Practice*, In Clinical Practice,
https://doi.org/10.1007/978-3-030-53736-4_14

common findings are nonspecific inflammation or fibrosis of the pericardium [4, 5]. With regards to pericardial effusions, most are small and asymptomatic, with large effusions presenting uncommonly and tamponade very rarely [3]. Large effusions are typically associated with concomitant renal disease and/or pulmonary hypertension and carry a poor prognosis with a mortality rate up to 55% [2, 3]. Effusions are typically exudative, with a high protein content, high LDH, and low white blood cell count [2, 6].

Pericardial disease is not associated with disease duration, and is seen in both diffuse and limited disease, though tends to be slightly more common in diffuse disease [1, 7]. Pericardial effusions can appear before skin involvement, and are more likely to occur in men, where they also tend to develop more rapidly [2, 7]. Serologically, patients with pericardial effusions are more likely to be anti-topoisomerase or anti-centromere antibody positive [7]. Pulmonary arterial hypertension is an important risk factor and has a poor prognosis when combined with a hemodynamically significant effusion [4]. Moderate to large effusions associated with EKG changes are also associated with higher mortality [1].

Presenting symptoms for SSc associated pericardial effusions overlap significantly with the symptoms of pericardial effusions not due to connective tissue diseases. Dyspnea is almost universal, with the next most common features being chest pain and temperature greater than 37.8 °C [8]. Physical exam findings in SSc and connective tissue disease-unrelated pericardial effusions are similar, with pedal edema, distended neck veins, liver enlargement, pulsus paradoxus, pulsus alternans, tachycardia, liver enlargement, Kussmaul's sign, and pericardial friction rub (only in acute pericarditis) [8]. Associated laboratory findings are leukocytosis and high ESR [8]. Electrical manifestations are typically T-wave changes and low EKG voltages [8]. Most common imaging findings apart from pericardial effusion seen on echocardiography were increased interstitial markings and pleural effusion on chest imaging [9]. Massive pericardial effusions are very uncommon and are defined as fluid volume of more then 200 mL [6]. These effusions are associated with diffuse disease, wide areas of skin hyperpigmentation, flexion contractures, esophageal hypomotility, pulmonary fibrosis, and antibodies against anti-topoisomerase-1 [6]. The most common complication of large to massive effusions is renal failure [6].

Pleural Disease: The main lung findings in SSc are bibasilar interstitial infiltrates and basilar changes related to aspiration pneumonias, with pleural findings such as thickening and effusion representing minor contributors [9]. Pleural effusions are uncommon in scleroderma, with one study estimating only 7% of patients had an effusion not attributable to causes other than their systemic sclerosis [10]. This finding is more common in patients with a diffuse phenotype [10]. There are no reports of large or symptomatic pleural effusions due to SSc alone. The profile of the fluid is exudative, although drainage for purposes other than diagnostic is uncommon [5]. Management is typically medical and does not differ substantially from that of pericardial effusions outlined above.

Clinical Case

Our patient was a 38-year-old female known for SSc with diffuse skin involvement and arthritis for over 5 years. She was followed at an academic centre subspecialty clinic in systemic sclerosis. She was ANA and Scl-70 positive and maintained on methotrexate with no end-organ complications on screening echocardiography and lung imaging. Her disease was generally well-controlled, with no flares or hospitalizations. She did not have previously evident pericardial or pleural involvement.

She had insidious onset of shortness of breath and central chest pain over several weeks, and eventually presented to the emergency department due to significant shortness of breath limiting ambulation to less than 10 m. She had a normal respiratory exam, but a significant pericardial friction rub. BP was normal. Also evident on exam were sclerodactyly, diffuse skin thickening over the arms, legs, and chest, calcinosis of the digits and extensor surfaces of the elbows, and reduced mouth opening. No synovitis was detectable on exam. Chest X-ray showed small bilateral pleural effusions, and bedside echocardiography demonstrated a small circumferential pericardial effusion. She did not have electrical changes on her EKG. Laboratory testing disclosed a slightly elevated CRP, WBC count, with normal kidney function. Viral screening on nasal swab was negative.

She was treated with colchicine 0.6 mg BID and ASA 650 mg daily initially for acute pericarditis and had some improvement in her breathlessness over 3 days of treatment. Her acute pericarditis was felt to be due to her SSc due to absence of evidence for viral or other common trigger. She was discharged home with close follow-up by her rheumatologist, who saw her in clinic 2 weeks later. Corticosteroids were initially avoided due to concern for precipitating renal crisis, however given her ongoing chest pain that had not responded to colchicine and ASA, she was subsequently treated with prednisone 15 mg PO followed by a taper. Her ASA dose was reduced to 80 mg daily. She had some improvement in her pain, but at an Internal Medicine clinic visit 3 days later was experiencing increased dyspnea and chest pain. She was febrile at 38.1 °C, with a large pericardial effusion with evidence of pre-tamponade physiology on directed echocardiogram and increased left pleural effusion. She was admitted for drainage of both effusions, and discharged home on her previous doses of ASA and colchicine with augmentation of her prednisone dose to 25 mg daily. Laboratory testing of both effusions revealed an exudate without evidence of infection or malignancy. Her symptoms had markedly improved when she saw her rheumatologist 2 weeks later, and she was subsequently successfully tapered to 10 mg of prednisone over the next two months with further taper by 2.5 mg every 2 weeks .

Treatment: Pericardial disease is usually treated according to the severity of symptoms and presence/absence plus size of pericardial effusion. Most commonly, patients receive corticosteroids, ASA, NSAIDs, and colchicine [2]. Where aggressive intervention is indicated, it usually consists of pericardiectomy or pericardial window [2]. Methotrexate is commonly used for chronic effusions [1]. In one study of SSc patients hospitalized for any cause, 7% had clinically symptomatic pericardial effusions [2]. The mean age of this population was 60, with over 80% female [2]. Most were treated with medical therapy alone, while 22% required an intervention such as pericardiocentesis or pericardial window [2]. If the patient has PAH and an effusion causing hemodynamic compromise, they should be cautiously managed by medically optimizing right ventricular function with pulmonary vasodilators, and only have their effusion drained with caution if drainage is absolutely necessary [4]. Rapid or large volume drainage of a pericardial effusion in this situation prior to cardiac optimization can result in cardiovascular collapse. If therapeutic anticoagulation is being considered for a patient with systemic sclerosis, an echocardiogram prior to starting is recommended as there have been case reports of patients with chronic pericardial effusions progressing to hemodynamically significant effusions due to bleeding into the effusion [1].

Summary: Symptomatic pericardial disease in SSc is uncommon. Our patient's case is fairly typical for most described symptomatic cases; the pleural and pericardial effusions with significant dyspnea are similar to cases described in the literature. Slightly atypical was her suboptimal response to colchicine, and most patients do not require corticosteroids. Treatment depends on the symptomatic and hemodynamic severity and chronicity. Although uncommon, clinicians should be aware that pericardial disease does occur in SSc, can occasionally be associated with other serious complications such as PAH and scleroderma renal crisis and can, on its own, be the cause of serious hemodynamic compromise.

References

1. Wooten MD, Reddy GV, Johnson RD. Cardiac tamponade in systemic sclerosis: a case report and review of 18 reported cases. J Clin Rheumatol. 2000;6:35–40.
2. Hosoya H, Derk CT. Clinically symptomatic pericardial effusions in hospitalized systemic sclerosis patients: demographics and management. Biomed Res Int. 2018;2018:6812082.
3. Nabatian S, Kantola R, Sabri N, Broy S, Lakier JB. Recurrent pericardial effusion and pericardial tamponade in a patient with limited systemic sclerosis. Rheumatol Int. 2007;27:759–61.
4. Desai CS, Lee DC, Shah SJ. Systemic sclerosis and the heart: current diagnosis and management. Curr Opin Rheumatol. 2011;23:545–54.
5. Kitchongcharoenying P, Foocharoen C, Mahakkanukrauh A, Suwannaroj S, Nanagara R. Pericardial fluid profiles of pericardial effusion in systemic sclerosis patients. Asian Pac J Allergy Immunol. 2013;31:314–9.
6. Satoh M, Tokuhira M, Hama N, et al. Massive pericardial effusion in scleroderma: a review of five cases. Br J Rheumatol. 1995;34:564–7.
7. Jaeger VK, Wirz EG, Allanore Y, et al. Incidences and risk factors of organ manifestations in the early course of systemic sclerosis: a longitudinal EUSTAR study. PLoS One. 2016;11:e0163894.
8. McWhorter JE, LeRoy EC. Pericardial disease in scleroderma (systemic sclerosis). Am J Med. 1974;57:566–75.
9. Leslie KO, Trahan S, Gruden J. Pulmonary pathology of the rheumatic diseases. Semin Respir Crit Care Med. 2007;28:369–78.
10. Thompson AE, Pope JE. A study of the frequency of pericardial and pleural effusions in scleroderma. Br J Rheumatol. 1998;37:1320–3.

Chapter 15
Constipation, Bloating and Abdominal Pain

Stamatia-Lydia Chatzinikolaou and Charles Murray

Introduction

GI involvement occurs in more than 90% of patients in systemic sclerosis (SSc). Any part of the GI tract can be involved, and the disease is progressive in nature [1]. Patients may be asymptomatic or present with a range of GI symptoms attributed to different etiologies. Bloating and abdominal pain are common among scleroderma patients. Gastric involvement manifesting as gastroparesis is reported in 38–50% of SSc patients [2] and small intestinal participation occurs in 40–70%. Colonic involvement leading to constipation is observed in 20–50% of scleroderma cases [3]. Symptoms of abdominal distension, pain and constipation can be a major source of poor quality of life and their management can prove challenging [4].

S.-L. Chatzinikolaou · C. Murray (✉)
Department of Gastroenterology, Royal Free London NHS Foundation Trust and Institute of Liver and Diigestive Health, University College London, London, UK
e-mail: stamatia.chatzinikolaou@nhs.net; charlesmurray1@nhs.net

© Springer Nature Switzerland AG 2021

M. Matucci-Cerinic, C. P. Denton (eds.), *Practical Management of Systemic Sclerosis in Clinical Practice*, In Clinical Practice,
https://doi.org/10.1007/978-3-030-53736-4_15

Clinical Case

VK is a 37-year-old patient of afro-caribbean origin, diagnosed with diffuse systemic sclerosis and dermatomyositis overlap. She has severe upper and lower GI involvement. She presented to the gastroenterology scleroderma clinic with symptoms of severe bloating, central abdominal pain, heartburn, dysphagia, constipation alternating with diarrhoea and weight loss.

VK has undergone several investigations to assess GI involvement. A barium swallow revealed a dilated esophagus, a sliding hiatus hernia and a patulous LES. A gastric emptying study confirmed gastroparesis. Upper GI endoscopy showed ulcerative esophagitis, and no gastric outlet obstruction. Colonoscopy was normal. A barium meal and follow-through pointed to the characteristic "accordion-like" appearance of the small bowel, with dilation of the distal duodenum and proximal jejunum. In addition, slow transit times were noted. A hydrogen breath test was positive for small intestinal bacterial overgrowth (SIBO).

VK's treatment in terms of her GI symptoms is mainly symptomatic. She is on dual acid suppression therapy and she uses metoclopramide (previously domperidone) to aid with gastric emptying and intestinal motility. She has been on cyclical antibiotic courses for SIBO (rifaximin, doxycycline and ciprofloxacin). She is on a longstanding combination of laxatives (movicol, bisacodyl, senna), but lately symptoms improved following the addition of prucalopride to her treatment.

Constipation

Constipation has been reported in up to 50% of scleroderma patients. In practice, fewer patients may complain of decreased bowel frequency and symptoms may not appear until later in the disease process.

Pathophysiology

Colonic involvement is common in GI scleroderma. There is initially patchy muscle atrophy which is followed by fibrosis, mainly affecting the circular muscle layer. The predominant atrophic changes, in combination with hypomotility, impaired peristalsis and loss of gastro-colic reflex, lead to slow-transit times observed in scleroderma patients [5].

Diagnosis

Constipation is most commonly due to dysmolity and slow transit, but may also be the result of functional anorectal outlet obstruction or side effects of medication (e.g. opiates, iron supplements). Metabolic causes, e.g. hypothyroidism and diabetes mellitus, should be considered in the initial assessment. Detailed history, clinical assessment and investigations should aim to establish diagnosis and tailor treatment accordingly. Patients may complain of decreased bowel frequency, abdominal pain and discomfort, hard stool, straining, sense of incomplete bowel emptying, bloating and the need to use manual manoeuvres. Symptoms are usually longstanding and there is gradual deterioration.

Acute onset constipation, or presence of red flags, should be urgently investigated to exclude mechanical obstruction, malignancy or acute colonic pseudo-obstruction, which is a medical emergency requiring hospital care [6]. Other severe but rare complications are volvulus, colonic stenosis and stercoral ulceration.

Investigations

Slow transit constipation can be demonstrated with the use of radiopaque markers [7]. Plain abdominal radiographs and CT scans can be used to exclude mechanical obstruction, assess for colonic dilation and the presence of faecal impaction or wide-mouthed diverticula at the antimesenteric colonic border. Endoscopic assessment is recommended to exclude malignancy and endoluminal pathology, and should be considered in scleroderma patients with recent change in bowel habits.

Treatment

Dietary modifications can be initially adopted, however they have limited effect in slow transit constipation and high-fibre diets may exacerbate symptoms, particularly in the presence of gastroparesis and SIBO. The same applies for bulk-forming laxatives. Stimulant (e.g. bisacodyl, senna, lubiprostone) and osmotic (e.g. macrogol, lactulose) laxatives, and stool softeners form the mainstay of constipation management. They are usually more effective in the initial stages of the disease and combinations of different agents are usually employed, particularly in the long-term setting [8]. Prokinetic agents, like metoclopramide and domperidone, have been shown to have some effect on colonic motility [9]. Prucalopride is a 5-HT4 receptor agonist that promotes colonic transit and it has been used successfully in cases of SSc [10]. It is currently approved for patients failing laxative treatment.

In addition to the pharmacologic management of constipation, other techniques such as biofeedback may be useful [3]. Surgery should be reserved as a last resort for emergency cases, as it carries a high risk of complications and is of limited therapeutic value. Limiting medications that promote constipation should be considered as part of the overall management, alongside correction of possible metabolic defects (e.g. hypercalcemia, hypothyroidism). Assessment of anorectal function should be considered. Figure 15.1 provides an algorithm for the overall management of constipation in SSc.

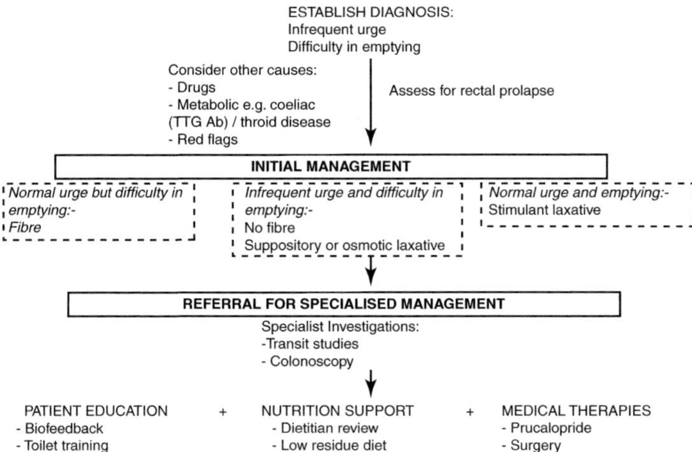

Figure 15.1 Algorithm for management of constipation (Ref. [3])

Bloating and Abdominal Pain

The main causes of abdominal pain and bloating in scleroderma patients are gastroparesis, SIBO and small intestinal pseudo-obstruction. Colonic pseudo-obstruction and true mechanical obstruction (e.g. tumour, volvulus) are rarer causes of abdominal pain and distention that have a more acute onset and require prompt medical attention and in-hospital care.

Pathophysiology

Smooth muscle atrophy followed by fibrosis and anatomic and neurovascular changes in the GI tract are characteristic processes of GI scleroderma. The dysmotility together with autonomic dysfunction contribute to impaired gastric accommodation and compliance, resulting in gastroparesis [11, 12]. In the small intestine, hypomotility, loss of Migrating Motor

Complexes (MMC), the presence of diverticula and chronic PPI use, lead to stasis of intestinal contents and migration of colonic bacteria in the small intestine, creating ideal conditions for bacterial overgrowth [5]. Intestinal pseudo-obstruction is a result of the established dysmotility in combination with the uncoordinated contractile activity and failure to produce a successful propagatory movement of intestinal contents to the colon, in the absence of mechanical obstruction.

Diagnosis

Gastroparesis is reported in up to 50% of patients with SSc. Apart from abdominal pain and bloating, symptoms include early satiety, postprandial fullness, nausea, vomiting, exacerbation of reflux symptoms. Gastric outlet obstruction should be initially ruled out. Co-morbidities (e.g. diabetes mellitus) and medications that contribute to delayed gastric emptying (e.g. opiates, anti-cholinergics) should be considered and the presence of Helicobacter Pylori infection may exacerbate symptoms [6].

SIBO is reported in 43–55% of SSc patients [13, 14]. Patients complain of abdominal distention, pain, excessive flatulence, nausea, vomiting, early satiety, diarrhoea, and in more severe cases malabsorption and weight loss become evident. There is a marked symptomatic overlap between SIBO and gastroparesis, and in some cases chronic intestinal pseudo-obstruction (CIPO) (obstructive symptoms for >6 months), making the diagnostic distinction challenging. CIPO presents with very similar symptoms as SIBO, however it is much less frequent, with one centre reporting a 3.9% prevalence [15].

Acutely presenting or rapidly deteriorating abdominal pain and distention should prompt for immediate investigations to exclude mechanical obstruction and volvulus.

Investigations

Investigating abdominal pain and bloating in scleroderma should be initially tailored by history and clinical findings, and it should be remembered that symptoms may be also attributed to non-scleroderma causes. Gastroparesis is diagnosed with a scintigraphic gastric emptying study [16]. Upper GI endoscopy helps ruling out gastric outlet obstruction and assessing for H.Pylori.

The gold-standard for the diagnosis of SIBO is culture of jejunal aspirates collected during upper GI endoscopy. The test however has limitations and is not widely used in clinical practice. The glucose and lactulose hydrogen breath tests are non-invasive methods, that rely on the metabolism of ingested carbohydrates by intestinal bacteria to produce hydrogen and methane [17, 18, 19]. Fecal calprotectin has been found to increase in scleroderma patients with SIBO [20]. Although it cannot confirm diagnosis, it can be used as a tool to identify patients for further testing, and also assess treatment outcomes. In the same content, a low vitamin B12 level and a raised serum folate and/or vitamin K should raise clinical suspicion for SIBO. Bacteria in the small intestine consume vitamin B12 and produce folic acid and vitamin K, providing an indirect indication for further assessment [5, 21].

Imaging modalities should be employed to exclude mechanical obstruction and assess for CIPO. A plain abdominal radiograph may reveal dilated small bowel loops, with or without air-fluid levels. The small bowel loops may have the characteristic "accordion-like" appearance (on contrast studies), owing to the tightly packed volvulae convinantes. Cross-sectional imaging helps differentiate between CIPO and true mechanical obstruction. In CIPO, there is intestinal dilatation, in the absence of a transition point. Transient intussusceptions may also be observed and are associated with chronic abdominal distention and pain.

Treatment

Dietary and lifestyle modifications can be employed as a first approach in the management of gastroparesis. Low-residue and low-fat diets, in combination with small frequent meals and avoidance of recumbinant position following food ingestion, may provide some symptomatic control [22]. Prokinetic agents work in early disease stages, before muscle atrophy and fibrosis are well-established. Metoclopromide, domperidone and erythromycin have been used successfully in scleroderma patients, however potential side effects should be borne in mind [6, 23]. Enteral and parenteral nutrition may be the only options in advanced disease.

Management of SIBO relies in the empirical use of antibiotics. Antibiotics commonly used include ciprofloxacin, metronidazole, doxycycline, co-amoxiclav, norfloxacin, tetracycline and rifaximin [24, 25]. Cyclical courses of different compounds may be needed to achieve eradication and minimize resistance. Side effects, safety, effectiveness and availability usually determine the choice of antibiotics. In advanced disease states, continual rotating courses may be needed. Probiotics have been shown to provide some symptomatic relief, however there are no clear recommendations regarding their use [26].

Treatment of CIPO is conservative, comprising bowel rest, IV hydration, bowel decompression and use of prokinetic agents. Metoclopromide and domperidone may increase small intestinal motility. Octreotide has been successfully used in scleroderma patients to improve intestinal motility, however side effects and cost limit its long-term use [27, 28]. Surgery carries a high risk in these patients and should only be reserved for emergency cases (e.g. in bowel perforation, volvulus). Figure 15.2 provides an algorithm for the management of abdominal pain and distension in SSc.

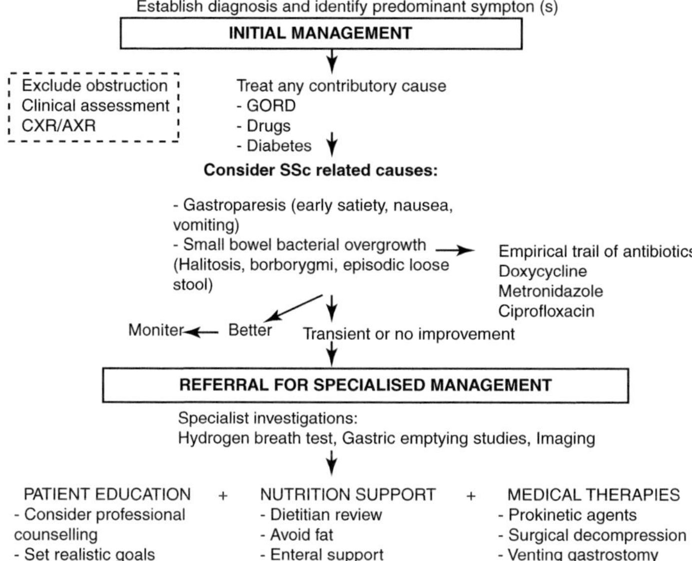

FIGURE 15.2 Algorithm for management of bloating and abdominal pain (Ref. [3])

References

1. Kumar S, Singh J, Rattan S, DiMarino J, Cohen S, Jimenez SA. Review article: pathogenesis and clinical manifestations of gastrointestinal systemic sclerosis. Aliment Pharmacol Ther. 2017;45(7):883–98.
2. Savarino E, Mei F, Parodi A, Ghio M, Furnari M, Gentile A, et al. Gastrointestinal motility disorder assessment in systemic sclerosis. Rheumatology. 2013;52(6):1095–100.
3. Hansi N, Thoua N, Carulli M, Chakravarty K, Lal S, Smyth A, et al. Consensus best practice pathway of the UK scleroderma study group: gastrointestinal manifestations of systemic sclerosis. Clin Exp Rheumatol. 2014;32(6Suppl 86):S-214-21.

4. Khanna D, Nagaraja V, Gladue H, Chey W, Pimentel M, Frech T. Measuring response in the gastrointestinal tract in systemic sclerosis. Curr Opin Rheumatol. 2013;25(6):00–6. doi: 10.1097/01
5. Harrison E, Murray C, Lal S. Small and large intestinal involvement and nutritional issues. In: Varga J, Denton CP, Wigley FM, Allanore Y, Kuwana M, editors. Scleroderma: from pathogenesis to comprehensive management. New York: Springer; 2017. p. 443–58.
6. Shreiner AB, Murray C, Denton C, Khanna D. Gastrointestinal manifestations in systemic sclerosis. J Scleroderma Relat Disord. 2016;1(3):247–56. https://doi.org/10.5301/jsrd.5000214.
7. Basilico G, Barbera R, Vanoli M, Bianchi P. Anorectal dysfunction and delayed colonic transit in patients with progressive systemic sclerosis. Dig Dis Sci. 1993;38:1525–9.
8. Wald A. Is chronic use of stimulant laxatives harmful to the colon? J Clin Gastroenterol. 2003;36(5):386–9.
9. Emmanuel AV, Tack J, Quigley EM, Talley NJ. Pharmacological management of constipation. Neurogastroenterol Motil. 2009;21(Suppl 2):41–54. https://doi.org/10.1111/j.1365-2982.
10. Boeckxstaens GE, Bartelsman JF, Lauwers L, Tytgat GN. Treatment of GI dysmotility in scleroderma with the new enterokinetic agent prucalopride. Am J Gastroenterol. 2002;97:194–7.
11. Iovino P, Valentini G, Ciacci C, De Luca A, Tremolaterra F, Sabbatini F, et al. Proximal stomach function in systemic sclerosis: relationship with autonomic nerve function. Dig Dis Sci. 2001;46(4):723–30.
12. Savarino E, Furnari M, de Bortoli N, Martinucci I, Bodini G, Ghio M, et al. Gastrointestinal involvement in systemic sclerosis. Presse Med. 2014;43(10 Pt 2):e279–91. https://doi.org/10.1016/j.lpm.2014.03.029.
13. Marie I, Ducrotte P, Denis P, Menard JF, Levesque H. Small intestinal bacterial overgrowth in systemic sclerosis. Rheumatology. 2009;48(10):1314–9. https://doi.org/10.1093/rheumatology/kep226.
14. Bures J, Cyrany J, Kohoutova D, Förstl M, Rejchrt S, Kvetina J, et al. Small intestinal bacterial overgrowth syndrome. World J Gastroenterol. 2010;16(24):2978–90.
15. Muangchan C, Canadian Scleroderma Research Group, Baron M, Pope J. The 15% rule in scleroderma: the frequency of severe organ complications in systemic sclerosis. A systematic

review. J Rheumatol. 2013;40(9):1545–56. https://doi.org/10.3899/jrheum.121380.
16. Nagaraja V, McMahan ZH, Getzug T, Khanna D. Management of gastrointestinal involvement in scleroderma. Curr Treatm Opt Rheumatol. 2015;1(1):82–105.
17. Romagnuolo J, Schiller D, Bailey RJ. Using breath tests wisely in a gastroenterology practice: an evidence-based review of indications and pitfalls in interpretation. Am J Gastroenterol. 2002;97(5):1113–26.
18. Khoshini R, Dai SC, Lezcano S, Pimentel M. A systematic review of diagnostic tests for small intestinal bacterial overgrowth. Dig Dis Sci. 2008;53(6):1443–54.
19. Braun-Moscovici Y, Braum M, Khanna D, Balbir-Gurman A, Furst DE. What tests should you use to assess small intestinal bacterial overgrowth in systemic sclerosis? Clin Exp Rheumatol. 2015;33(4 Suppl 91):S117–22.
20. Marie I, Leroi AM, Menard JF, Levesque H, Quillard M, Ducrotte P. Fecal calprotectin in systemic sclerosis and review of the literature. Autoimmun Rev. 2015;14(6):547–54. https://doi.org/10.1016/j.autrev.2015.01.018.
21. Kaye SA, Lim SG, Taylor M, Patel S, Gillespie S, et al. Small bowel bacterial overgrowth in systemic sclerosis: detection using direct and indirect methods and treatment outcome. Br J Rheumatol. 1995;34:265–9.
22. Frech TM, Mar D. Gastrointestinal and hepatic disease in systemic sclerosis. Rheum Dis Clin N Am. 2018;44(1):15–28.
23. McFarlane IM, Bharma MS, Kreps A, Iqbal S, Al-Ani F, Saladini-Aponte C, et al. Gastrointestinal manifestations of systemic sclerosis. Rheumatology. 2018;8(1). pii: 235 https://doi.org/10.4172/2161-1149.1000235.
24. Baron M, Bernier P, Cote LF, Delegge MH, Falovitch G, Friedman G, et al. Screening and therapy for malnutrition and related gastro-intestinal disorders in systemic sclerosis: recommendations of a north American expert panel. Clin Exp Rheumatol. 2010;28(2 Suppl 58):S42–6.
25. Gatta L, Scarpignato C. Systematic review with meta-analysis: rifaximin is effective and safe for the treatment of small instestine bacterial overgrowth. Aliment Pharmacol Ther. 2017;45(5):604–6016.
26. Frech TM, Khanna D, Maranian P, Frech EJ, Sawitzke AD, Murtaugh MA. Probiotics for the treatment of systemic

sclerosis-associated gastrointestinal bloating/ distention. Clin Exp Rheumatol. 2011;29(2 Suppl 65):S22–5.

27. Nikou GC, Toumpanakis C, Katsiari C, Charalambopoulos D, Sfikakis PP. Treatment of small intestinal disease in systemic sclerosis with octreotide: a prospective study in seven patients. J Clin Rheumatol. 2007;13(3):119–23.
28. Perlemuter G, Cacoub P, Chaussade S, Wechsler B, Couturier D, Piette JC. Octreotide treatment of chronic intestinal pseudoobstruction secondary to connective tissue diseases. Arthritis Rheum. 1999;42(7):1545–9.

Chapter 16
Gastroesophageal Reflux

Amir Masoud and Monique Hinchcliff

Clinical Vignette

Case 1: A 35-year old woman with a 5-year history of Raynaud phenomenon and 6 months of puffy hands that prohibits her from wearing rings presents to the emergency department with complaints of substernal chest pain and inability to catch her breath. The patient endorses smoking cigarettes (10 cigarettes per day for 20 years). She takes no medications. Her family history is significant for a maternal cousin with systemic lupus erythematosus. On exam, the skin on her fingers bilaterally appears shiny and tight. Digital pitting is noted on the finger pulps. ECG abnormalities and elevated troponins are not noted. Chest computed tomography for pulmonary emboli reveals no evidence for emboli, but ground glass opacities especially in the right middle lobe and at the lung bases bilaterally are noted. She is discharged

A. Masoud
Department of Medicine, Section of Gastroenterology, Yale School of Medicine, New Haven, CT, USA

M. Hinchcliff (✉)
Department of Medicine, Section of Rheumatology, Allergy & Immunology, Yale School of Medicine, New Haven, CT, USA
e-mail: monique.hinchcliff@yale.edu

© Springer Nature Switzerland AG 2021

M. Matucci-Cerinic, C. P. Denton (eds.), *Practical Management of Systemic Sclerosis in Clinical Practice*, In Clinical Practice,
https://doi.org/10.1007/978-3-030-53736-4_16

home on daily omeprazole daily and told to follow-up with her primary care physician for gastroesophageal reflux.

Case 2: A 45-year old woman with diffuse cutaneous systemic sclerosis (dcSSc) for 1 year complicated by polymyositis presents with severe epigastric pain. She was initially prescribed prednisone 60 mg PO QD with steroid taper and weekly oral alendronate pills to prevent steroid-induced osteoporosis along with calcium, vitamin D and weight-bearing exercise. She notes midline pain just inferior to the xiphoid process. She presents to a rheumatologist who urges her to stop taking weekly alendronate and refers the patient to a gastroenterologist who performs an upper endoscopy (EGD). During the EGD, a large white tablet, likely alendronate, is extracted from the upper esophageal 1/3 and proton pump inhibition is prescribed. Three weeks later the patient endorses complete resolution of pain.

Epidemiology

Reflux of gastric contents into the esophagus resulting in symptoms or esophageal damage is referred to as gastroesophageal reflux disease (GERD). Gastroesophageal reflux disease is highly prevalent in patients with systemic sclerosis (SSc/scleroderma) and can be associated with impairments in health-related quality of life especially sleep [1, 2]. Abnormal esophageal motility on diagnostic testing is reported in 75–90% of patients with SSc, highlighting an additional pathophysiologic component [3]. The prevalence of SSc-GERD depends upon the detection modality that includes barium swallow, high-resolution manometry, pH reflux and impedance testing and upper endoscopy/ esophagogastroduodenoscopy (EGD). SSc subtype (limited versus diffuse cutaneous), age, race and sex do not appear to strongly influence SSc-GERD development, but longer SSc duration and the presence of interstitial lung disease have been associated with more manometric esophageal abnormalities [4, 5].

Pathogenesis

Gastroesophageal reflux (GER) is a physiologic process whereby gastric contents flow retrograde into the esophagus [6]. Patients with SSc can experience acid and/or non-acid GER (discussed below). In the postprandial period, gastric acid floats atop undigested food forming what is called the gastric acid pocket that functions as a gastric acid reservoir [6]. The higher the location of the gastric acid pocket relative to the crural diaphragm, the more acidic the refluxate [6]. Additionally, impairment of normal esophageal peristalsis in SSc also contributes to GERD development. Abnormal esophageal function in SSc has been attributed to a four-stage process that mirrors SSc skin changes: (1) an early vasculopathy that manifests as mild changes in intestinal permeability, transport, and absorption, (2) neural dysfunction, (3) smooth muscle atrophy, and (4) end-stage fibrosis [7]. Autopsy studies demonstrate that the major pathology is likely smooth muscle atrophy as opposed to fibrosis [8–11]. Additionally, anti-myenteric autoantibodies have been described in SSc patients that may contribute to neural dysfunction [12]. The end result is a flaccid esophagus and lower esophageal sphincter (LES) that permit GER.

Clinical Presentation

Patients with SSc-GERD may spontaneously report typical reflux symptoms including the sensation of intermittent regurgitation of stomach contents into the chest, throat or mouth especially following meals, or during forward flexion or recumbency. In most cases, patients will only endorse typical GERD symptoms during a detailed review of systems. Atypical GERD symptoms include atypical chest pain (Case 1), hoarseness, pharyngitis, halitosis, dental and periodontal issues, and nasopharyngeal complaints (ear and sinus fullness). In these instances, a high index of suspicion is required for accurate diagnosis. The presence of extraesophageal

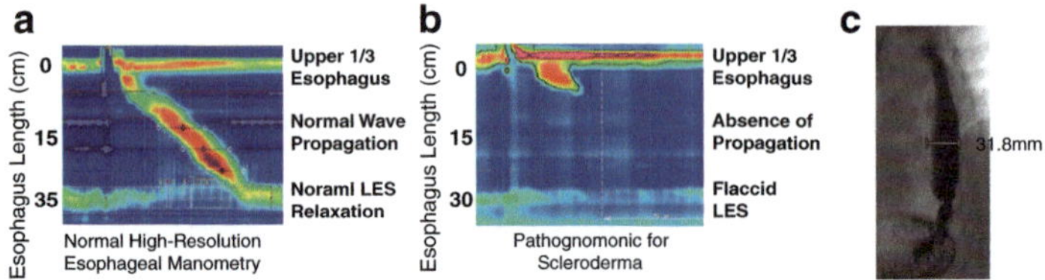

FIGURE 16.1 High-resolution esophageal manometry. (**a**) Image from a normal exam showing the initiation of a swallow and normal esophageal peristalsis and lower esophageal sphincter relaxation. (**b**) Image from an abnormal exam from a patient with SSc showing absent esophageal peristalsis and lack of lower esophageal sphincter relaxation. (**c**) Esophagram or barium swallow exam that demonstrates esophageal dilation as well as peptic stricture formation, a consequence of uncontrolled gastroesophageal reflux disease

symptoms such as cough, throat irritation, hoarseness, laryngitis or pharyngitis should prompt consideration of additional diagnostic testing including esophageal reflux testing and manometry (Fig. 16.1a and b) or barium swallow (Fig. 16.1c). Long standing, uncontrolled GERD commonly results in peptic stricture formation with resultant dysphagia.

Diagnostic Evaluation

Twenty-four-hour ambulatory pH testing with multichannel intraluminal impedance (MII) is the current state-of-the-art GERD assessment tool (Fig. 16.2). Patients record timing of meals, medications and sleep and note reflux symptoms by depressing a button on an event recorder worn around the waist or over the shoulder. The nose is anesthetized prior to placement of the catheter that is swallowed into the stomach, and no sedation is provided to enable patient participation. The catheter consists of impedance recording channels intermittently spaced as well as pH electrodes placed at different points in the esophagus. The impedance recording channels detect liquid, semisolid, or gas GER episodes based on elec-

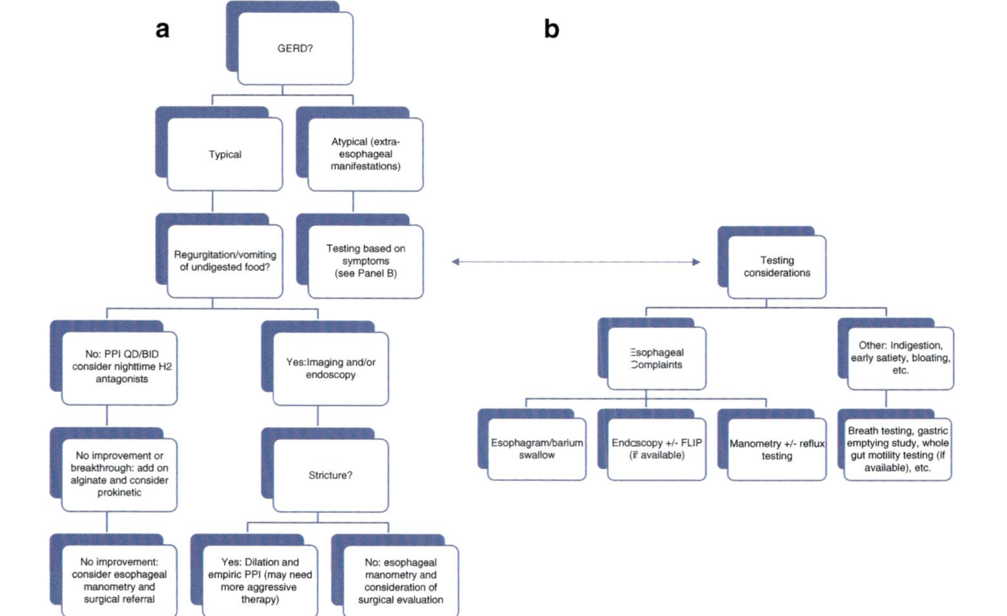

Figure 16.2 Approach to the SSc patient with gastroesophageal reflux disease (GERD). (**a**) SSc patient with typical GERD symptoms. (**b**) SSc patient with atypical GERD symptoms. *FLIP* Functional Lumen Imaging Probe

trical resistance changes (measured in ohms), to electrical current flow, between adjacent electrodes along the length of the MII probe [13]. Reflux events by impedance are defined as a ≥ 50% reduction in impedance values. Refluxate is considered acidic, mildly acidic and nonacidic with pH ≤4, 4–<7 and ≥7 respectively. Acid exposure time (AET) is defined as the total time that the esophageal mucosa is exposed to a refluxate with pH < 4. A total AET ≥ 4.5% during a 24 period is considered abnormal. The proportion of the time spent with acid exposure in supine and upright positions is also determined. The Demeester score is also calculated with any score greater than 14.72 signifying abnormal esophageal acid exposure. The score is calculated using six variables including the percent of total time with pH <4, supine and upright time with pH <4, number of episodes lasting at least 5 min, longest episodes (minutes), and total number of episodes with pH <4. Impedance testing enables measurement of the proximal height of the refluxate that may be associated with concomitant SSc-interstitial lung disease (ILD) [14].

Esophageal manometry evaluates the form and vigor of esophageal contractions in response to a swallow. Expected abnormalities in SSc include weak contractions, ineffective esophageal motility, and absent peristalsis (Fig. 16.1). Resting LES pressure is also expected to be low, particularly in advanced disease (Fig. 16.1). The impedance portion of the exam evaluates for clearance of the saline bolus used to initiate the swallow. Of note, absent peristalsis is not specific for SSc and can be found in patients with overlap syndromes, systemic lupus erythematosus, polymyositis, etc. [15].

At some institutions the multiple rapid swallow (MRS) test, performed during esophageal manometry, is used to evaluate peristaltic reserve. The patient repetitively swallows sips of saline spaced several seconds apart in the supine position. The normal response in a person with intact esophageal neural mechanisms and muscular integrity is an initial diminution and subsequent augmentation of esophageal body and LES contractions [16]. Patients with SSc, regardless of manometric motility diagnosis, demonstrated impaired esophageal peristalsis and LES contractions compared to healthy controls [16]. These data suggest that abnormal response to MRS may be the most common esophageal manometric abnormality in patients with SSc.

A barium swallow, another out-patient procedure that provides a simple assessment of esophageal structure and diameter, can be performed prior to consideration of esophageal endoscopy or manometry. Some institutions favor endoscopy with manometry in all patients with SSc and avoid barium swallow exams. This is due to the concern that concomitant gastric and intestinal hypomotility can lead to barium retention that may extravasate into the peritoneum in patients with pneumatosis cystoides intestinalis. The risk is very low and the decision to perform esophageal manometry versus barium swallow is best made in close consultation between the treating rheumatologist and gastroenterologist.

Esophagogastroduodenoscopy (EGD) is an essential tool to evaluate for esophagitis and esophageal strictures that can complicate uncontrolled GER. It is also useful for assessing for candida esophagitis and other forms of infectious esophagitis, ulcer formation and esophageal metaplasia (Barrett's esophagus).

Treatment

The management of SSc-related GERD starts with aggressive lifestyle modifications including smoking cessation, head of bed elevation, attainment and maintenance of ideal body weight. Dietary modification is essential and involves avoidance of food and drink before periods of recumbency, avoidance of excess alcohol consumption, and eating small frequent, as opposed to large infrequent, meals. Pharmacologic treatments include agents that reduce gastric acid secretion, such as proton pump inhibitors (PPI) (best taken 30 min prior to the largest meal), histamine H2 receptor antagonists, antacids, physical LES barriers (alginic acid formulations) and prokinetic agents (Table 16.1 and Fig. 16.2). Compared with

Table 16.1 GERD pharmacologic treatments

Histamine H2 antagonists	
Cimetidine	
Famotidine	
Loxtidine	
Lamitidine	
Proton pump inhibitors (in order of increasing potency)	**Relative potency**
Pantoprazole	0.23
Lansoprazole	0.90
Dexlansoprazole	Not studied
Omeprazole	1.00
Esomeprazole	1.60
Rabeprazole	1.82
Antacids	
Calcium carbonate	
Magnesium trisilicate	
Aluminum hydroxide	
Alginic acid formulations	
Sodium alginate and potassium bicarbonate	
Promotility agents	
Domperidone	
Metoclopramide	
Macrolide antibiotics Azithromycin [6] Erythromycin	

Based on the mean 24-h gastric pH, the relative potencies of the five PPIs compared to omeprazole [17].

healthy volunteers, patients with GERD need a 1.9-fold higher PPI dose to achieve a given increase in mean 24-h intragastric pH [17]. Prior to increasing PPI dose or frequency, physicians should counsel patients regarding proper PPI administration (30 min before meals) and/or consider trialing a different PPI (e.g. higher potency PPI) (Table 16.1). Lifestyle modifications, in addition to once or twice daily PPIs, can be insufficient for symptom control [18]. Recent results of a 4-week randomized trial of alginic acid (n = 37) versus domperidone (n = 38) in SSc patients with partial response to twice daily omeprazole failed to discern which of these add-on therapies is superior [18].

Invasive interventions including laparoscopic fundoplication, and Roux-en-Y gastric bypass (gastrojejunostomy) are performed in select patients with SSc, but only after a comprehensive multidisciplinary evaluation including esophageal manometry and nutritional status assessment [19]. Esophageal dysmotility on manometry consisting of ineffective, weak or absent peristalsis increases the risk for post-operative dysphagia. However, study results have shown that the degree of pre-operative esophageal dysmotility manometry parameters does not adequately predict post-operative dysphagia [19].

Gastroesophageal reflux complicating lung transplantation is a concern in patients with SSc [20, 21]. Thus, transplantation centers have developed protocols for addressing this potential complication including aggressive PPI, head of bed elevation to 45° and anti-reflux surgical interventions such as fundoplication. Peri-transplant anti-reflux surgery has been shown to improve 1- and 3-year survival in lung transplant recipients, though this has not been specifically studied in SSc patients. Analysis of the United Network for Organ Sharing (UNOS) data from 229 adults with SSc, 201 with pulmonary arterial hypertension (PAH), and 3333 with ILD who underwent lung transplantation in the US between May 4, 2005 and September 14, 2012 demonstrated no difference in 30-day post-transplant survival between patients with SSc and those with ILD (HR 0.65[95% CI 0.27–1.58]) [22]. Moreover, in the patients who survived 1-year, the 3-year survival among SSc patients exceeded PAH survival rates suggesting that lung transplantation should not be refused to SSc patients out of concern for GERD [22].

Incomplete Response to Proton Pump Inhibition in SSc Patients

The results of a recent retrospective case-control study of 38 non-SSc patients and 38 SSc patients who were taking PPI BID and underwent 24-hour ambulatory impedance pH testing found that 58% of SSc patients had manometric findings of the "scleroderma esophagus" defined as hypotensive esophagogastric junction tone and absent contractility (Fig. 16.1b) [23]. Additionally, SSc patients had significantly higher total acid exposure time (AET) 6.8% (2.4–18.7) compared to 1.8% (0.5–3.8) in non-SSc controls ($p < .001$). 72% of SSc patients had absent esophageal contractility compared to none of the controls ($p < .001$). Moreover, SSc patients had substantially reduced mean nocturnal baseline impedance 492 ohms (257–915) compared to 2783 ohms (1050–3275) in controls ($p < .001$), suggestive of more liquid reflux and potentially impaired esophageal clearance. Thus, patients with SSc may experience more GERD symptoms due to delayed esophageal content and refluxate clearance.

Exacerbating Factors

The high prevalence of asymptomatic GERD warrants caution, and, if possible, the avoidance of pharmacotherapies that are often associated with pill esophagitis whereby pills lodge in the upper or mid 1/3 of the esophagus and can cause erosions. Oral bisphosphonates (as described in Case 2), some antibiotics such as doxycycline, oral iron or potassium and some NSAIDs are common culprits [24, 25]. When possible, liquid, intramuscular or parenteral formulations should be prescribed. Noncompliance with lifestyle modifications, listed above, may also worsen GERD symptoms.

Summary

Gastroesophageal reflux disease is common in patients with SSc. Lifestyle and medication modifications coupled with newer diagnostic and treatment modalities help inform medical decision-making and improve health-related quality of life.

Acknowledgements The authors thank Darren Brenner, MD for providing the high-resolution manometry images.

References

1. Yang H, Xu D, Li MT, Yao Y, Jin M, Zeng XF, et al. Gastrointestinal manifestations on impaired quality of life in systemic sclerosis. J Dig Dis. 2019;20(5):256–61.
2. Horsley-Silva JL, Umar SB, Vela MF, Griffing WL, Parish JM, DiBaise JK, et al. The impact of gastroesophageal reflux disease symptoms in scleroderma: effects on sleep quality. Dis Esophagus. 2019;32(5)
3. Gyger G, Baron M. Systemic sclerosis: gastrointestinal disease and its management. Rheum Dis Clin N Am. 2015;41(3):459–73.
4. Ntoumazios SK, Voulgari PV, Potsis K, Koutis E, Tsifetaki N, Assimakopoulos DA. Esophageal involvement in scleroderma: gastroesophageal reflux, the common problem. Semin Arthritis Rheum. 2006;36(3):173–81.
5. Crowell MD, Umar SB, Griffing WL, DiBaise JK, Lacy BE, Vela MF. Esophageal motor abnormalities in patients with scleroderma: heterogeneity, risk factors, and effects on quality of life. Clin Gastroenterol Hepatol. 2017;15(2):207–13. e1
6. Rohof WO, Bennink RJ, de Ruigh AA, Hirsch DP, Zwinderman AH, Boeckxstaens GE. Effect of azithromycin on acid reflux, hiatus hernia and proximal acid pocket in the postprandial period. Gut. 2012;61(12):1670–7.
7. Gyger G, Baron M. Gastrointestinal manifestations of scleroderma: recent Progress in evaluation, pathogenesis, and management. Curr Rheumatol Rep. 2012;14(1):22–9.
8. Treacy WL, Baggenstoss AH, Slocumb CH, Code CF. Scleroderma of the esophagus. A correlation of histologic and physiologic findings. Ann Intern Med. 1963;59:351–6.
9. D'Angelo WA, Fries JF, Masi AT, Shulman LE. Pathologic observations in systemic sclerosis (scleroderma). A study of fifty-

eight autopsy cases and fifty-eight matched controls. Am J Med. 1969;46(3):428–40.
10. Roberts CG, Hummers LK, Ravich WJ, Wigley FM, Hutchins GM. A case-control study of the pathology of oesophageal disease in systemic sclerosis (scleroderma). Gut. 2006;55(12):1697–703.
11. Ebert EC. Esophageal disease in scleroderma. J Clin Gastroenterol. 2006;40(9):769–75.
12. Howe S, Eaker EY, Sallustio JE, Peebles C, Tan EM, Williams RC Jr. Antimyenteric neuronal antibodies in scleroderma. J Clin Invest. 1994;94(2):761–70.
13. Mousa HM, Rosen R, Woodley FW, Orsi M, Armas D, Faure C, et al. Esophageal impedance monitoring for gastroesophageal reflux. J Pediatr Gastroenterol Nutr. 2011;52(2):129–39.
14. Savarino E, Bazzica M, Zentilin P, Pohl D, Parodi A, Cittadini G, et al. Gastroesophageal reflux and pulmonary fibrosis in scleroderma: a study using pH-impedance monitoring. Am J Respir Crit Care Med. 2009;179(5):408–13.
15. Kimmel JN, Carlson DA, Hinchcliff M, Carns MA, Aren KA, Lee J, et al. The association between systemic sclerosis disease manifestations and esophageal high-resolution manometry parameters. Neurogastroenterol Motil. 2016;28(8):1157–65.
16. Carlson DA, Crowell MD, Kimmel JN, Patel A, Gyawali CP, Hinchcliff M, et al. Loss of peristaltic reserve, determined by multiple rapid swallows, is the Most frequent esophageal motility abnormality in patients with systemic sclerosis. Clin Gastroenterol Hepatol. 2016;14(10):1502–6.
17. Kirchheiner J, Glatt S, Fuhr U, Klotz U, Meineke I, Seufferlein T, et al. Relative potency of proton-pump inhibitors-comparison of effects on intragastric pH. Eur J Clin Pharmacol. 2009;65(1):19–31.
18. Foocharoen C, Chunlertrith K, Mairiang P, Mahakkanukrauh A, Suwannaroj S, Namvijit S, et al. Effectiveness of add-on therapy with domperidone vs alginic acid in proton pump inhibitor partial response gastro-oesophageal reflux disease in systemic sclerosis: randomized placebo-controlled trial. Rheumatology (Oxford). 2017;56(2):214–22.
19. Bakhos CT, Petrov RV, Parkman HP, Malik Z, Abbas AE. Role and safety of fundoplication in esophageal disease and dysmotility syndromes. J Thorac Dis. 2019;11(Suppl 12):S1610–s7.
20. Perez Rivera CJ, Kadamani Abiyomaa A, Gonzalez-Orozco A, Ocampo MA, Caicedo I, Mosquera MS. Total gastrectomy in systemic scleroderma when anti-reflux surgery is not viable: a case report. Int J Surg Case Rep. 2019;62:103–7.

21. Panchabhai TS, Abdelrazek HA, Bremner RM. Lung transplant in patients with connective tissue diseases. Clin Chest Med. 2019;40(3):637–54.
22. Bernstein EJ, Peterson ER, Sell JL, D'Ovidio F, Arcasoy SM, Bathon JM, et al. Survival of adults with systemic sclerosis following lung transplantation: a nationwide cohort study. Arthritis Rheumatol. 2015;67(5):1314–22.
23. Stern EK, Carlson DA, Falmagne S, Hoffmann AD, Carns M, Pandolfino JE, et al. Abnormal esophageal acid exposure on high-dose proton pump inhibitor therapy is common in systemic sclerosis patients. Neurogastroenterol Motil. 2018;30(2):e13247.
24. Kikendall JW, Friedman AC, Oyewole MA, Fleischer D, Johnson LF. Pill-induced esophageal injury. Case reports and review of the medical literature. Dig Dis Sci. 1983;28(2):174–82.
25. Kikendall J. Pill-induced esophageal injury. In: Castell DORJ, editor. The esophagus. Third ed. Philadelphia: Lippincott Williams & Wilkins; 1999. p. 527–37.

Chapter 17
Management Diarrhea in Systemic Sclerosis

Elizabeth R. Volkmann

Introduction

Gastrointestinal tract (GIT) dysfunction is a leading cause of morbidity and mortality in patients with systemic sclerosis (SSc). The majority of patients with SSc (over 90%) have some involvement of their GIT over the course of their disease [1, 2]. Unlike other features of SSc, such as cutaneous sclerosis, the course of GIT involvement is often progressive over time. The various manifestations of SSc-GIT dysfunction can evolve late into the SSc disease course, even when other aspects of this condition (e.g., interstitial lung disease [ILD]) are quiescent.

Despite the disease burden of GIT dysfunction in SSc, this dimension of SSc remains poorly understood from both a pathological and treatment perspective. Lower GIT dysfunction, in particular, adversely affects quality of life [3], is associated with depressive symptoms [4], can cause profound malnourishment and weight loss [5, 6], and in certain cases, can lead to death [7].

E. R. Volkmann (✉)
Department of Medicine, University of California, Los Angeles, David Geffen School of Medicine, Los Angeles, CA, USA
e-mail: evolkmann@mednet.ucla.edu

© Springer Nature Switzerland AG 2021
M. Matucci-Cerinic, C. P. Denton (eds.), *Practical Management of Systemic Sclerosis in Clinical Practice*, In Clinical Practice,
https://doi.org/10.1007/978-3-030-53736-4_17

Diarrhea is a common manifestation of SSc-GIT dysfunction [1]. The present chapter summarizes the clinical presentation and management of diarrhea in SSc. Through highlighting two demonstrative clinical vignettes, this chapter presents strategies for ameliorating diarrhea and improving nutritional status in patients with SSc.

Pathogenesis of Lower GIT Dysfunction in SSc

As described above, our understanding of the pathogenesis of lower GIT dysfunction is limited [8]. Historical studies demonstrated that patients with SSc-GIT involvement had evidence of vasculopathy, smooth muscle atrophy, as well as neural dysfunction and fibrosis [8]. However, these early studies focused primarily on upper GIT pathology [9, 10]. Subsequent reports demonstrated that auto-antibodies may contribute in specific manifestations of SSc-GIT dysfunction, such as dysmotility [11–13]. Smoking has also been associated with increased GIT symptoms as described in one large (N = 606) observational cohort study in Canada [14].

More recent studies have suggested that changes in the lower GIT microbiota may contribute to SSc-GIT dysfunction [15, 16]. Observational studies have demonstrated microbial community differences between patients with SSc and healthy controls [17–22]. These studies have described depletions in beneficial commensal genera (e.g., *Faecalibacterium*, *Clostridium*, and *Bacteroides*), as well as enrichments in potentially pathobiont genera (e.g., *Fusobacterium*, *Prevotella*, *Ruminococcus Akkermansia*) in the lower GIT in SSc patients [17–19]. In addition, these reports have demonstrated important connections between lower GIT microbial composition and specific SSc disease features (e.g., ILD [17, 18]), as well as SSc-GIT symptoms [17–19]. The aforementioned investigations into the GIT microbiome in SSc have stimulated new research efforts in this area that may ultimately reveal important treatment targets for managing SSc-GIT dysfunction.

However, in clinical practice, the etiology of diarrhea is often multi-factorial. While the SSc disease state itself can contribute to diarrhea, a plethora of other factors may also contribute to these symptoms (Table 17.1). While caring for patients with SSc, health care providers need to explore and address all possible causes of diarrhea.

Table 17.1 Common causes of diarrhea in patients with SSc

Cause	Diagnostic clues
SSc-related dysmotility	Alternating cycles of distention/ constipation with periods of diarrhea, or loose stools
Small intestine bacterial overgrowth (SIBO) with malabsorption	Bloating/distension are common, as is increased flatulence. Constipation can also occur. Symptoms are often temporarily alleviated with antibiotics.
Intestinal pseudo-obstruction	Pain and cramping are more prominent than with other causes of diarrhea. Nausea and vomiting can occur. While constipation and distention are the predominant symptoms of pseudo-obstruction, overflow diarrhea can occur.
Antibiotic use	Diarrhea onset/worsening is within 3–4 days of initiation of antibiotics.
Medication side effects (e.g. mycophenolate)	Diarrhea improves upon cessation of the offending medication.
Food intolerances (e.g., dairy, gluten)	Diarrhea improves after eliminating the offending food and recurs once the food is reintroduced.
Overlap syndrome with inflammatory bowel disease (IBD)	SSc-diarrhea symptoms can be indistinguishable from IBD-diarrhea symptoms. Further gastrointestinal testing (e.g., colonoscopy) is often necessary to detect IBD.

(continued)

Table 17.1 (continued)

Cause	Diagnostic clues
Overlap syndrome with irritable bowel syndrome (IBS)	Careful history taking reveals an emotional component to symptoms. Diarrhea alternating with constipation is common. Stress is often a trigger for symptoms. Further gastrointestinal testing (e.g., colonoscopy) is often necessary to rule out IBD.
Excessive consumption of sugar alcohols	Food intake diary reveals consumption of sugar-free foods, including soda, gum and other foods that contain substances, such as sorbitol, maltitol.
Gastrointestinal infection	Suspicion is raised in an immunocompromised host.[a] extra-intestinal signs of infection may be present, such as fevers, chills, and weight loss.
Foodborne illness	Acute onset of symptoms; history of intake of foods commonly associated with foodborne illnesses (e.g. fried rice, raw milk, raw seafood, undercooked meat, lettuce, sprouts); exposure to daycares; or travel history.

[a]An immunocompromised state can be induced by medications (e.g., mycophenolate, cyclophosphamide, etc.), but it can also be caused by malnutrition

Assessment of Lower GIT Dysfunction in SSc

In clinical practice, self-reported symptoms of lower GIT dysfunction are the cornerstone to monitoring disease progression and treatment response. Whereas pulmonary function tests (PFT) are employed to monitor progression of ILD, no valid, objective measures of disease activity exist for SSc-GIT dysfunction. Patients may be reluctant to share intimate details of their bowel habits; therefore, the provider should solicit this history with sensitivity and compassion. Using a metric, such as the UCLA SCTC GIT 2.0 [23], may help the provider understand the clinical course of symptoms. The GIT 2.0 is a 34-item self-administered questionnaire that contains 7 domains; one of which is diarrhea [23]. The GIT 2.0 provides a total score of GIT severity (summation of all scales except constipation) and has relatively good reliability and validity across different SSc cohorts [24–26].

Additional tools may also be helpful in assessing diarrhea in patients with SSc, such as the Subjective Global Assessment (SGA) [27]. This metric combines clinical history data (e.g., weight changes, gastrointestinal symptoms, dietary intake, functionality) with physical examination findings [27]. The Patient-Reported Outcomes Measurement Information System (PROMIS) GIT symptom item bank assesses GIT-specific symptoms and correlates well with the GIT 2.0 [28]. The Malnutrition Universal Screen Tool (MUST) can help identify patients who are at risk for malnutrition due to diarrhea and has been evaluated in SSc [5, 29].

Assessment of SSc lower GIT symptoms can also include a variety of imaging and diagnostic procedures that are often orchestrated through a consulting gastroenterologist [8]. Table 17.2 summarizes commonly performed studies in SSc patients with diarrhea.

Table 17.2 Diagnostic testing in patients with SSc suffering from diarrhea

Diagnostic test	Purpose
Colonoscopy	Detect obstructing lesions, mucosal inflammation, telangiectasias
CT or MR enterography	Evaluate for small bowel disease and extraluminal pathology
Barium study	Detect obstruction/pseudo-obstruction

(continued)

Table 17.2 (continued)

Diagnostic test	Purpose
Defecography	Evaluate for rectal outlet obstruction
Abdominal X-ray	Assess for pneumatosis intestinalis
Video capsule endoscopy	Assess for intraluminal small-bowel pathology
Breath tests (hydrogen, bile acids, nonradioactive glucose, lactulose)	Diagnose SIBO[a]
Fecal fat, pH tests; measurements for fat soluble vitamin levels	Diagnose malabsorption
Anorectal manometry	Detect anorectal motility problems
Surface electromyography	Evaluate for sphincter fecal incontinence

[a]The gold standard for diagnosing SIBO is aspiration and culture of jejunal fluid, but this is rarely performed in clinical practice due to the invasive nature of the procedure

Clinical Cases: Focus on Diarrhea in SSc

Case 1: JK

Presentation

JK is a 76-year-old Caucasian female with a 30-year history of limited cutaneous systemic sclerosis. Her SSc-related disease manifestations include mild Raynaud's phenomenon, gastroesophageal reflux disease (GERD), and ILD. She is antinuclear antibody (ANA) positive, but negative for SSc-specific serologies, including centromere, anti-topoisomerase I and RNA Polymerase III. The patient has never received immunosuppressive therapy for her SSc.

Upon presentation, she described episodes of constipation alternating with episodes of diarrhea for the past few years. Specifically, over the course of 4–5 days, she developed increased bloating/distension and constipation. Subsequently, she experienced profuse, watery diarrhea for 1–2 days. She also reported decreased appetite and a 10-lb weight loss over the last year. She avoided eating out at restaurants and traveling by plane, as both caused her symptoms to worsen. She had no significant life stressors; however, her GIT symptoms caused her emotional distress.

On physical examination, she was a thin woman with a slightly distended abdomen that was non-tender and without rebound or guarding. Her laboratory testing revealed a mild anemia and hypovitaminosis D, without any signs of systemic inflammation. The patient underwent age-appropriate screening for colon cancer 3 years prior, and the colonoscopy was unremarkable. She refused to undergo another colonoscopy, or any other GIT testing at this time.

Detailed dietary history revealed that the patient consumed an abundance of raw fruits and vegetables for breakfast, lunch and dinner. She seldom ate meat, but did consume seafood on occasion. She consumed some dairy and wheat products. When she became constipated, she would drink an abundance polyethylene glycol. She took no other bowel medications.

Intervention

The initial management approach was to help the patient have a daily bowel movement. The patient's diarrhea was likely due to overflow diarrhea in combination with excessive use of polyethylene glycol during severe distension episodes. She was started on prucalopride, a pro-motility agent that is effective in the treatment of slow-transit constipation [30] and has been studied in patients with SSc [31]. She was instructed to use polyethylene glycol sparingly.

In addition, she was advised to limit her consumption of raw fruits and vegetables, particularly those high in

Fermentable Oligosaccharides, Disaccharides, Monosaccharides and Polyols (FODMAPs). These compounds can often worsen distention and bloating, especially when consumed raw. While some recommend avoiding all foods high in FODMAPs, it is the author's opinion that many patients can tolerate vegetables containing high FODMAPs, as long as they are cooked well. For example, steamed artichokes are generally well tolerated and are an excellent source of inulin, a natural prebiotic. Prebiotics are substances, which help promote the growth of healthy, commensal gut bacteria. Animal studies have demonstrated that consumption of Jerusalem artichoke tubers modified the microbiota ecology in the large intestine to a great extent than the consumption of probiotics [32].

Probiotics were not prescribed for this patient. Probiotics are live microorganisms (typically *Bifidobacterium* and *Lactobacillus*) that are administered as food or supplements [33]. A very small, open-label study (N = 10) of SSc patients with moderate to severe bloating symptoms demonstrated that the administration of *Bifidobacterium* and *Lactobacillus* led to a significant improvement of GIT symptoms as measured by the GIT 2.0 [34]. However, this study lacked a control group. There is no compelling evidence presently that probiotics exhibit meaningful disease-modifying effects on any human diseases [35, 36]. Furthermore, in several unique SSc cohorts, the abundance of *Lactobacillus* was actually increased compared with healthy controls [17–20].

She was also started on a natural fiber supplement after the prucalopride was introduced to increase the bulk of her stools. This was started slowly by adding a few tablespoons of ground flaxseed to her morning oatmeal. Eventually, she increased the amount of ground flaxseed to approximately one half a cup per day (mixed with either oatmeal and yogurt, primarily).

At her follow up visit 3 months later, the patient reported near resolution of her diarrhea. With the addition of prucalopride and the avoidance of raw foods high in FODMAPs, the patient was able to have a daily bowel movement. Instead of requiring large doses of polyethylene glycol 1–2 times per week, the patient only needed this medication once a month, and typically, this was after a day, during which she deviated from her dietary plan.

Lessons learned from Case 1

- Diarrhea is a not uncommon manifestation of slow transit constipation, especially when laxatives are used in excess or overflow diarrhea occurs.
- Adhering to a low FODMAP diet may help ameliorate GIT dysfunction; however, vegetables with high FODMAPs are often tolerated when cooked well.
- Pro-motility agents can help to regulate bowel movements even in patients with diarrhea, if the underlying cause of symptoms is dysmotility.

Case 2: SC

Presentation

SC is a 66 year old Caucasian female with a 12-year history of diffuse SSc with a history of renal crisis, ILD, Raynaud's phenomenon, digital ulcers and GERD (ANA positive, Scl-70 positive). She had been treated early in the course of her disease with multiple courses of intravenous cyclophosphamide administered approximately monthly over 2 years. She was then transitioned to azathioprine for another 5 years as maintenance therapy.

Upon presentation to the clinic, she had been off of immunosuppressant therapy for 4 years. Her main complaint was diarrhea, and she reported between 15 and 30 episodes of watery diarrhea daily. She also had frequent digital ulcer infections that required multiple courses of broad-spectrum antibiotic therapy.

The patient adhered to a low FODMAP diet, but had experienced profound weight loss (>30 lbs) over the past year. She also reported fatigue and depression due to the fact that her GIT symptoms prevented her from traveling to visit her grandchildren.

On physical examination, she was cachectic and had a flat, non-tender abdomen. Her laboratory testing revealed a low prealbumin, low hemoglobin, low albumin and multiple other vitamin deficiencies including carotene, vitamin B12, folate, and iron. Lactulose breath testing was positive. Stool examination demonstrated *Clostridium difficile* infection positivity. Colonoscopy showed non-specific inflammation in various parts of the colon.

Intervention

The cause of the patient's diarrhea was likely due to both *C. difficile* infection and small intestine bacterial overgrowth (SIBO) with malabsorption [37]. The patient did not recall having problems with constipation prior to the onset of her diarrhea. Chronic antibiotic use and her extensive history of immunosuppressive therapy may have contributed to SIBO.

The patient was treated with oral vancomycin for her *Clostridium difficile* infection. Her diarrhea improved, but she still had multiple episodes of loose, watery stools even after treatment of her infection. Shortly thereafter, she was given another course of antibiotics for a urinary tract infection and developed worsening diarrhea secondary to *C. difficile* recurrence. She was treated again with oral vancomycin, but her symptoms and the infection persisted upon repeat testing.

At this juncture, the patient was referred for fecal transplant for treatment-refractory *C. difficile* infection. The most common indication for fecal transplantation is recurrent *C. difficile* infection (typically three or more infections). Within a week of the transplant, the patient reported resolution of her diarrhea. For an entire year following the transplant, the patient experienced no diarrhea. With vitamin supplementation and referral to a nutritionist who specializes in SSc, her vitamin levels normalized and she regained weight.

Studies have demonstrated that administration of immunosuppressive agents can alter the GIT microbiome. For instance, cyclophosphamide (CYC) reduced the diversity and shifted the microbiota composition towards a reduction in *Bacteroidetes* in one animal study [38]. It is plausible that patients who receive immunosuppression may be at heightened risk for the development of SIBO independent of the SSc disease state.

Furthermore, repeated courses of antibiotics have profound effects on the GIT microbiome and can cause dysbiosis [39, 40]. While short courses of antibiotics can ameliorate GIT symptoms in patients with SIBO [41], the long-term use of rotating cycles of antibiotics is likely more harmful than beneficial given the enduring impact of antibiotics on the GIT microbiome. However, more research is needed in this area, particularly to understand the long-term effects of agents such as Rifaximin [42], which is used to treat irritable bowel syndrome (IBS) [43] and has been tested in small group of patients with SSc [44].

Lessons Learned from Case 2

- It is important to rule out infection in patients with SSc, even when SIBO is present.
- Frequent courses of antibiotics can drive dysbiosis in the GIT microbiota.
- Fecal transplantation may be a viable option in the future to treat dysbiosis in patients with SSc and studies assessing this intervention are underway.

Summary and Recommendations

Diarrhea is a common complication of SSc with diverse underlying etiologies. The most common causes of diarrhea directly attributable to SSc are SSc-related dysmotility and SIBO with malabsorption; however, other causes should be considered, as described in Table 17.1.

The treatment approach to managing diarrhea in SSc depends on the underlying cause(s) of symptoms and often involves a multi-disciplinary approach. Gastroenterology consultation is particularly helpful in complicated cases, when overlap GIT conditions (e.g., inflammatory bowel disease (IBD), IBS) are present, and/or when further diagnostic testing is indicated (Table 17.2). Anti-diarrheal medication should be used sparingly (after *C. difficile* infection has been ruled out), as these agents can cause severe constipation and rectal prolapse [45].

Nutritional consultation is also beneficial, especially since patients may develop highly restrictive diets when they suffer from diarrhea that can compromise their nutritional status. Table 17.3 highlights nutritional strategies that can be helpful to

Table 17.3 Nutritional strategies to explore when managing diarrhea in SSc

- Limit consumption of raw fruits and vegetables
- If raw fruits and vegetables are consumed, eat these foods in isolation, preferably early in the day
- Consider following the low FODMAP diet, or at least using it as a guide to determine what foods you can/cannot tolerate
- Cook vegetables well (steamed, roasted, sautéed). If diarrhea is severe, consume vegetables in soups and purees primarily.
- Trial of the elimination diet to identify dietary intolerances[a]
- Increase consumption of healthy fats (e.g., olive oil, avocado, flax seed [ground or oil])
- Gradually increase consumption of cultured foods (e.g., yogurt, milks- these can be derived from animals [cows, goats, sheep] or from nuts, oats, rice, or hemp for individuals who cannot tolerate dairy)
- Gradually increase consumption of fermented foods (e.g., sauerkraut, pickles, kombucha)
- Limit consumption of processed foods (i.e. food that comes in packages with more than 5–10 ingredients)

[a]The author rarely finds food allergy testing helpful. Instead, she recommends that patients try eliminating certain foods (e.g., gluten, dairy) for 1 month and then re-introducing them one at a time to determine whether symptoms subside during cessation and worsen during re-introduction. Elimination diets should only be performed under the close supervision of a medical professional to ensure that the patient is receiving an adequate source of key vitamins, minerals and calories during the elimination phase of this process.

explore in patients with SSc. Often, patients need to be followed closely to observe how their symptoms change and evolve with specific dietary modifications. While the low FODMAP diet is used frequently in clinical practice, no controlled trials have evaluated its impact on SSc-GIT dysfunction. Furthermore, consuming a low FODMAP diet can alter the gut microbiota and metabolome, and it is unclear how these alterations affect immune function and health [46, 47]. Fiber supplementation should be used judiciously in patients with diarrhea as it can lead to constipation and fecal impaction [48, 49]. I therefore recommend introducing a natural fiber supplement (e.g., ground flaxseed) in small amounts initially.

Since changes in the microbiome likely underlie the symptomatic improvement that patients experience with diet changes [50–52], it is important to recognize that adherence to dietary changes is critical. Studies have demonstrated that the GIT shifts in microbial composition occur rapidly in response to dietary changes [53]. One study found that switching mice from a low-fat, plant polysaccharide-rich diet to a high-fat, high-sugar "Western" diet altered the composition of the microbiome in just 1 day [54]. Therefore, both the patient and the health care provider need to understand that sustainable improvements in GIT function will only occur when the patient is fully committed to adhering to their dietary plan.

If the patient has anxiety, depression, and/or any component of IBS, these issues also require attention. Various modalities can be helpful in these cases including psychotherapy, psychoactive medication, biofeedback, and meditation [55, 56].

In summary, diarrhea is a troubling complication of SSc that adversely affects quality of life and can lead to malnutrition and in severe cases, death. No disease-modifying treatments exist to manage this feature of SSc, but new research on the GIT microbiome will hopefully help uncover novel targets for therapeutic intervention.

Acknowledgements The author thanks her patients with systemic sclerosis.

References

1. Thoua NM, Bunce C, Brough G, Forbes A, Emmanuel AV, et al. Assessment of gastrointestinal symptoms in patients with systemic sclerosis in a UK tertiary referral Centre. Rheumatology (Oxford). 2010;49:1770–5.
2. Lock G, Zeuner M, Lang B, Hein R, Scholmerich J, Holstege A. Anorectal function in systemic sclerosis: correlation with esophageal dysfunction? Dis Colon Rectum. 1997;40:1328–35.
3. Sallam H, McNearney TA, Chen JD. Systematic review: pathophysiology and management of gastrointestinal dysmotility in systemic sclerosis (scleroderma). Aliment Pharmacol Ter. 2006;23:691–712.
4. Bodukam V, Hays RD, Maranian P, Furst DE, Seibold JR, Impens A, et al. Association of gastrointestinal involvement and depressive symptoms in patients with systemic sclerosis. Rheumatology (Oxford). 2011;50(2):330–4.
5. Baron M, Hudson M, Steele R. Canadian scleroderma research group. Malnutrition is common in systemic sclerosis: results from the Canadian scleroderma research group database. J Rheumatol. 2009;36(12):2737–43.
6. Krause L, Becker MO, Brueckner CS, Bellinghausen CJ, Becker C, Schneider U, et al. Nutritional status as marker for disease activity and severity predicting mortality in patients with systemic sclerosis. Ann Rheum Dis. 2010;69(11):1951–7.
7. Steen VD, Medsger TA Jr. Severe organ involvement in systemic sclerosis with diffuse scleroderma. Arthritis Rheum. 2000;43:2437–44.
8. Kumar S, Singh J, Rattan S, DiMarino AJ, Cohen S, Jimenez SA. Review article: pathogenesis and clinical manifestations of gastrointestinal involvement in systemic sclerosis. Aliment Pharmacol Ther. 2017;45(7):883–98.
9. Piasecki C, Chin J, Greenslade L, McIntyre N, Burroughs AK, McCormick PA. Endoscopic detection of ischaemia with a new probe indicates low oxygenation of gastric epithelium in portal hypertensive gastropathy. Gut. 1995;36(5):654–6.
10. Malandrini A, Selvi E, Villanova M, Berti G, Sabadini L, Salvadori C, et al. Autonomic nervous system and smooth muscle cell involvement in systemic sclerosis: ultrastructural study of 3 cases. J Rheumatol. 2000;27(5):1203–6.

11. Goldblatt F, Gordon TP, Waterman SA. Antibody-mediated gastrointestinal dysmotility in scleroderma. Gastroenterology. 2002;123(4):1144–50.
12. Singh J, Mehendiratta V, Del Galdo F, Jimenez SA, Cohen S, DiMarino AJ, et al. Immunoglobulins from scleroderma patients inhibit the muscarinic receptor activation in internal anal sphincter smooth muscle cells. Am J Physiol Gastrointest Liver Physiol. 2009;297(6):G1206–13.
13. Singh J, Cohen S, Mehendiratta V, Mendoza F, Jimenez SA, DiMarino AJ, et al. Effects of scleroderma antibodies and pooled human immunoglobulin on anal sphincter and colonic smooth muscle function. Gastroenterology. 2012;143(5):1308–18.
14. Hudson M, Lo E, Lu Y, Hercz D, Baron M, Steele R. Canadian scleroderma research group. Arthritis Rheum. 2011;63(1):230–8.
15. Bellocchi C, Volkmann ER. Update on the gastrointestinal microbiome in systemic sclerosis. Curr Rheumatol Reports. 2018;20:49.
16. Volkmann ER. Intestinal microbiome in scleroderma: Recent progress. Curr Opin Rheumatol. 2017;29:553–60.
17. Volkmann ER, Chang Y-L, Barroso N, Furst DE, Clements PJ, Gorn AH, et al. Association of Systemic Sclerosis with a unique colonic microbial consortium. Arthritis Rheumatol. 2016;68:1483–92.
18. Volkmann ER, Hoffmann-Vold A-M, Chang Y-L, Jacobs JP, Tillisch K, Mayer EA, et al. Systemic sclerosis is associated with specific alterations in gastrointestinal microbiota in two independent cohorts. BMJ Gastroenterol. 2017;4:e000134.
19. Andréasson K, Alrawi Z, Persson A, Jönsson G, Marsal J. Intestinal dysbiosis is common in systemic sclerosis and associated with gastrointestinal and extraintestinal features of disease. Arthritis Res Ther. 2016;18:278.
20. Bosello S, Paroni Sterbini F, Natalello G, Canestrari G, Parisi F, Sanguinetti M, et al. The intestinal involvement in systemic sclerosis is characterized by a peculiar gut microbiota [abstract]. Arthritis Rheumatol. 2016;68(suppl. 10)
21. Patrone V, Puglisi E, Cardinali M, Schnitzler TS, Svegliati S, Festa A, et al. Gut microbiota profile in systemic sclerosis patients with and without clinical evidence of gastrointestinal involvement. Sci Rep. 2017;7:14874.

22. Bellocchi C, Fernández-Ochoa Á, Montanelli G, Vigone B, Santaniello A, Milani C, et al. Microbial and metabolic multi'omic correlations in systemic sclerosis patients. Ann N Y Acad Sci. 2018;1421(1):97–109.
23. Khanna D, Furst DE, Maranian P, Seibold JR, Impens A, Mayes MD, et al. Minimally important differences of the UCLA scleroderma clinical trial consortium gastrointestinal tract instrument. J Rheumatol. 2011;38(9):1920–4.
24. Bae S, Allanore Y, Coustet B, Maranian P, Khanna D. Development and validation of French version of the UCLA scleroderma clinical trial consortium gastrointestinal tract instrument. Clin Exp Rheumatol. 2011;29(2 Suppl 65):S15–21.
25. Baron M, Hudson M, Steele R, Lo E. Canadian scleroderma research G. validation of the UCLA scleroderma clinical trial gastrointestinal tract instrument version 2.0 for systemic sclerosis. J Rheumatol. 2011;38(9):1925–30.
26. Pope J. Measures of systemic sclerosis (scleroderma): health assessment questionnaire (HAQ) and scleroderma HAQ (SHAQ), physician- and patient-rated global assessments, symptom burden index (SBI), University of California, los Angeles, scleroderma clinical trials consortium gastrointestinal scale (UCLA SCTC GIT) 2.0, baseline dyspnea index (BDI) and transition dyspnea index (TDI) (Mahler's index), Cambridge pulmonary hypertension outcome review (CAMPHOR), and Raynaud's condition score (RCS). Arthritis Care Res. 2011;63(Suppl 11):S98–111.
27. Murtaugh MA, Frech TM. Nutritional status and gastrointestinal symptoms in systemic sclerosis patients. Clin Nutr. 2013;32(1):130–5.
28. Nagaraja V, Hays RD, Khanna PP, Spiegel BM, Chang L, Melmed GY, et al. Construct validity of the patient-reported outcomes measurement information system gastrointestinal symptom scales in systemic sclerosis. Arthritis Care Res. 2014;66(11):1725–30.
29. Harrison E, Herrick AL, McLaughlin JT, Lal S. Malnutrition in systemic sclerosis. Rheumatology (Oxford). 2012;51(10):1747–56.
30. Camilleri M, Kerstens R, Rykx A, Vandeplassche L. A placebo-controlled trial of prucalopride for severe chronic constipation. N Engl J Med. 2008;358(22):2344–54.
31. Vigone B, Caronni M, Severino A, Bellocchi C, Baldassarri AR, Fraquelli M, et al. Preliminary safety and efficacy profile of prucalopride in the treatment of systemic sclerosis (SSc)-related

intestinal involvement: results from the open label cross-over PROGASS study. Arthritis Res Ther. 2017;19(1):145.
32. Barszcz M, Taciak M, Skomiał J. The effects of inulin, dried Jerusalem artichoke tuber and a multispecies probiotic preparation on microbiota ecology and immune status of the large intestine in young pigs. Arch Anim Nutr. 2016;70(4):278–92.
33. Hill C, Guarner F, Reid G, Gibson GR, Merenstein DJ, Pot B, et al. Expert consensus document. The international scientific Association for Probiotics and Prebiotics consensus statement on the scope and appropriate use of the term probiotic. Nat Rev Gastroenterol Hepatol. 2014;11:506–14.
34. Frech TM, Khanna D, Maranian P, Frech EJ, Sawitzke AD, Murtaugh MA. Probiotics for the treatment of systemic sclerosis-associated gastrointestinal bloating/ distention. Clin Exp Rheumatol. 2011;29(2 Suppl 65):S22–5.
35. Gupta P, Andrew H, Kirschner BS, Guandalini S. Is lactobacillus GG helpful in children with Crohn's disease? Results of a preliminary, open-label study. J Pediatr Gastroenterol Nutr. 2000;31:453–7.
36. Hayes SR, Vargas AJ. Probiotics for the prevention of pediatric antibiotic-associated diarrhea. Explor J Sci Heal. 2016;12:463–6.
37. Marie I, Ducrotté P, Denis P, Menard JF, Levesque H. Small intestinal bacterial overgrowth in systemic sclerosis. Rheumatology (Oxford). 2009;48:1314–9.
38. Xu X, Zhang X. Effects of cyclophosphamide on immune system and gut microbiota in mice. Microbiol Res. 2015;171:97–106.
39. Ferrer M, Mendez-Garcia RD, Barbas C, Moya A. Antibiotic use and microbiome function. Biochem Pharmacol. 2017;134:114–26.
40. Francino MP. Antibiotics and the human gut microbiome: Dysbioses and accumulation of resistances. Front Microbiol. 2016;12(6):1543.
41. Pittman N, Rawn SM, Wang M, Masetto A, Beattie KA, Larché M. Treatment of small intestinal bacterial overgrowth in systemic sclerosis: a systematic review. Rheumatology (Oxford). 2018;57(10):1802–11.
42. Lopetuso LR, Petito V, Scaldaferri F, Gasbarrini A. Gut microbiota modulation and mucosal immunity: focus on Rifaximin. Mini Rev Med Chem. 2015;16(3):179–85.
43. Chang C. Short-course therapy for diarrhea-predominant irritable bowel syndrome: understanding the mechanism, impact on gut microbiota, and safety and tolerability of rifaximin. Clin Exp Gastroenterol. 2018;11:335–45.

44. Parodi A, Sessarego M, Greco A, Bazzica M, Filaci G, Setti M, et al. Small intestinal bacterial overgrowth in patients suffering from scleroderma: clinical effectiveness of its eradication. Am J Gastroenterol. 2008;103(5):1257–62.
45. Sallam H, McNearney TA, Chen JD. Systematic review: pathophysiology and management of gastrointestinal dysmotility in systemic sclerosis (scleroderma). Aliment Pharmacol Ther. 2006;23:691–712.
46. McIntosh K, Reed DE, Schneider T, Dang F, Keshteli AJ, De Palma G, et al. FODMAPs alter symptoms and the metabolome of patients with IBS: a randomised controlled trial. Gut. 2017;66:1241–51.
47. Staudacher HM, Whelan K. The low FODMAP diet: recent advances in understanding its mechanisms and efficacy in IBS. Gut. 2017;66:1517–27.
48. Butt S, Emmanuel A. Systemic sclerosis and the gut. Expert Rev Gastroenterol Hepatol. 2013;7:331–9.
49. Emmanuel AV, Tack J, Quigley EM, Talley NJ. Pharmacological management of constipation. Neurogastroenterol Motil. 2009;21:41–54.
50. Sandhu KV, Sherwin E, Schellekens H, Stanton C, Dinan TG, Cryan JF. Feeding the microbiota-gut-brain axis: diet, microbiome, and neuropsychiatry. Transl Res. 2017;179:223–44.
51. Valdes AM, Walter J, Segal E, Spector TD. Role of the gut microbiota in nutrition and health. BMJ. 2018;361:k2179.
52. Singh RK, Chang H-W, Yan D, Lee KM, Uemak D, Abrouk M, et al. Influence of diet on the gut microbiome and implications for human health. J Transl Med. 2017;15:73.
53. David LA, Maurice CF, Carmody RN, Gootenberg DB, Button JE, Wolfe BE, et al. Diet rapidly and reproducibly alters the human gut microbiome. Nature. 2013;505(7484):559–63.
54. Turnbaugh PJ, Ridaura VK, Faith JJ, Re FE, Knight R, Gordon JI. The effect of diet on the human gut microbiome: a metagenomic analysis in humanized Gnotobiotic mice. Sci Transl Med. 2009;1(6):6ra14.
55. Kearney DJ, Brown-Chang J. Complementary and alternative medicine for IBS in adults: mind-body interventions. Nat Clin Pract Gastroenterol Hepatol. 2008;5(11):624–36.
56. Grundmann O, Yoon SL. Complementary and alternative medicines in irritable bowel syndrome: an integrative view. World J Gastroenterol. 2014;20(2):346–62.

Chapter 18
Gastric Antral Vascular Ectasia (GAVE)

Devis Benfaremo, Lucia Manfredi, and Armando Gabrielli

Clinical Vignette
A 65-year-old woman with limited cutaneous systemic sclerosis (lcSSc) was admitted for the evaluation of worsening fatigue. Routine blood tests showed a hemoglobin level of 9.4 g/dL, with a ferritin level of 4 ng/mL. The fecal occult blood test was positive. Esophagogastroduodenoscopy revealed diffuse gastric vascular ectasias involving the antrum and converging towards the pylorus (Fig. 18.1). How should this case be managed?

Introduction

Gastric antral vascular ectasia (GAVE) is a rare acquired vascular disease involving the antral mucosa of the stomach [1]. The disease is also known as *watermelon stomach* because of its striking endoscopic appearance, characterized by multiple longitudinal stripes of red vessels originating

D. Benfaremo · L. Manfredi · A. Gabrielli (✉)
Dipartimento di Scienze Cliniche e Molecolari,
Clinica Medica, Università Politecnica delle Marche, Ancona, Italy
e-mail: d.benfaremo@pm.univpm.it;
lucia.manfredi@ospedaliriuniti.marche.it; a.gabrielli@staff.univpm.it
© Springer Nature Switzerland AG 2021

M. Matucci-Cerinic, C. P. Denton (eds.), *Practical Management of Systemic Sclerosis in Clinical Practice*, In Clinical Practice,
https://doi.org/10.1007/978-3-030-53736-4_18

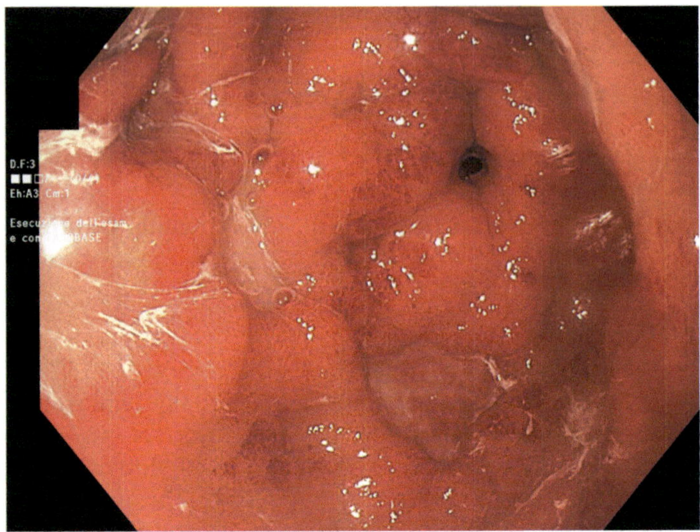

FIGURE 18.1 Endoscopic appearance of gastric antral vascular ectasia (GAVE): multiple longitudinal stripes of red vessels involving the gastric antrum and converging to the pylorus

from the pylorus and involving the antrum. The macroscopic appearance of GAVE is related to the underlying pathogenic mechanisms and microscopic features, characterized by capillary dilatation, small vessel fibrin deposition and microthrombosis [2].

Although GAVE is a known complication of cirrhosis, only a third of patients with GAVE actually have a chronic liver disease [3]. Among non-cirrhotic patients, GAVE can be mostly observed in patients with autoimmune connective tissue disorders, bone marrow transplantation and chronic renal failure [3]. Despite the rarity of both diseases, the association of GAVE and systemic sclerosis (SSc) has been clearly established in recent years, and several studies have shed light upon the prevalence, significance and prognosis of such an association.

Epidemiology

After *Jabbari et al* accurately described it in 1984 [1], GAVE has increasingly been associated with scleroderma and SSc-related features in the subsequent years [4–6].

To date, the prevalence of GAVE in patients with SSc is estimated between 1% and 22.3%, varying largely according to the different studies [7, 8]. The differences may be mostly accounted to the design of the study (i.e. retrospective or prospective) and the selection of the patients (i.e. whether patients were systematically screened or not regardless of the presence of symptoms).

Overall, retrospective studies report a lower prevalence (1–5.7%) [7, 8] than the prospective Scleroderma Cyclophosphamide Or Transplant (SCOT) trial that systematically assessed all patients by endoscopy regardless of clinical symptoms (22.3%) [9].

In most of the studies, GAVE appears to be an early complication of SSc, since on average it occurs within the first 18–36 months after the diagnosis of SSc [8, 10]. In 15–20% of the cases, the diagnosis of GAVE may precede or be concurrent to that of SSc [7, 11]. Finally, in up to a third of SSc patients GAVE may represent the first non-Raynaud symptom [8].

Pathogenesis

The etiology of GAVE is still largely unknown [3]. However, several mechanisms have been suspected to be involved in the pathogenesis of watermelon stomach, including altered motility of the gastric antrum and mucosal trauma secondary to mechanical stress [3]. The role of vasoactive substances is uncertain, but locally released neurotransmitters may be responsible for vasodilatation and hence the propensity to bleed [12].

The microscopic features of GAVE further suggest that vascular ectasia is acquired rather than congenital. Several histopathological aspects have been described, including dilatation of mucosal capillaries with focal fibrin thromboses and fibromuscular hyperplasia of the lamina propria [13].

In SSc, GAVE may represent a complication belonging to the spectrum of vascular alterations, along with Raynaud's phenomenon, telangiectasias, pulmonary and renal vascular involvements [8].

Clinical Aspects

The clinical presentation of GAVE is related to its pathological aspects. Submucosal ectasic vessels can erode through the gastric mucosa, leading to chronic blood loss and substantial iron deficiency anemia. GAVE is responsible for around 4% of non-variceal upper gastrointestinal bleedings [14], with a substantial proportion of patients (60–70%) requiring blood transfusions due to recurrent anemia despite iron supplementation.

In SSc-associated GAVE, clinically meaningful anemia may develop in about 80–90% of patients, with half of them requiring blood transfusions [8]. Acute hemorrhage in the form of melena or hematemesis may be the first presentation of GAVE in few cases [7].

Several studies reported significant clinical associations between GAVE and SSc features. SSc patients with GAVE appear to have a low prevalence of anti-topoisomerase I antibodies [8–10], and a lower proportion of them exhibit pulmonary fibrosis on chest CT scan [8].

Conversely, anti-RNA polymerase III (RNAP III) positivity appears to be significantly associated to GAVE, as confirmed by several studies [8, 10, 15]. Patients that are positive to anti-RNAP III antibodies carry a significant higher risk of developing GAVE (OR 4.6, 95%CI 1.2–21.1) and other vascular events such as scleroderma renal crisis and pulmonary hypertension [8], and are more likely to have a shorter disease duration, a more rapid disease onset (defined as the interval from appearance of Raynaud's phenomenon to first symptom other than Raynaud's) and faster skin thickening in the first months after SSc onset, compared to anti-topoisomerase I positive patients [10, 15]. Furthermore, patients with early diffuse cutaneous subset (dcSSc) seems to have a higher risk of developing GAVE [9, 10], although this has not been confirmed in all studies [8].

Finally, SSc patients with GAVE have a higher prevalence of telangiectasias and systemic hypertension [7, 8, 10].

At the functional level, patients with GAVE more frequently exhibit a diminished diffusing capacity (DLCO) with a low DLCO/alveolar volume (DLCO/AV) ratio at pulmonary function tests, suggesting an underlying vascular pulmonary involvement in these patients [8, 9]. Taken together, these data indicate that GAVE may be a significant manifestation of the "vascular phenotype" of SSc, along with renal, pulmonary and cutaneous vascular complications [8, 9].

Diagnosis

The diagnosis of GAVE is usually supported by the endoscopic appearance [14]. In long-standing diseases, gastroscopy may disclose the typical watermelon stomach characterized by prominent, erythematous stripes, radiating in a spoke-like fashion from the antrum to the pylorus, but in early stages the findings may be limited to multiple red spots or linear red stripes in the antrum (Fig. 18.1) [11].

Routine histopathological examination is not required for a definite diagnosis, but it may be useful for cases in which the diagnosis is uncertain, or when other diseases (i.e. antral gastritis) need to be investigated.

Management

Although in the last two decades several therapeutic options have become available for GAVE-related gastrointestinal bleeding, the management of watermelon stomach remains a challenging issue. Therapeutic options include medical, endoscopic and surgical procedures [14].

Medical Management

Different medical treatments have been proposed for the management of GAVE-related bleeding, though evidence is weak. Corticosteroids [16], thalidomide [17], tranexamic acid [18], octreotide [19] and hormone replacement [20] have been occasionally reported to be successful, mostly in individual case reports, but their efficacy may be limited because of the development of adverse events.

Cyclophosphamide (CYC), with or without intravenous methylprednisolone, may be effective for the resolution of GAVE-related bleeding in SSc patients as reported by several case reports and case series [21–25]. These patients were mostly refractory to conventional endoscopic treatments, and CYC was able to achieve stable hemoglobin levels. Due to its unfavorable safety profile, CYC should be reserved for patients with refractory disease.

Autologous hematopoietic stem cell transplantation (HSCT), that recently became a treatment option for SSc patients [26], may also be effective for SSc-related GAVE. In a series of three patients with persistent bleeding despite multiple endoscopic treatments, HSCT was successful to achieve transfusion independence and maintain stable hemoglobin at 1 year. Interestingly, the surveillance endoscopy showed significant improvement of vascular ectasia [27].

Endoscopic Management

Endoscopy is the treatment of choice for the management of GAVE-related gastrointestinal bleeding [14]. Endoscopic techniques have also been successfully applied in patients with SSc [7, 8].

Treatments modalities that have been proven to be useful in GAVE include thermal and mechanical methods, with meaningful success rates and acceptable safety profiles (Table 18.1).

Table 18.1 Endoscopic treatment for gastric antral vascular ectasia

Method	Bleeding cessation rate[a]	Mean number of sessions	Complications[b]
Cryotherapy	50–71%	2–6	Major: ~0%; minor 0–8%
Nd: YAG laser	60–100%	1–5	Major 0–13%; minor ~0%
Argon plasma coagulation	30–100%	2–6	Major: ~0%; minor ~0%
Endoscopic band ligation	65–95%	2–3	Major: ~0%; minor 8–12%
Radiofrequency ablation	67–86%	2–3	Major ~0%; minor 1–2%

Reproduced from Hsu WH, Wang YK, Hsieh MS, Kuo FC, Wu MC, Shih HY, et al. Insights into the management of gastric antral vascular ectasia (watermelon stomach). Therap Adv Gastroenterol. 2018;11:1–9

Nd: YAG, neodymium-yttrium-aluminium garnet

[a]Definition of bleeding cessation: rising hemoglobin level and no requirement for blood transfusion

[b]Major complication: death, perforation, stenosis; minor complication: gastrointestinal upset

Endoscopic treatments are usually considered effective if they are able to improve gastrointestinal bleeding, achieving bleeding cessation, a condition in which hemoglobin levels rise and blood transfusions are no longer required [14].

Cryotherapy is an endoscopic technique using nitrous oxide to apply an extremely cold temperature on affected tissue and achieve hemostasis by thermal destruction or necrosis of the mucosa [14].

Two small studies demonstrated limited efficacy of cryotherapy on GAVE-related bleeding, with a cessation rate of 50–71% after a median of 2–6 sessions of treatment [28, 29].

Neodymium-yttrium-aluminum garnet laser coagulation (Nd: YAG) laser is a thermal device that causes tissue destruction by absorption of laser light without direct contact [14]. The efficacy of Nd: YAG laser in stopping bleeding and decreasing the requirement for blood transfusions ranges between 60% and 100% after a median of 1–4 sessions [30–32]. However, Nd: YAG lasers have been largely replaced by other treatment modalities because of higher cost and serious complications, such as perforation, antral narrowing, and mortality, compared to other treatment modalities [14].

Argon plasma coagulation (APC) is another thermal method that has gradually become the treatment of choice for GAVE. APC produces high frequency electrical current flows to achieve tissue coagulation by using ionized argon gas (plasma) as a medium. Compared with Nd: YAG lasers, APC is easier to apply and safer due to its favorable side-effect profile, and less expensive [14].

Several studies demonstrated that APC is effective in GAVE, with variable bleeding cessation rates (30–100%), but also reported that usually repeated endoscopic sessions are warranted [33–35]. APC may be unsatisfactory in long-term follow-up and yield high bleeding recurrence rates [36–38]. The recurrent bleeding following APC may be related to its limited depth of mucosal coagulation [14]. Although APC presumably has a favorable side effect profile due to its non-contact method and limited depth of mucosal injury, some major complications are still a concern. Gastric outlet obstruction and hyperplastic polyps were reported as serious adverse events after APC treatment [39, 40].

Radiofrequency ablation (RFA) is another thermal technique that has been recently proposed as treatment modality for GAVE. The principle of RFA is to apply high-energy coaptive coagulation to destroy the superficial mucosal capillary ectasia with the subsequent regeneration of epithelium composed of a normal capillary structure [14]. RFA has a success rate of 67–86% in achieving bleeding cessation after a median of 2–3 sessions, with a low rate of minor complications [41–43]. The minimal time interval of 6 weeks between each treatment session is recommended and proton pump inhibitors should be prescribed. RFA appears to be a well-tolerated and feasible method for patients with GAVE with poor response to other treatment modalities [14].

Among mechanical methods, endoscopic band ligation (EBL), usually used for the treatment of esophageal varices, may be also effective for GAVE-related bleeding [14]. In retrospective studies, EBL showed higher rates of bleeding cessation and fewer treatment sessions compared to APC, whereas in prospective studies EBL reached a 95% success rate for bleeding cessation [44–47]. EBL appears to be safe and well tolerated and thus it may be an option for the treatment of patients refractory to thermoablative methods.

Surgical Treatments

With the advances of endoscopic techniques, surgery is now reserved for patients that fail to improve despite medical and endoscopic treatments [14]. Surgical approaches include antrectomies (with Billroth I, II, and Roux-en-Y reconstructions), partial gastrectomy, total gastrectomy and esophagogastrectomy [48]. The results of surgical hemostasis are usually satisfying but several complications may develop, such as late dumping syndrome, nutritional deficiencies and death [14].

Prognosis

The natural history of SSc-associated GAVE has not been fully elucidated given the paucity of data. Bleeding recurrence and transfusion dependence are common issues in patients with long-standing disease [7, 8, 11]. The median time of GAVE recurrence is 10 months after the initial diagnosis [7].

These issues may be overcome by planning re-treatment endoscopic sessions or integrating different endoscopic techniques and medical therapy [7].

Although frequently associated with the positivity of anti-RNAP III antibody, that is burdened with substantial morbidity, characterized by the rapid evolution of skin thickening and the occurrence of scleroderma renal crisis, the presence of GAVE does not appear to impact on mortality of SSc patients, at least in the study with the longer follow-up (30 months) [8].

Conclusion

GAVE is a rare but burdensome complication that appears to belong to the broad spectrum of vascular alterations of SSc. The presence of watermelon stomach should be considered when unexplained iron-deficiency anemia occurs in SSc patients, especially in patients with early diffuse skin involvement. Given the close association of GAVE and anti-RNA polymerase III antibodies, screening these high risk patients with endoscopy should be considered even in absence of anemia or gastric-related symptoms. Endoscopic treatment is effective, safe and well tolerated in patients with SSc-related GAVE with significant bleeding.

References

1. Jabbari M, Cherry R, Lough JO, Daly DS, Kinnear DG, Goresky CA. Gastric Antral vascular Ectasia: the watermelon stomach. Gastroenterology. 1984;87(5):1165–70.
2. Ruhl GH, Schnabel R, Peiseler M, Seidel D. Gastric antral vascular ectasia: a case report of a 10 year follow-up with special consideration of histopathological aspects. Z Gastroenterol. 1994;32(3):160–4.
3. Burak KW, Lee SS, Beck PL. Portal hypertensive gastropathy and gastric antral vascular ectasia (GAVE) syndrome. Gut. 2001;49(6):866 LP-872.
4. Jouanolle H, Bretagne JF, Ramée MP, Lancien G, Le Jean-Colin I, Heresbach D, et al. Antral vascular ectasia and scleroderma. Endoscopic, radiologic and anatomopathologic aspects of an uncommon association. Gastroenterol Clin Biol. 1989;13(2):217–21.
5. Murphy FT, Enzenauer RJ, Cheney CP. Watermelon stomach. Arthritis Rheum. 1999;42(3):573.
6. Watson M, Hally RJ, McCue PA, Varga J, Jiménez SA. Gastric antral vascular ectasia (watermelon stomach) in patients with systemic sclerosis. Arthritis Rheum. 1996;39(2):341–6.
7. Marie I, Ducrotte P, Antonietti M, Herve S, Levesque H. Watermelon stomach in systemic sclerosis: its incidence and management. Aliment Pharmacol Ther. 2008;28(4):412–21.
8. Ghrénassia E, Avouac J, Khanna D, Derk CT, Distler O, Suliman YA, et al. Prevalence, correlates and outcomes of gastric antral vascular ectasia in systemic sclerosis: a eustar case-control study. J Rheumatol. 2014;41(1):99–105.
9. Hung EW, Mayes MD, Sharif R, Assassi S, Machicao VI, Hosing C, et al. Gastric Antral vascular Ectasia and its clinical correlates in patients with early diffuse systemic sclerosis in the SCOT trial. J Rheumatol. 2013;40(4):455 LP-460.
10. Ingraham KM, O'Brien MS, Shenin MAX, Derk CT, Steen VD. Gastric Antral vascular Ectasia in systemic sclerosis: demographics and disease predictors. J Rheumatol. 2010;37(3):603–7.
11. El-Gendy H, Shohdy KS, Maghraby GG, Abadeer K, Mahmoud M. Gastric antral vascular ectasia in systemic sclerosis: where do we stand? Int J Rheum Dis. 2017;20(12):2133–9.

12. Lowes JR, Rode J. Neuroendocrine cell proliferations in gastric antral vascular ectasia. Gastroenterology. 1989;97(1):207–12.
13. Suit PF, Petras RE, Bauer TW, Petrini JL. Gastric antral vascular ectasia. A histologic and morphometric study of "the watermelon stomach". Am J Surg Pathol. 1987;11(10):750–7.
14. Hsu WH, Wang YK, Hsieh MS, Kuo FC, Wu MC, Shih HY, et al. Insights into the management of gastric antral vascular ectasia (watermelon stomach). Ther Adv Gastroenterol. 2018;11:1–9.
15. Ceribelli A, Cavazzana I, Airò P, Franceschini F. Anti-RNA polymerase III antibodies as a risk marker for early gastric Antral vascular Ectasia (GAVE) in systemic sclerosis. J Rheumatol. 2010;37(7):1544.
16. Calès P, Voigt JJ, Payen JL, Bloom E, Berg P, Vinel JP, et al. Diffuse vascular ectasia of the antrum, duodenum, and jejunum in a patient with nodular regenerative hyperplasia. Lack of response to portosystemic shunt or gastrectomy. Gut. 1993;34(4):558–61.
17. Dunne KA, Hill J, Dillon JF. Treatment of chronic transfusion-dependent gastric antral vascular ectasia (watermelon stomach) with thalidomide. Eur J Gastroenterol Hepatol. 2006;18(4):455–6.
18. McCormick PA, Ooi H, Crosbie O. Tranexamic acid for severe bleeding gastric antral vascular ectasia in cirrhosis. Gut. 1998;42(5):750 LP-752.
19. Nardone R, Balzano B. The efficacy of octreotide therapy in chronic bleeding due to vascular abnormalities of the gastrointestinal tract. Aliment Pharmacol Ther. 1999;13(11):1429–36.
20. Tran A, Villeneuve J-P, Bilodeau M, Willems B, Marleau D, Fenyves D, et al. Treatment of chronic bleeding from gastric Antral vascular Ectasia (Gave) with estrogen-progesterone in cirrhotic patients: an open pilot study. Am J Gastroenterol. 1999;94(10):2909–11.
21. Lorenzi AR, Johnson AH, Davies G, Gough A. Gastric antral vascular ectasia in systemic sclerosis: complete resolution with methylprednisolone and cyclophosphamide. Ann Rheum Dis. 2001;60(8):796 LP-798.
22. Azam J, Caperon A, Lawson CA, Gough A. Medical versus laser therapy for gastric antral vascular ectasia: comment on the clinical images by Thonhofer et al. Arthritis Rheum. 2010;62(11):3517.
23. Schulz SW, O'Brien M, Maqsood M, Sandorfi N, Del Galdo F, Jimenez SA. Improvement of severe systemic sclerosis-associated gastric antral vascular ectasia following immunosuppressive treatment with intravenous cyclophosphamide. J Rheumatol. 2009;36(8):1653–6.

24. Papachristos DA, Nikpour M, Hair C, Stevens WM. Intravenous cyclophosphamide as a therapeutic option for severe refractory gastric antral vascular ectasia in systemic sclerosis. Intern Med J. 2015;45(10):1077–81.
25. Sawada T, Mizuuchi T, Hayashi H, Tsubouchi S, Yasuda T, Tahara K, et al. Intravenous cyclophosphamide for gastric Antral vascular Ectasia associated with systemic sclerosis refractory to endoscopic treatment: a case report and review of the pertinent literature. Intern Med. 2018;58(1):135–9.
26. Del Papa N, Pignataro F, Zaccara E, Maglione W, Minniti A. Autologous hematopoietic stem cell transplantation for treatment of systemic sclerosis. Front Immunol. 2018;9:2390.
27. Bhattacharyya A, Sahhar J, Milliken SAM, Ma D, Tymms K, Danta M, et al. The Journal of Rheumatology Autologous Hematopoietic Stem Cell Transplant for Systemic Sclerosis Improves Anemia from Gastric Antral Vascular Ectasia The Journal of Rheumatology is a monthly international serial edited by Earl D . in rheumatology and rela. 2015;42(3).
28. Kantsevoy SV, Cruz-Correa MR, Vaughn CA, Jagannath SB, Pasricha PJ, Kalloo AN. Endoscopic cryotherapy for the treatment of bleeding mucosal vascular lesions of the GI tract: a pilot study. Gastrointest Endosc. 2003;57(3):403–6.
29. Cho S, Zanati S, Yong E, Cirocco M, Kandel G, Kortan P, et al. Endoscopic cryotherapy for the management of gastric antral vascular ectasia. Gastrointest Endosc. 2008;68(5):895–902.
30. Potamiano S, Carter CR, Anderson JR. Endoscopic laser treatment of diffuse gastric antral vascular ectasia. Gut. 1994;35(4):461–3.
31. Calamia KT, Scolapio JS, Viggiano TR. Endoscopic YAG laser treatment of watermelon stomach (gastric antral vascular ectasia) in patients with systemic sclerosis. Clin Exp Rheumatol. 2000;18(5):605–8.
32. Mathou NG, Lovat LB, Thorpe SM, Bown SG. Nd:YAG laser induces long-term remission in transfusion-dependent patients with watermelon stomach. Lasers Med Sci. 2004;18(4):213–8.
33. Fuccio L, Zagari RM, Serrani M, Eusebi LH, Grilli D, Cennamo V, et al. Endoscopic argon plasma coagulation for the treatment of gastric Antral vascular Ectasia-related bleeding in patients with liver cirrhosis. Digestion. 2009;79(3):143–50.
34. Boltin D, Gingold-Belfer R, Lichtenstein L, Levi Z, Niv Y. Long-term treatment outcome of patients with gastric vascular ectasia

treated with argon plasma coagulation. Eur J Gastroenterol Hepatol. 2014;26(6):588–93.
35. Rosenfeld G, Enns R. Argon photocoagulation in the treatment of gastric antral vascular ectasia and radiation proctitis. Can J Gastroenterol. 2009;23(12):801–4.
36. Naga M, Esmat S, Naguib M, Sedrak H. Long-term effect of argon plasma coagulation (APC) in the treatment of gastric antral vascular ectasia (GAVE). Arab J Gastroenterol. 2011;12(1):40–3.
37. Sebastian S, McLoughlin R, Qasim A, O'Morain CA, Buckley MJ. Endoscopic argon plasma coagulation for the treatment of gastric antral vascular ectasia (watermelon stomach): long-term results. Dig Liver Dis. 2004;36(3):212–7.
38. Kwan V, Bourke MJ, Williams SJ, Gillespie PE, Murray MA, Kaffes AJ, et al. Argon plasma coagulation in the Management of Symptomatic Gastrointestinal Vascular Lesions: experience in 100 consecutive patients with long-term follow-up. Am J Gastroenterol. 2006;101:58–63.
39. Shah N, Cavanagh Y, Kaswala DH, Shaikh S. Development of hyperplastic polyps following argon plasma coagulation of gastric antral vascular ectasia. J Nat Sci Biol Med. 2015;6(2):479–82.
40. Farooq FT, Wong RCK, Yang P, Post AB. Gastric outlet obstruction as a complication of argon plasma coagulation for watermelon stomach. Gastrointest Endosc. 2007;65(7):1090–2.
41. Gross SA, Al-Haddad M, Gill KRS, Schore AN, Wallace MB. Endoscopic mucosal ablation for the treatment of gastric antral vascular ectasia with the HALO90 system: a pilot study. Gastrointest Endosc. 2008;67(2):324–7.
42. McGorisk T, Krishnan K, Keefer L, Komanduri S. Radiofrequency ablation for refractory gastric antral vascular ectasia (with video). Gastrointest Endosc. 2013;78(4):584–8.
43. Markos P, Bilic B, Ivekovic H, Rustemovic N. Radiofrequency ablation for gastric antral vascular ectasia and radiation proctitis. Indian J Gastroenterol. 2017;36(2):145–8.
44. Wells CD, Harrison ME, Gurudu SR, Crowell MD, Byrne TJ, DePetris G, et al. Treatment of gastric antral vascular ectasia (watermelon stomach) with endoscopic band ligation. Gastrointest Endosc. 2008;68(2):231–6.
45. Keohane J, Berro W, Harewood GC, Murray FE, Patchett SE. Band ligation of gastric antral vascular ectasia is a safe and effective endoscopic treatment. Dig Endosc. 2013;25(4):392–6.

46. Sato T, Yamazaki K, Akaike J. Endoscopic band ligation versus argon plasma coagulation for gastric antral vascular ectasia associated with liver diseases. Dig Endosc. 2012;24(4):237–42.
47. Zepeda-Gómez S, Sultanian R, Teshima C, Sandha G, Van Zanten S, Montano-Loza AJ. Gastric antral vascular ectasia: a prospective study of treatment with endoscopic band ligation. Endoscopy. 2015;47(6):538–40.
48. Novitsky YW, Kercher KW, Czerniach DR, Litwin DEM. Watermelon stomach: pathophysiology, diagnosis, and management. J Gastrointest Surg. 2003;7(5):652–61.

Chapter 19
Management of Orofacial Complications

Rawen Smirani, Raphaël Devillard, and Marie-Elise Truchetet

Introduction

Oropharyngeal features are frequent but understated in the treatment guidelines of systemic sclerosis (SSc) in spite of important consequences on comfort, aesthetics, nutrition and daily life [1]. Patients do not easily express their needs in dental care and this aspect may be left out when other serious systemic symptoms appear, minimising the impact of oral involvement on the quality of life and long-term life expectancy.

Moreover, literature showed that significant depressive syndromes among SSc patients reduced daily oral upkeep, suggesting the fact that significant oral neglect can alert clinicians [2].

R. Smirani (✉) · R. Devillard
Université de Bordeaux, Laboratoire Bioingénierie Tissulaire (BioTis), INSERM U1026, Bordeaux cedex, France
e-mail: rawen.smirani@u-bordeaux.fr; raphael.devillard@u-bordeaux.fr

M.-E. Truchetet
Univ. Bordeaux, CNRS, Laboratoire ImmunoConCEpT, UMR 5164, CHU Bordeaux, Bordeaux, France
e-mail: marie-elise.truchetet@chu-bordeaux.fr

© Springer Nature Switzerland AG 2021

M. Matucci-Cerinic, C. P. Denton (eds.), *Practical Management of Systemic Sclerosis in Clinical Practice*, In Clinical Practice,
https://doi.org/10.1007/978-3-030-53736-4_19

The three main features reported in literature and clinical practice are a severe limitation of mouth opening, periodontal diseases and an increased xerostomia (sometimes due to secondary Sjögren's syndrome). The other disorders reported, although less frequently, are temporomandibular joint symptoms, high caries experience and oral cavity/ pharynx cancer.

Limitation of Mouth Opening

Description

Microstomia is defined as an abnormally small oral orifice: an inter-labial distance less than 45 mm or an inter-incisor distance less than 40 mm [3, 4] (Fig. 19.1). It is the most frequently reported oral consequence of SSc in literature [1]. Mouth-related disability was proven to contribute to 35% of the variance in global disability [5]. Mouth opening seems to be the main factor implicated in this global assessment.

Mouth opening limitation is due to the interaction of various mechanisms (fibrosis, atrophy, …) on different tissues (temporomandibular joints, lips, tongue, …). A thorough analysis of all criteria is required to specify the aetiology.

Although temporomandibular joint involvement is common in SSc, it is difficult to determine which role it exactly plays in the limitation. Limitation of mouth opening and reduced movement of the cheeks and tongue usually leads to a poor oral health [6, 7].

Reported Symptoms

Patients complain of difficulties for opening the mouth and restricted mouth widening, talking (difficulty to speak clearly), closing the lips. Night oral inocclusion leads to an indirect increase in xerostomia.

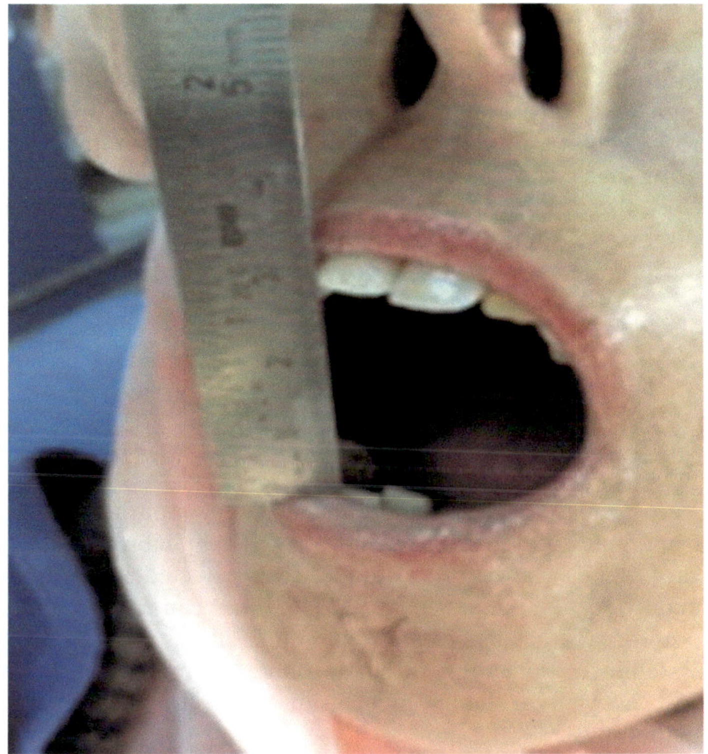

FIGURE 19.1 Microstomia

Performing oral self-care becomes challenging and painful; professional oral care can be complicated as well [8].

Clinical Signs

Tightening of perioral skin and inocclusion of the lips at rest are the most obvious signs. Most patients exhibit difficulty during movements, and a reduced inter-incisor distance [6, 9]. Masseter atrophy can be observed as well, associated with a modification of the muscle and bone morphology [10].

Management

Multidisciplinary programmes might improve mouth opening: they consist of mouth and hand exercises combined with regular dental check-ups (52–53). Physiotherapy could bring back some elasticity, less discomfort, possibility to close the lips. Hydrating lips before an oral examination or surgery is a simple but effective measure to limit discomfort during care.

Xerostomia

Description

Xerostomia is a symptom defined by a dry mouth, resulting from reduced or absent saliva flow [9, 11–15]. Fibrosis of salivary glands leads to xerostomia. It is detected in approximately 70% of patients with SSc [16, 17]. It can worsen in the presence of gastro-oesophageal reflux disease (GERD), a systemic complication often encountered in patients with SSc, as well as labial inocclusion (due to perioral skin tightening).

Biochemical modifications of the saliva were pinpointed by a statistically significant decrease in the specific peroxidase of the unstimulated saliva (ranging from 0.00003 to 0.00011 IU/100 mg) (14, 17).

Secondary Sjögren's syndrome (SS) was found in 10.4%–33.9% of SSc patients (10, 21, 24).

Reported Symptoms

Xerostomia or dry mouth syndrome is often reported by patients with the following criteria: a sticky and dry feeling in the mouth, swallowing difficulties, need to drink a lot, instability of dentures, burning sensation in the mouth, difficulty to eat acidic or spicy foods, troubles with tasting and speak-

Table 19.1 Questionnaire assessing xerostomia (initially made by Fox et al. 1987)

1. "Do you sip liquids to aid in swallowing dry foods?"
2. "Does your mouth feel dry when eating a meal?"
3. "Do you have difficulties swallowing any foods?"
4. "Does the amount of saliva in your mouth seem to be too little?"
The presence of dry mouth is indicated by a positive response to at least one question.

ing. Many patients also report the need to often wake up at night to drink.

A few simple questions can assess xerostomia (Table 19.1).

Clinical Signs

Dry and red tongue and mucosa are often observed and lips may stick together. Remaining saliva is usually thick and sticky.

Objective measures show significant low unstimulated flow rate (<1.5 mL/15 min).

According to the American-European Consensus Group (AECG) classification, in patients with another connective tissue disease, the presence of item I (ocular symptoms) or II (oral symptoms) plus any two from among items III (ocular signs), IV (histopathology) and V (objective evidence of salivary gland involvement) may be considered as indicative of secondary Sjögren's syndrome (25).

Inadequate salivary flow compromises the buffering within the oral cavity and allows:

- Erosion (acidity coming from extrinsic sources such as alimentation or intrinsic sources such as gastro-oesophageal reflux) (Fig. 19.2).
- Caries to develop (acidity produced by bacterial metabolism) (Fig. 19.2).
- Candidiasis [15].

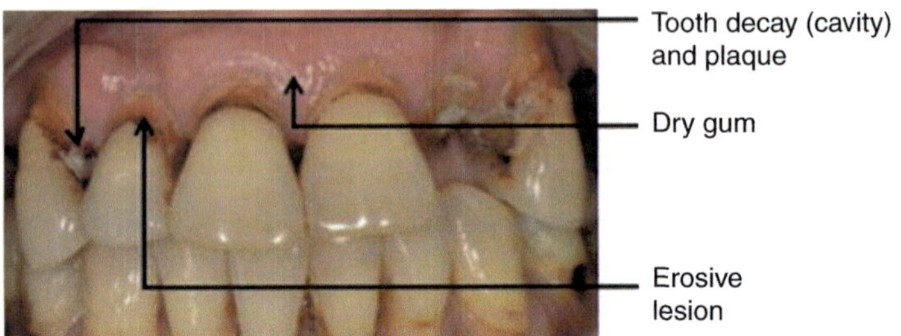

FIGURE 19.2 Oral consequences of xerostomia

Management

The main purpose of xerostomia management is to improve patients' oral comfort. Salivary substitutes containing hyaluronic acid are available in different presentations (gels, mouth sprays, mouthwashes) to accompany the patient throughout the day.

Nutritional advice to avoid irritant foods such as coffee, spices or alcohol can limit aggression of an already fragile mucosa (lack of salivary film protection).

Hyposialia can be managed by the prescription of oral pilocarpine hydrochloride [18]. The starting dose is 4 mg and is progressively increased to reach a maximum of 12 mg/day. A systematic follow-up at 4 to 8 weeks is necessary to confirm the efficacy of the treatment and avoid side effects.

Periodontal Diseases

Description

Periodontitis is a chronic multifactorial inflammatory disease associated with dysbiotic plaque biofilms and characterised by progressive destruction of tooth-supporting tissues [19].

This is to be distinguished from gingivitis, which is a reversible superficial gum inflammation without attachment loss (does not lead to tooth loss).

Gum inflammation and periodontitis in SSc patients may result from difficulties in ensuring a good oral hygiene (because of microstomia as well as handgrip impairment induced by sclerodactyly), altered capillary vascularisation [20] and dry mouth.

First, periodontitis and SSc have many similarities: a chronic and progressive course,

comparable pathogenesis pathways such as microvascular abnormalities, inflammation and fibrosis with a major impact on soft and hard tissues, and elevated levels of pro-inflammatory cytokines such as TNFα, IL-6 and IL-1 [21].

Furthermore, a correlation was found between the plaque index (PI) and sclerodactyly [22]. These results imply that sclerodactyly complicates oral hygiene and leads to an accumulation of plaque, accelerating the progression of periodontitis.

This multifactorial relationship between periodontitis and SSc remains of uncertain aetiology and requires further research to specify underlying mechanisms.

Reported Symptoms

Patients usually report discomfort, gum bleeding when toothbrushing or flossing, tooth mobility or flaring, halitosis, teeth that look longer than normal, and in extreme situations spontaneous tooth loss.

Clinical Signs

Clinical signs include red and swollen gums due to the accumulation of plaque and calculus (especially in interdental spaces), gum recessions exposing the roots, gums that bleed easily and tooth mobility (Fig. 19.3). Periodontal examination using a periodontal probe highlights the presence of periodontal pockets and clinical attachment loss which are indicators of periodontitis.

A list of criteria is provided in Table 19.2.

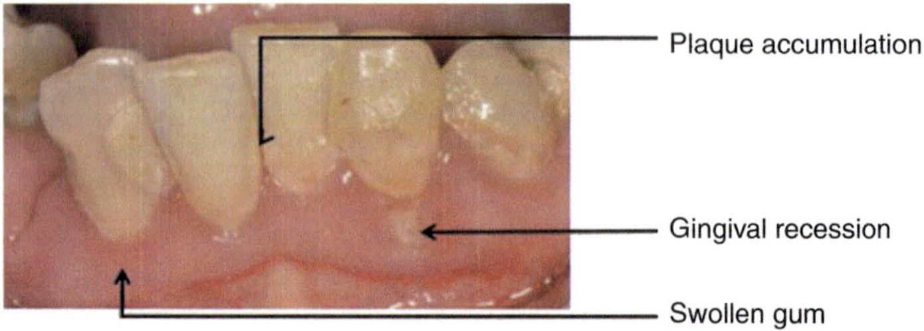

FIGURE 19.3 Clinical signs of periodontal disease

TABLE 19.2 Signs and symptoms of periodontal disease

1. Red, swollen gums.
2. Bleeding provoked by brushing, flossing, eating or spontaneous.
3. Pus between gum and teeth.
4. Persistent bad breath.
5. Lengthening of the teeth (gum recession).
6. Tooth mobility, tooth displacement, loose permanent tooth.

Management

The main purpose is to ensure daily oral hygiene to avoid the accumulation of plaque. SSc patients often have difficulties mainly because of microstomia and sclerodactyly. Specific products are available such as manual toothbrushes with large handles. Electric toothbrushes (also called power toothbrush) enable less wrist movement thanks to an oscillating and rotating technology of the head combined with a larger handle (Fig. 19.4).

General dental practitioners can provide professional care of periodontal disease with scaling, a careful periodontal assessment and specific periodontitis treatment if needed (non-surgical root planing). Periodontists are practitioners who specialise in the prevention, diagnosis and treatment of periodontal disease, as well as in the placement of dental implants. SSc patients should be referred to periodontists since they often display severe periodontal disease as well as a complex medical history.

Regular periodontal maintenance (every 3 months) prevents the progression of existing disease and provides a regular check-up of dental structures (prevention of tooth decay).

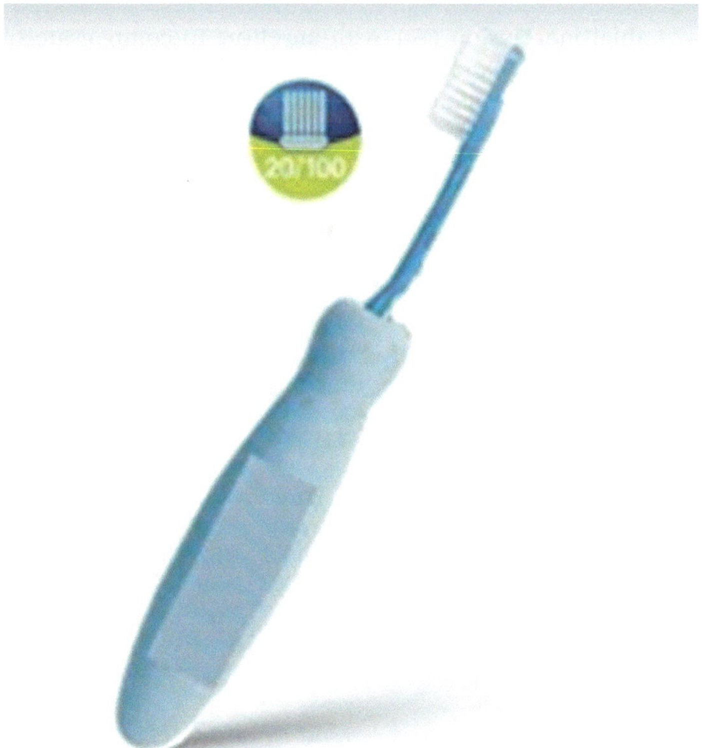

FIGURE 19.4 An example of manual toothbrush with a large foam handle

Clinical Case

We report the case of a 50-year-old woman presenting a diffuse systemic sclerosis for 10 years.

She reports dental pain when eating or drinking cold food as well as difficulties to eat, swallow and brush her teeth. Since she lost posterior teeth, mastication is difficult and sometimes painful. She also describes a significant aesthetic prejudice and only smiles by putting her hand in front of her mouth.

The oral features are:

- Labial inocclusion (A), with an effort to compensate by contracting chin muscles.
- Swollen gums, plaque accumulation signing the presence of periodontal disease (B).
- Tooth loss and decayed teeth (C).

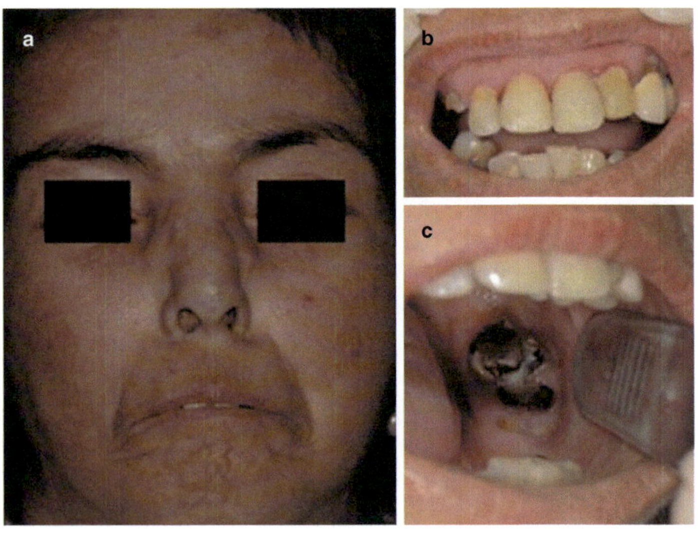

These are the steps of the multidisciplinary management:

- Microstomia: physiotherapy to soften perioral skin and obtain labial occlusion.
- Xerostomia (due to labial inocclusion): hyaluronic acid-based mouth gel.
- Periodontal disease: Professional cleaning and prescription of specific material (brush with larger handle, interdental brushes with grips, ...).
- Tooth decay: Non-restorable teeth were removed.
- Impaired mastication and Aesthetics: To enable the realisation of dentures (prosthetic space), it was decided to remove the remaining teeth and realise removable complete dentures (D, E, F).

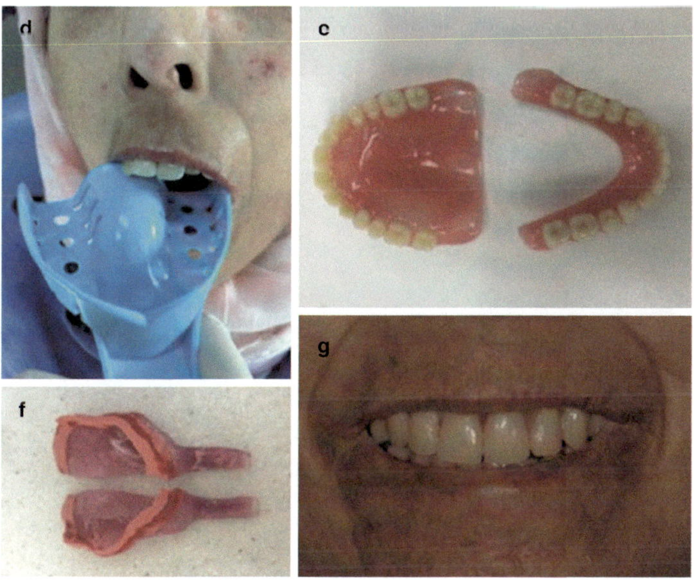

Thanks to all these steps, the patient was able to get comfort (no more dental pain), mastication and aesthetics by having her smile back (G).

Conclusion

Poor oral health is common in SSc and a major source of pain and discomfort. It was shown that oropharyngeal features critically impair patients' already altered quality of life with a major impact on confidence, daily life and nutrition [23].

Nutrition involvement is led by the vicious circle initiated by salivary secretion (Fig. 19.5).

Specialised physicians should be able to recognise patients needing oral care to address them quickly. A dental examination following the diagnosis of systemic sclerosis could be systematic and be part of the annual check-up in the same time as cardiac and pulmonary assessment. Early management of oral consequences, using a multi-disciplinary approach, avoids traumatic and invasive treatments.

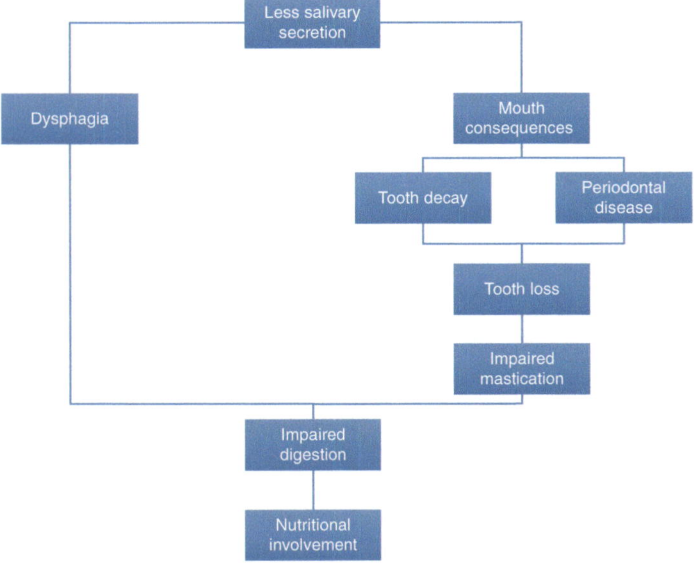

FIGURE 19.5 Vicious circle linking oral involvement in systemic sclerosis and malnutrition

Oral and facial manifestations associated with sclerodactyly may result in rapid decline. Maintenance of existing dentition is important because microstomia can make prosthetic replacement difficult.

References

1. Smirani R, Poursac N, Naveau A, Schaeverbeke T, Devillard R, Truchetet M-E. Orofacial consequences of systemic sclerosis: a systematic review. J Scleroderma Relat Disord. 2018;3:81–90.
2. Yuen HK, Hant FN, Hatfield C, Summerlin LM, Smith EA, Silver RM. Factors associated with oral hygiene practices among adults with systemic sclerosis. Int J Dent Hyg. 2014;12:180–6.
3. The glossary of prosthodontic terms. J Prosthet Den.t 2005 94:10–92.
4. Naylor WP, Douglass CW, Mix E. The nonsurgical treatment of microstomia in scleroderma: a pilot study. Oral Surg Oral Med Oral Pathol. 1984;57:508–11.
5. Mouthon L, Rannou F, Bérezné A, et al. Development and validation of a scale for mouth handicap in systemic sclerosis: the mouth handicap in systemic sclerosis scale. Ann Rheum Dis. 2007;66:1651–5.
6. Aliko A, Ciancaglini R, Alushi A, Tafaj A, Ruci D. Temporomandibular joint involvement in rheumatoid arthritis, systemic lupus erythematosus and systemic sclerosis. Int J Oral Maxillofac Surg. 2011;40:704–9.
7. Cazal C, Sobral APV, Neves RFSN, Freire Filho FWV, Cardoso AB, da Silveira MMF. Oral complaints in progressive systemic sclerosis: two cases report. Med Oral Patol Oral Cir Bucal. 2008;13:E114–8.
8. Comstedt LR, Svensson A, Troilius A. Improvement of microstomia in scleroderma after intense pulsed light: a case series of four patients. J Cosmet Laser Ther Off Publ Eur Soc Laser Dermatol. 2012;14:102–6.
9. Vincent C, Agard C, Barbarot S, et al. Orofacial manifestations of systemic sclerosis: a study of 30 consecutive patients. Rev Stomatol Chir Maxillofac. 2010;111:128–34.
10. Marcucci M, Abdala N. Analysis of the masseter muscle in patients with systemic sclerosis: a study by magnetic resonance imaging. Dento Maxillo Facial Radiol. 2009;38:524–30.

11. Baron M, Hudson M, Dagenais M, et al. The Canadian systemic sclerosis Oral health study V: relationship between disease characteristics and Oral radiologic findings in systemic sclerosis. Arthritis Care Res. 2015;68:673–80. https://doi.org/10.1002/acr.22739.
12. Baron M, Hudson M, Tatibouet S, et al. The Canadian systemic sclerosis oral health study: orofacial manifestations and oral health-related quality of life in systemic sclerosis compared with the general population. Rheumatol Oxf Engl. 2014;53:1386–94.
13. Knaś M, Zalewska A, Waszkiewicz N, Szulimowska J, Dziezcioł J, Sierakowski S, Waszkiel D. Salivary: flow and proteins of the innate and adaptive immunity in the limited and diffused systemic sclerosis. J Oral Pathol Med Off Publ Int Assoc Oral Pathol Am Acad Oral Pathol. 2014;43:521–9.
14. Chu CH, Yeung CMK, Lai IA, Leung WK, Mok MY. Oral health of Chinese people with systemic sclerosis. Clin Oral Investig. 2011;15:931–9.
15. Aliko A, Alushi A, Tafaj A, Lela F. Oral mucosa involvement in rheumatoid arthritis, systemic lupus erythematosus and systemic sclerosis. Int Dent J. 2010;60:353–8.
16. Avouac J, Sordet C, Depinay C, Ardizonne M, Vacher-Lavenu MC, Sibilia J, Kahan A, Allanore Y. Systemic sclerosis-associated Sjögren's syndrome and relationship to the limited cutaneous subtype: results of a prospective study of sicca syndrome in 133 consecutive patients. Arthritis Rheum. 2006;54:2243–9.
17. Shah AA, Wigley FM. Often forgotten manifestations of systemic sclerosis. Rheum Dis Clin N Am. 2008;34:221–38. ix
18. Salum FG, de AC M-JF, MAZ F, Cherubini K. Salivary hypofunction: an update on therapeutic strategies. Gerodontology. 2018;35:305–16.
19. Papapanou PN, Sanz M, Buduneli N, et al. Periodontitis: consensus report of workgroup 2 of the 2017 world workshop on the classification of periodontal and Peri-implant diseases and conditions: classification and case definitions for periodontitis. J Clin Periodontol. 2018;45:S162–70.
20. Scardina GA, Pizzigatti ME, Messina P. Periodontal microcirculatory abnormalities in patients with systemic sclerosis. J Periodontol. 2005;76:1991–5.
21. Nagy G, Kovács J, Zeher M, Czirják L. Analysis of the oral manifestations of systemic sclerosis. Oral Surg Oral Med Oral Pathol. 1994;77:141–6.

22. Elimelech R, Mayer Y, Braun-Moscovici Y, Machtei EE, Balbir-Gurman A. Periodontal conditions and tumor necrosis factor-alpha level in gingival Crevicular fluid of scleroderma patients. Isr Med Assoc J IMAJ. 2015;17:549–53.
23. Smirani R, Truchetet M-E, Poursac N, Naveau A, Schaeverbeke T, Devillard R. Impact of systemic sclerosis oral manifestations on patients' health-related quality of life: a systematic review. J Oral Pathol Med. 2018;47:808–15. https://doi.org/10.1111/jop.12739.

Chapter 20
Practical Approach to Malnutrition and Weight Loss in SSc

Gianluca Bagnato and Francesco Del Galdo

Prevalence of Malnutrition in Systemic Sclerosis

Prevalence of malnutrition in SSc was reported to be variable with a range between 10.9 and 55.6% and these differences are mainly linked to the detection method used. The most used tool to define malnutrition in SSc research was the Malnutrition Universal Screening Tool (MUST). MUST is a risk score which assigns the value ranging from 0 to 2 to body mass index (BMI), specifically BMI > 20.0 = 0, 18.5–20.1 = 1, < 18.5 = 2. A second set of 0 to 2 values are assigned to weight loss defined as unplanned weight loss in the past 3–6 months. A weight loss <5% = 0; 5%–10% = 1: >10% = 2. The values for BMI and weight loss are then summed for the total score, which is interpreted as follows: risks for malnutrition are low

G. Bagnato · F. Del Galdo (✉)
Leeds Institute of Rheumatic and Musculoskeletal Medicine, University of Leeds, Leeds, West Yorkshire, UK

NIHR BRC and Institute of Rheumatic and Musculoskeletal Medicine, University of Leeds, Leeds, West Yorkshire, UK
e-mail: g.bagato@leeds.ac.iuk; f.delgaldo@leeds.ac.uk

© Springer Nature Switzerland AG 2021
M. Matucci-Cerinic, C. P. Denton (eds.), *Practical Management of Systemic Sclerosis in Clinical Practice*, In Clinical Practice,
https://doi.org/10.1007/978-3-030-53736-4_20

for MUST score of 0, moderate for MUST score = 1, and high for MUST score ≥ 2 [1]. Independently of BMI and weight loss the MUST also includes a value of 2 and therefore high risk of malnutrition if there has been or is likely to be no nutritional intake for 5 days or more.

According to the studies that used MUST, a high risk of malnutrition is detected in 10.9/29.2% of SSc patients [2–6].

Another study assessed malnutrition by bioelectrical impedance analysis (BIA), which detects electrical conductivity of fat and lean tissue and measures the resistance (R) and reactance (Xc), and their relationship to acquire the Phase Angle (PhA). A PhA <5° was reported to reflect malnutrition [7] .According to this method, Krause et al. found that 55.6% of SSc patients are affected by malnutrition [7].

The prevalence of malnutrition remained similar (50%) when another tool has been used, the Subjective Global Assessment (SGA), which is based on history of recent intake, weight change, gastrointestinal symptoms and a clinical evaluation [5].

Other studies used an arbitrary BMI to define malnutrition in SSc (<19 or < 20 kg/m^2) with a reported prevalence between 13.7 and 19.2%. Also weight loss was used as an outcome, still with arbitrary measures (≥5% in the previous 3 months or ≥ 10% in the previous 6 months) providing again very wide disagreement in the clear definition of the prevalence of malnutrition is SSc [4, 8]. This indeed was proven by the low rate of prevalence (8.3%) [9] of malnutrition found in a study that used the combination of FFM and BMI to define malnutrition according to the most recent evidence provided by the ESPEN consensus (unintentional weight loss > 10% indefinite of time, or >5% over the last 3 months combined with either BMI <20 kg/m^2 if <70 years of age, or <22 kg/m^2 if >70 years of age or fat free mass index (FFMI) <15 and 17 kg/m^2 in women and men, respectively [10].

The heterogeneity of tools assessed and the recent standardisation by ESPEN clearly define the need for studies assessing malnutrition in SSc according to the recent international standards.

Gastrointestinal Involvement and Malnutrition in Systemic Sclerosis

The most commonly reported cause of malnutrition independently of the tool assessed to define it is severe gastrointestinal involvement.

The gastrointestinal (GI) tract involvement occurs in 75–90% of SSc patients, or even 98% according to a recent study [11], and is second in frequency only to the cutaneous involvement [12]. GI motility, digestion, absorption, continence and excretion can all be affected in SSc patients. GI symptoms, including pain, dysphagia, vomiting, diarrhoea, constipation, faecal incontinence and substantial weight loss, represent one of the main complaints in clinical practice and drivers of poor quality of life [13].

Severe GI involvement is usually defined as malabsorption, repeated episodes of pseudoobstruction, or severe problems requiring hyperalimentation. It affects only 8% of scleroderma patients, but when present carries a high mortality with only 15% of such patients surviving after 9 years [14]. In addition, 3–12% of overall SSc-deaths are related to gastrointestinal complications and severe malnutrition confers an HR of 3.77 for mortality [15, 16].

The most common GI manifestations reported as causes of malnutrition included oropharyngeal disorders, such as xerostomia or microstomia, a reduced mouth opening due to severe skin thickening which hinders food intake [17]. Indeed, Baron et al. reported on a cohort of 586 Canadian SSc patients a significant correlation between oral aperture size and malnutrition risk [3]. Another interesting study reported that xerostomia, in association with a reduced range of motion of the hands, was also linked to malnutrition because of reduced effective dental hygiene and mastication while promoting oral bacterial infections, dental caries and subsequent tooth loss [18].

Interstingly, despite the most frequently reported GI symptoms are linked to esophageal dysmotility [19], the same Canadian study mentioned above, showed no association between esophageal involvement symptoms including dysphagia or reflux and malnutrition risk, as assessed by the Malnutrition Universal Screening Tool (MUST) score [3].

On the contrary, dysmotility affecting the stomach and causing symptoms such as early saziety, nausea and vomiting, was significantly associated with malnutrition risk on bivariate analysis [3].

In this view, the scope of prokinetics, commonly used in clinical practice [20–22] and recently included in the most recent EULAR recommendations for the treatment of GI manifestations of SSc [23], could extend to the prevention of malnutrition, although there are no specific studies in this regard.

SSc may involve the colon and anorectum leading to a delayed colonic transit. Colonic dysmotility might eventually provoke severe pseudo-obstruction which impairs eating by inducing postprandial symptoms requiring parenteral nutrition support [24].

Another GI complication of SSc is exocrine pancreatic insufficiency and in a study involving 16 consecutive patients (dcSSc), 4 had a clinically relevant reduced exocrine function [25]. Untreated pancreatic insufficiency causes malabsorption, steatorrhea and results in weight loss [24].

The occurrence of autoimmune GI comorbities in SSc, such as primary biliary cirrhosis (PBC), which has an increased prevalence in SSc, especially in lcSSc [26], and the resultant cholestasis, can impair the absorption of fat and induce liposoluble vitamin deficiency [27]. However, there are no reports of associated nutritional compromise in SSc related to these group of comorbidities.

SIBO and Malnutrition

Small intestinal bacterial overgrowth (SIBO) is a common manifestation in SSc with a reported prevalence of 18–55% [28]. The diagnosis should be suspected with a clinical presentation characterized by abdominal pain or discomfort, bloating, diarrhoea, constipation and abdominal tenderness and it could lead, if untreated, eventually to malnutrition due to malabsorption [29].

No connection was found between the occurrence of SIBO and the disease form of SSc (diffuse vs. limited), while it was reported that antibodies against topoisomerase I (Scl-70) were less frequent in SSc patients with SIBO [30].

In one study comprising 37 SSc patients with GI complaints, 14 patients were affected by SIBO. These SIBO SSc patients had a longer disease duration than those who were unaffected with a median of 11 vs. 7 years, respectively ($P = 0.02$) [30]. The same patients also experienced significant weight loss within 6 months, 2 died for severe malnutrition and scored higher on the University of California Los Angeles Scleroderma Clinical Trial Consortium Gastrointestinal Tract Instrument 2.0, a questionnaire, which includes 34 items and 7 multi-item scales (reflux, distention/bloating, diarrhea, fecal soilage, constipation, emotional well-being, and social functioning) and provides a total GIT score to assess health-related quality of life and GIT symptoms severity in SSc.

The actual role of SIBO in malnutrition or weight loss could be underestimated because of the low sensitivity of the most commonly diagnostic methods.

The gold standard for SIBO diagnosis is the aspiration of small bowel fluid for culture and following bacterial count. In this context SIBO is diagnosed when there are ≥ 105 (CFU)/ml (colony forming units). However, this diagnostic tool is flawed by false-positives due to the potential contamination with oral and oesophageal flora and false-negatives due to the limitation to reach the relevant portion of the small bowels.

More commonly, the diagnosis of SIBO is primary made using breath testing being a non-invasive and relatively inexpensive alternative. This is done by ingesting various carbohydrate substrates such as glucose (sensitivity 20–93%, specificity 30–86%) or lactulose (sensitivity 31–68%, specificity 44–100%), which are then broken down by intestinal microbes, producing gases like hydrogen and methane. These gases enter the circulatory system and are expired via the lungs where they can be measured and the concentrations can be compared before and after the meal.

Antibiotics and prokinetics should be avoided, for 4 weeks and 1 week respectively, as they can alter the results of the test, while proton pump inhibitors (PPIs) prior to testing are believed to not alter the results.

The most recent EULAR recommendations suggest to prescribe prokinetics for symptomatic motility issues and rotating antibiotics for malabsorption due to SIBO, despite data for the treatment of SIBO in SSc are limited and guidelines have been extrapolated from SIBO in other populations [31]. Metronidazole, amoxicillin with clavulanic acid, cotrimoxazole, ciprofloxacin, norfloxacin and rifaximin are medications being used for the treatment of SIBO. A common approach is based on the oral administration of amoxicillin during the first month (500 mg 3×/24 h), ciprofloxacin during the second month (500 mg 2×/24 h) and metronidazole during the third month (500 mg 3×/24 h). Particular interest and high expectations are coming from rifaximin, nonabsorbable in the digestive tract and with bactericidal activity, which is currently under evaluation in SSc.

Apart from SIBO, also dysbiosis was recently studied in SSc and linked to malnutrition. In this study, dysbiosis has been defined by generating genomic data on the intestinal microbiota composition by using 54 bacterial ribosomal RNA probes specific for various intestinal bacterial species or clades [32]. In this study, among 19 patients at risk for malnutrition according to the MUST score, 18 exhibited dysbiosis, while only one patient out of 24 with a negative dysbiosis test was at risk for malnutrition.

Clinical Features of SSc Patients at Risk of Malnutrition

Many factors may contribute to the development of nutritional impairment in SSc.

Baron et al. reported in the larger study (n = 586) on malnutrition in SSc research that diffuse disease subset, shorter disease duration, the number of GI complaints (poor appetite, early satiety, nausea, constipation, and diarrhea), oral aperture and hemoglobin together with physician assessment of disease severity and possible malabsorption, and abdominal distension at examination were predictors of malnutrition risk based on MUST score [3].

Several studies have suggested that depression and anxiety, altering the control of appetite, might influence nutritional intake and consequently might contribute to malnutrition or weight loss. The prevalence of depression in SSc is variably reported to affect 19–69% of patients with SSc [33, 34]. Indeed, depression is more frequent in SSc when compared to the adult populations (2.6–3.2%), and also compared to individuals with two or more common chronic physical diseases (23%) [35]. Similarly, up to 80% of patients with SSc, reports anxiety compared with 4.4% of the general adult population.

Depression and/or anxiety may impair nutrition by decreasing appetite or by negatively impacting on crucial activities, such as food preparation.

The occurrence of digital ulcers, observed in up to 58% of patients [36], may also influence food intake and preparation, by causing pain, which subsequently alters functional status and the ability to eat [37]. In addition, the severity of lung involvement, fatigue and myalgia are all factors that influence global disability, further worsening the functional status of SSc patients [3] [6].

Clinical Management of Malnutrition in SSc

It seems reasonable, according to the evidence that malnutrition has multifactorial causes and increases the risk of mortality, that all patients with SSc should be screened for malnutrition. An history of weight loss should be investigated to identify unintentional events.

A general rule of thumb was identified by the North American expert panel for a relevant weight loss: 1–2% in the previous week, >5% in the previous month, >7.5% in the previous 3 months and > 10% in the previous year [38].

SSc patients should be screened using a questionnaire such as the MUST questionnaire, but it appears more appropriate to evaluate weight changes compared to last visit, and measure body mass index (BMI). If BMI cannot be measured, it may be estimated by measuring mid upper arm circumference (MUAC). A MUAC less than 23.5 cm estimates BMI to be less than 20 kg/m^2 (underweight).

This evaluation should be paralleled by the assessment of GI involvement by using the most widely accepted questionnaire developed at the University of California at Los Angeles [39]. Laboratory assessment should include: hemoglobin, vitamin A, B, folic acid and ferritin. A recent study showed that malnourished SSc patients have lower FVC and DLCo values, longer disease duration and lower haemoglobin levels [40]. Haemoglobin may indicate nutritional deficiency such as iron, folic acid or vitamin B12, while serum carotene might be indicative of fat malabsorption and serum folate might be elevated in bacterial overgrowth. Measurement of pre-albumin is more reliable (due to long-term protein stores) since albumin has a quick turnover and indeed, low levels of pre-albumin is an independent predictor of mortality [41].

In addition, if malabsorption is suspected, the following tests should confirm the diagnosis: high levels of serum methylmalonic acid (MMA), decreased zinc levels, 25-OH vitamin D levels, vitamin K level or prothrombin time (PT).

Finally, oral health, saliva production and depressive symptom should be screened. Specific comorbidities should be promptly treated to reduce the impact of malnutrition contributors, such as xerostomia (artificial saliva or biotine products or pilocarpine in selected cases), esophageal disease (PPI with the possibility to double the dose and/or add ranitidine), gastric emptying disorders (domperidone or metoclopramide). Dietist and gastroenterologist consult should be requested in order to address comorbidities and drive appropriate supplement therapy. Parenteral and enteral therapy is the last source for resistant cases.

References

1. Stratton RJ, Hackston A, Longmore D, et al. Malnutrition in hospital outpatients and inpatients: prevalence, concurrent validity and ease of use of the 'malnutrition universal screening tool'

('MUST') for adults. Br J Nutr. 2004;92(5):799–808. https://doi.org/10.1079/Bjn20041258.
2. Cereda E, Codullo V, Klersy C, et al. Disease-related nutritional risk and mortality in systemic sclerosis. Clin Nutr. 2014;33(3):558–61. https://doi.org/10.1016/j.clnu.2013.08.010.
3. Baron M, Hudson M, Steele R, et al. Malnutrition is common in systemic sclerosis: results from the Canadian scleroderma research group database. J Rheumatol. 2009;36(12):2737–43. https://doi.org/10.3899/jrheum.090694.
4. Caporali R, Caccialanza R, Bonino C, et al. Disease-related malnutrition in outpatients with systemic sclerosis. Clin Nutr. 2012;31(5):666–71. https://doi.org/10.1016/j.clnu.2012.02.010.
5. Murtaugh MA, Frech TM. Nutritional status and gastrointestinal symptoms in systemic sclerosis patients. Clin Nutr. 2013;32(1):130–5. https://doi.org/10.1016/j.clnu.2012.06.005.
6. Preis E, Franz K, Siegert E, et al. The impact of malnutrition on quality of life in patients with systemic sclerosis. Eur J Clin Nutr. 2018;72:504–10. https://doi.org/10.1038/s41430-018-0116-z.
7. Krause L, Becker MO, Brueckner CS, et al. Nutritional status as marker for disease activity and severity predicting mortality in patients with systemic sclerosis. Ann Rheum Dis. 2010;69(11):1951–7. https://doi.org/10.1136/ard.2009.123273.
8. Rosato E, Gigante A, Gasperini ML, et al. Nutritional status measured by BMI is impaired and correlates with left ventricular mass in patients with systemic sclerosis. Nutrition. 2014;30(2):204–9. https://doi.org/10.1016/j.nut.2013.07.025.
9. Spanjer MJ, Bultink IEM, de van der Schueren MAE, et al. Prevalence of malnutrition and validation of bioelectrical impedance analysis for the assessment of body composition in patients with systemic sclerosis. Rheumatology (Oxford). 2017;56(6):1008–12. https://doi.org/10.1093/rheumatology/kex014.
10. Cederholm T, Bosaeus I, Barazzoni R, et al. Diagnostic criteria for malnutrition - an ESPEN consensus statement. Clin Nutr. 2015;34(3):335–40. https://doi.org/10.1016/j.clnu.2015.03.001. [published Online First: 2015/03/24]
11. Schmeiser T, Saar P, Jin D, et al. Profile of gastrointestinal involvement in patients with systemic sclerosis. Rheumatol Int. 2012;32(8):2471–8. https://doi.org/10.1007/s00296-011-1988-6.
12. Clements PJ, Becvar R, Drosos AA, et al. Assessment of gastrointestinal involvement. Clin Exp Rheumatol. 2003;21(3 Suppl 29):S15–8.

13. Gyger G, Baron M. Gastrointestinal manifestations of scleroderma: recent progress in evaluation, pathogenesis, and management. Curr Rheumatol Rep. 2012;14(1):22–9. https://doi.org/10.1007/s11926-011-0217-3.
14. Steen VD, Medsger TA Jr. Severe organ involvement in systemic sclerosis with diffuse scleroderma. Arthritis Rheum. 2000;43(11):2437–44. https://doi.org/10.1002/1529-0131(200011)43:11<2437::AID-ANR10>3.0.CO;2-U.
15. Cruz-Dominguez MP, Garcia-Collinot G, Saavedra MA, et al. Malnutrition is an independent risk factor for mortality in Mexican patients with systemic sclerosis: a cohort study. Rheumatol Int. 2017;37(7):1101–9. https://doi.org/10.1007/s00296-017-3753-y.
16. Tyndall AJ, Bannert B, Vonk M, et al. Causes and risk factors for death in systemic sclerosis: a study from the EULAR scleroderma trials and research (EUSTAR) database. Ann Rheum Dis. 2010;69(10):1809–15. https://doi.org/10.1136/ard.2009.114264.
17. Mouthon L, Rannou F, Berezne A, et al. Development and validation of a scale for mouth handicap in systemic sclerosis: the mouth handicap in systemic sclerosis scale. Ann Rheum Dis. 2007;66(12):1651–5. https://doi.org/10.1136/ard.2007.070532.
18. Poole JL, Brewer C, Rossie K, et al. Factors related to oral hygiene in persons with scleroderma. Int J Dent Hyg. 2005;3(1):13–7. https://doi.org/10.1111/j.1601-5037.2004.00108.x.
19. Thoua NM, Bunce C, Brough G, et al. Assessment of gastrointestinal symptoms in patients with systemic sclerosis in a UK tertiary referral Centre. Rheumatology (Oxford). 2010;49(9):1770–5. https://doi.org/10.1093/rheumatology/keq147.
20. Sridhar KR, Lange RC, Magyar L, et al. Prevalence of impaired gastric emptying of solids in systemic sclerosis: diagnostic and therapeutic implications. J Lab Clin Med. 1998;132(6):541–6.
21. Marie I, Levesque H, Ducrotte P, et al. Gastric involvement in systemic sclerosis: a prospective study. Am J Gastroenterol. 2001;96(1):77–83. https://doi.org/10.1111/j.1572-0241.2001.03353.x.
22. Manetti M, Milia AF, Benelli G, et al. The gastric wall in systemic sclerosis patients: a morphological study. Ital J Anat Embryol. 2010;115(1–2):115–21.
23. Kowal-Bielecka O, Fransen J, Avouac J, et al. Update of EULAR recommendations for the treatment of systemic sclerosis. Ann Rheum Dis. 2017;76(8):1327–39. https://doi.org/10.1136/annrheumdis-2016-209909.

24. Jaovisidha K, Csuka ME, Almagro UA, et al. Severe gastrointestinal involvement in systemic sclerosis: report of five cases and review of the literature. Semin Arthritis Rheum. 2005;34(4):689–702. https://doi.org/10.1016/j.semarthrit.2004.08.009.
25. Hendel L, Worning H. Exocrine pancreatic function in patients with progressive systemic sclerosis. Scand J Gastroenterol. 1989;24(4):461–6.
26. Norman GL, Bialek A, Encabo S, et al. Is prevalence of PBC underestimated in patients with systemic sclerosis? Dig Liver Dis. 2009;41(10):762–4. https://doi.org/10.1016/j.dld.2009.01.014.
27. Phillips JR, Angulo P, Petterson T, et al. Fat-soluble vitamin levels in patients with primary biliary cirrhosis. Am J Gastroenterol. 2001;96(9):2745–50. https://doi.org/10.1111/j.1572-0241.2001.04134.x.
28. Polkowska-Pruszynska B, Gerkowicz A, Szczepanik-Kulak P, et al. Small intestinal bacterial overgrowth in systemic sclerosis: a review of the literature. Arch Dermatol Res. 2019;311(1):1–8. https://doi.org/10.1007/s00403-018-1874-0.
29. Kowal-Bielecka O, Landewe R, Avouac J, et al. EULAR recommendations for the treatment of systemic sclerosis: a report from the EULAR scleroderma trials and research group (EUSTAR). Ann Rheum Dis. 2009;68(5):620–8. https://doi.org/10.1136/ard.2008.096677.
30. Tauber M, Avouac J, Benahmed A, et al. Prevalence and predictors of small intestinal bacterial overgrowth in systemic sclerosis patients with gastrointestinal symptoms. Clin Exp Rheumatol. 2014;32(6 Suppl 86):S-82-7.
31. outcome. Sbboissdudaimat.
32. Andreasson K, Alrawi Z, Persson A, et al. Intestinal dysbiosis is common in systemic sclerosis and associated with gastrointestinal and extraintestinal features of disease. Arthritis Res Ther. 2016;18(1):278. https://doi.org/10.1186/s13075-016-1182-z.
33. Baubet T, Ranque B, Taieb O, et al. Mood and anxiety disorders in systemic sclerosis patients. Presse Med. 2011;40(2):e111–9. https://doi.org/10.1016/j.lpm.2010.09.019.
34. Ostojic P, Zivojinovic S, Reza T, et al. Symptoms of depression and anxiety in Serbian patients with systemic sclerosis: impact of disease severity and socioeconomic factors. Mod Rheumatol. 2010;20(4):353–7. https://doi.org/10.1007/s10165-010-0285-7.
35. Singleton N, Bumpstead R, O'Brien M, et al. Psychiatric morbidity among adults living in private households, 2000. Int Rev

Psychiatry. 2003;15(1–2):65–73. https://doi.org/10.1080/0954026021000045967.

36. Hughes M, Herrick AL. Digital ulcers in systemic sclerosis. Rheumatology (Oxford). 2017;56(1):14–25. https://doi.org/10.1093/rheumatology/kew047.
37. Berezne A, Seror R, Morell-Dubois S, et al. Impact of systemic sclerosis on occupational and professional activity with attention to patients with digital ulcers. Arthritis Care Res. 2011;63(2):277–85. https://doi.org/10.1002/acr.20342.
38. Baron M, Bernier P, Cote LF, et al. Screening and therapy for malnutrition and related gastro-intestinal disorders in systemic sclerosis: recommendations of a north American expert panel. Clin Exp Rheumatol. 2010;28(2 Suppl 58):S42–6.
39. Khanna D, Hays RD, Maranian P, et al. Reliability and validity of the University of California, los Angeles scleroderma clinical trial consortium gastrointestinal tract instrument. Arthritis Rheum. 2009;61(9):1257–63. https://doi.org/10.1002/art.24730.
40. Caimmi C, Caramaschi P, Venturini A, et al. Malnutrition and sarcopenia in a large cohort of patients with systemic sclerosis. Clin Rheumatol. 2018;37(4):987–97. https://doi.org/10.1007/s10067-017-3932-y.
41. Codullo V, Cereda E, Klersy C, et al. Serum prealbumin is an independent predictor of mortality in systemic sclerosis outpatients. Rheumatology. 2016;55(2):315–9. https://doi.org/10.1093/rheumatology/kev322.

Chapter 21
Calcinosis

Ariane L. Herrick and Muditha Samaranayaka

Introduction

Systemic sclerosis (SSc)-related calcinosis is painful, disabling and disfiguring. At present there is no effective treatment. Approximately 20–40% of patients with SSc are affected [1–8] and develop 'lumps' of subcutaneous or intracutaneous deposits of calcium salts (mainly hydroxyapatite and carbonated apatite [9–11]). Calcinosis occurs mainly over pressure points (for example in the fingers, and over the extensor aspects of the elbow/forearm and knee) but can occur in other areas, for example the spine [12–14]. Areas of calcinosis can become infected, especially when they ulcerate

A. L. Herrick (✉)
Centre for Musculoskeletal Research, The University of Manchester, Salford Royal NHS Foundation Trust, Manchester Academic Health Science Centre, Manchester, UK

NIHR Manchester Biomedical Research Centre, Manchester University NHS Foundation Trust, Manchester, UK
e-mail: ariane.herrick@manchester.ac.uk

M. Samaranayaka
Rheumatology Department, Salford Royal NHS Foundation Trust, Salford, UK
e-mail: Muditha.Samaranayaka@srft.nhs.uk

© Springer Nature Switzerland AG 2021

M. Matucci-Cerinic, C. P. Denton (eds.), *Practical Management of Systemic Sclerosis in Clinical Practice*, In Clinical Practice,
https://doi.org/10.1007/978-3-030-53736-4_21

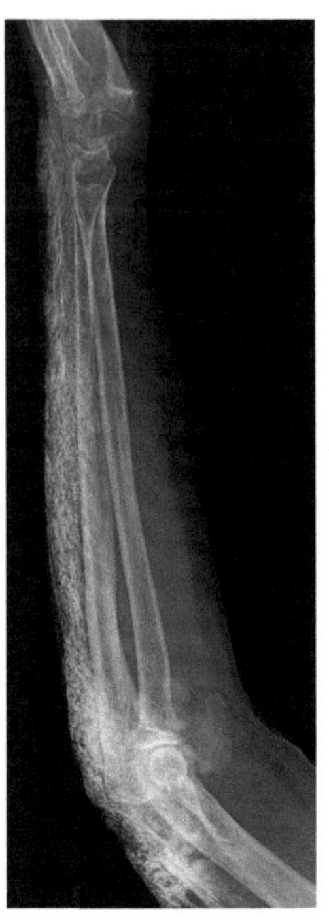

FIGURE 21.1 Plain radiograph showing extensive 'sheet' calcinosis of the forearm

through skin. Although the most common form of SSc-related calcinosis is 'nodular' or 'tumoral' (exemplified in the case history below) [15, 16], calcinosis can also occur in a linear pattern (in 'sheets') (Fig. 21.1).

The pathogenesis of SSc-related calcinosis is incompletely understood. It is not related to hypercalcaemia and is most likely dystrophic, with ischaemia [8] and mechanical pressures [17] most likely contributing.

Following a case history to 'set the scene', we shall discuss epidemiology (including associates) of calcinosis, clinical and imaging features, and management. Areas of current research will not be discussed, although it is worth highlighting that calcinosis is no longer a neglected area of research—studies of pathogenesis, measurement and treatment are ongoing.

Case History

A 57 year old woman was assessed on an urgent basis in November 2018 because of worsening painful calcinosis of her right thumb and right index finger. She also complained of pain related to her left knee calcinosis. She had been initially diagnosed in 2005 as having dermatomyositis (when symptoms included new onset Raynaud's phenomenon), treated with corticosteroids and azathioprine. In 2007 she developed features of SSc (puffy fingers, distal skin tightness and telangiectases) and was found to be anti-PM-Scl100 positive. Her calcinosis-related problems began around 2011 (Figs. 21.2 and 21.3), and she had had previous surgical debulking of fingertip and right elbow calcinosis which at the time had successfully reduced her pain. She also had osteoporosis.

Treatment comprised daily azathioprine 150 mg, prednisolone 5 mg, sildenafil 125 mg in divided doses (for digital ischaemia), omeprazole 20 mg, calcium and vitamin D supplements, and annual intravenous zoledronate infusions. Prior to assessment in November 2018 she had already had two recent courses of oral antibiotics for infection related to the finger calcinosis.

On examination, she was afebrile. The thumb and index finger had calcinosis exposed at the skin surface with a yellowish discharge and erythema, swelling and tenderness of the surrounding soft tissues. The left knee demonstrated hard irregular swelling typical of calcinosis (Fig. 21.3a). Other findings included digital pitting, mild sclerodactyly, and multiple telangiectases.

She was admitted for 5 days of intravenous iloprost as this had been symptomatically beneficial in the past for the finger tip pain (she had severe digital ischaemia in addition to the calcinosis). A further course of oral flucloxacillin was prescribed, with improvement in the soft tissue infection. On this occasion the hand surgeon advised a conservative approach. Plain radiograph of the left knee showed extensive calcinosis

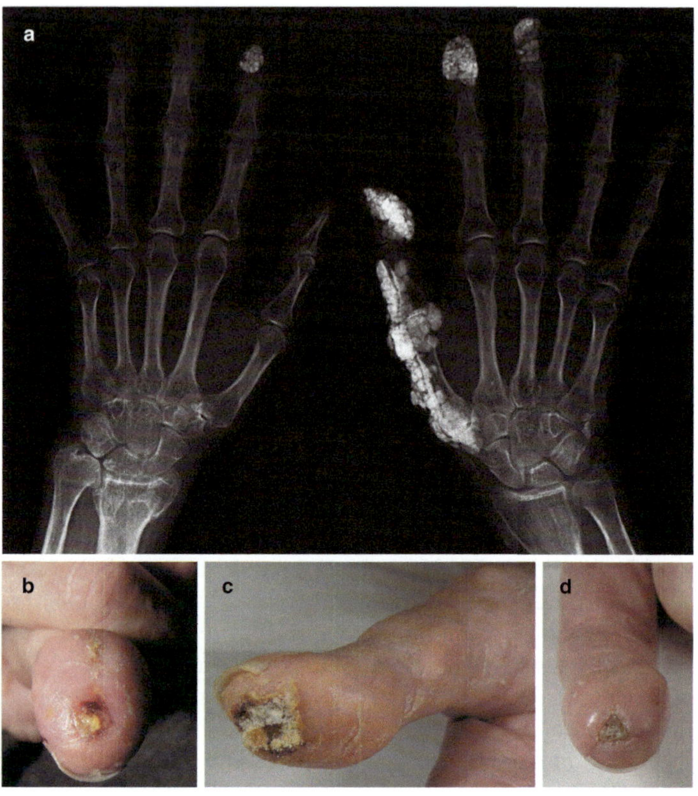

Figure 21.2 (**a**) Hand radiograph showing extensive soft tissue calcification including of the right thumb and index finger. (**b**) Infected calcinosis of right thumb. (**c**) Right thumb and (**d**) right index finger tip showing swelling due to calcinosis (which was hard on palpation) and extrusion of calcinotic material through skin (these photographs were taken 1 month following surgical debridement in March 2018: the lesions subsequently healed)

(Fig. 21.3b), previously well demonstrated on computerised tomography (CT) scanning (Fig. 21.3c).

Given the impact on her life of the calcinosis, the patient chose to commence once weekly intravenous infusions of

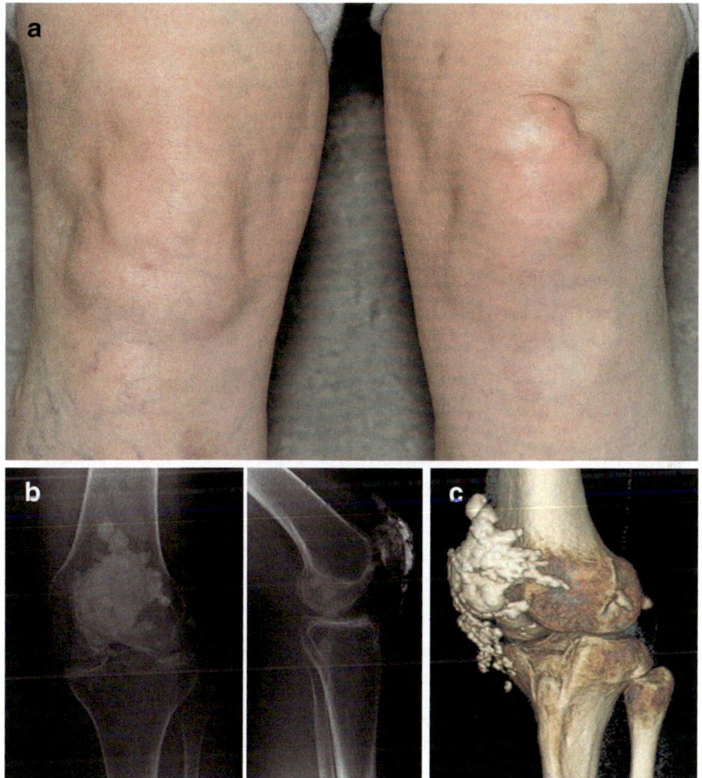

FIGURE 21.3 (**a**) Irregular swelling indicating calcinosis anterior to the left knee. (**b**) Radiographs of the left knee (anteroposterior and lateral views) showing extensive calcinosis. (**c**) Earlier CT scan (surface rendered reconstruction) demonstrating the extensive subcutaneous calcification anterior to the knee

25 g sodium thiosulphate. She knew that although there was no good evidence base for this approach, some patients had reported benefit. However this was discontinued after 2 doses due to severe nausea and vomiting unresponsive to cyclizine and ondansetron.

Epidemiology (Including Associates) of Calcinosis

Prevalence depends on how calcinosis is defined and how carefully it is searched for: in some patients it is subclinical (detected only on imaging). Although it was previously believed that calcinosis occurs mainly in the limited cutaneous subtype of SSc (hence the 'C' of 'CREST') patients with diffuse cutaneous SSc are also commonly affected [2, 8], especially later on in the disease course. The longer the disease duration, the more likely a patient is to have calcinosis [1, 5, 6, 18, 19]. Other reported associates of calcinosis in patients with SSc include:

1. Certain SSc-specific autoantibodies. Calcinosis is positively associated with anticentromere antibody [5, 6, 8, 20–22], anti-PM-Scl antibody [23–25] (as in the case history) and (in one recent report) with anti-RNA polymerase [8]. Calcinosis is negatively associated with anti-topoisomerase (Scl-70) antibody [5, 6, 21, 22].
2. Severe digital ischaemia, including digital ulceration [4, 6, 8, 26, 27], and acro-osteolysis [28]. An association with severity of microvascular abnormality on nailfold capillaroscopy has been reported in some studies [8, 22, 29]
3. Osteoporosis [6, 19].

Clinical Features

Patients are often themselves aware of hard lumps beneath the skin. These calcinotic lumps are frequently painful, especially when they enlarge, ulcerate through skin (patients often report extrusion of a toothpaste-like material) and/or become infected (Fig. 21.2b).

On examination, areas of calcinosis feel hard and often irregular, although sometimes they contain softer and/or fluctant areas representing liquid or semi-solid calcinosis. They may or may not be tender: tenderness should always raise suspicion that the calcinosis has become infected. If there is any clinical doubt as to whether or not a lesion is calcinotic, this can readily be confirmed with a plain radiograph.

Imaging of Calcinosis

Calcinosis is easily visible on plain radiographs (Figs. 21.1–21.3). Ultrasound has been reported to have similar sensitivity to plain radiography in detecting calcinosis in the hands and wrists [30]. CT scanning [32–34] produces three dimensional images which clearly demonstrate the extent of the calcinosis (as in the case history, Fig. 21.3c), although this is seldom required in the routine clinical setting.

A challenging question is how to measure calcinosis, in order to measure disease progression and treatment response in clinical trials. Scoring systems for assessing the extent of calcinosis on plain radiographs have been proposed [28, 31]. Although CT scanning can measure volumes [34], the radiation involved is a disadvantage when repeated (longitudinal) measurements over time are required.

Management

Although numerous treatments have been advocated over the years, it is generally accepted that there is no treatment with proven efficacy to either prevent or reduce calcinosis. However, antibiotics (for suspected infection) and surgery (in selected patients) have a role. Here we describe current approach to treatment, and some of the treatments which over the years have attracted interest on the basis of anecdotal reports or small series.

General Measures

Antibiotics and analgesia. A major concern with calcinosis is that lesions can become infected, and this can lead to spreading cellulitis, and even septicaemia. Also, lesions can become chronically infected. A key aspect of management (as demonstrated in the case history) is to emphasise to the patient the importance of seeking urgent medical advice if there is any suspicion that infection is developing. An oral antibiotic will often suffice, but in more severe situations intravenous antibiotics may be required. 'Flares' of calcinosis (with or without infection) are often very painful: adequate analgesia is also important.

Multidisciplinary team (MDT) input. Ulceration overlying calcinosis can be very difficult to heal and expert wound care [35] is integral to management. The podiatry team should be involved when calcinosis involves the toes/foot. Occupational therapy is indicated for patients with compromised hand function.

Surgical Debridement

Surgery is indicated for pain and loss of function, and when infected areas do not respond to antibiotic therapy then debridement and washout may be required [36, 37]. The patient must be advised that surgery will not completely remove calcinosis, but will only debulk it, and that the calcinosis may 'regrow'. A further problem is that calcinotic deposits are infiltrative: for example in the fingers the neurovascular bundle may run through the mass of calcified tissue. Surgery of the hand in patients with SSc is complex for other reasons including the poor blood supply to the fingers, and should be performed in specialist centres.

Specific Therapies Aimed at Reducing Calcinosis

Drug treatments. Calcinosis is difficult to study due to its heterogeneity, and essentially there have been no controlled clinical trials of therapy specifically for SSc-related calcinosis. When interpreting case reports and small series (some of which include patients with dermatomyositis-related calcinosis), it is important to bear in mind that symptoms of calcinosis sometimes improve spontaneously (for example after calcinosis discharges through skin) and the difficulties in measuring the 'burden' of calcinosis. Treatments which have attracted interest in the past (reviewed in [7, 38–43]) include warfarin [44, 45], colchicine [46] (which does have some rationale on the assumption that some 'flares' of calcinosis may be due to shedding of crystals into the surrounding soft tissues), diltiazem [46–48], minocycline [49], bisphosphonates [42, 50, 51], and biologic agents, specifically rituximab (but with conflicting results [39, 52–56]) and infliximab (one case report with SSc-myositis overlap) [57]. Intra-lesional corticosteroid injection, intravenous immunoglobulins, and aluminium hydroxide have also been tried.

Sodium thiosulphate has attracted some recent interest in calcinosis related to different conditions, although the evidence is contradictory and some reports have been in abstract form only [58–61]. Intravenous sodium thiosulphate was tried the patient described above. The use of topical sodium thiosulphate has also been described [62, 63]).

Procedural treatments (other than surgical debridement). Carbon dioxide laser [64, 65] and extracorporeal shock-wave lithotripsy [66–68] have both been advocated, but require further research.

Conclusions

Calcinosis is a major source of morbidity in patients with SSc. Increased understanding of pathogenesis and advances in imaging techniques are guiding research into new avenues of therapy. In the meantime the main thrust of treatment is relief of pain and early treatment of any infection.

Acknowledgements We are grateful to Professor Jonathan Harris for the CT image.

References

1. Steen VD, Zeigler GL, Rodnan GP, Medsger TA. Clinical and laboratory associations of anticentromere antibody in patients with progressive systemic sclerosis. Arthritis Rheum. 1984;27:125–31.
2. Akesson A, Wollheim FA. Organ manifestations in 100 patients with progressive systemic sclerosis: a comparison between the CREST syndrome and diffuse scleroderma. Br J Rheumatol. 1989;28:281–6.
3. Tager RE, Tikly M. Clinical and laboratory manifestations of systemic sclerosis (scleroderma) in black south Africans. Rheumatology. 1999;38:397–400.
4. Avouac J, Guerini H, Wipff J, et al. Radiological hand involvement in systemic sclerosis. Ann Rheum Dis. 2006;65:1088–92.
5. Mahmood M, Wilkinson J, Manning J, Herrick AL. History of surgical debridement, anticentromere antibody, and disease duration are associated with calcinosis in patients with systemic sclerosis. Scand J Rheumatol. 2015;45:114–7.
6. Valenzuela A, Baron M, the Canadian Scleroderma Research Group, et al. Calcinosis is associated with digital ulcers and osteoporosis in patients with systemic sclerosis: a scleroderma clinical trial consortium study. Semin Arthritis Rheum. 2016;46:344–9.
7. Herrick AL, Gallas A. Systemic sclerosis-related calcinosis. J Scleroderma Rel Disorders. 2016;1:194–203.
8. Baron M, Pope J, Robinson D, et al. Calcinosis is associated with digital ischaemia in systemic sclerosis-a longitudinal study. Rheumatology. 2016;55:2148–55.
9. Leroux J-L, Pernot F, Fedou P, et al. Ultrastructural and crystallographic study of calcifications from a patient with CREST syndrome. J Rheumatol. 1983;10:242–6.
10. Fei F, Gallas A, Chang Y-C, et al. Quartz crystal microbalance assay of clinical calcinosis samples and their synthetic models differentiates the efficacy of chelation-based treatments. ACS Appl Mater Inter. 2017;9:27544–52.
11. Hsu VM, Emge T, Schlesinger N. X-ray diffraction analysis of spontaneously draining calcinosis in scleroderma patients. Scand J Rheumatol. 2017;46:118–21.
12. Smucker JD, Heller JG, Bohlman HH, Whitesides TE. Surgical treatment of destructive calcific lesions of the cervical spine in scleroderma: case series and review of the literature. Spine. 2006;31:2002–8.

13. Bluett J, Davies C, Harris J, Herrick A. Cervical spine calcinosis in systemic sclerosis. J Rheumatol. 2013;40:1617–8.
14. Sambataro D, Sambataro G, Zaccara E, Maglione W, Vitali C, Del Papa N. Tumoral calcinosis of the spine in the course of systemic sclerosis: report of a new case and review of the literature. Clin Exp Rheumatol. 2015;33(Suppl. 91):S175–8.
15. Shahi V, Wetter DA, Howe BM, Ringler MD, Davis MD. Plain radiography is effective for the detection of calcinosis cutis occurring in association with autoimmune connective tissue disease. Br J Dermatol. 2014;170:1073–9.
16. Bartoli F, Fiori G, Braschi F, et al. Calcinosis in systemic sclerosis: subsets, distribution and complications. Rheumatology. 2016;55:1610–4.
17. Gauhar R, Wilkinson J, Harris J, Manning J, Herrick AL. Calcinosis preferentially affects the thumb compared to other fingers in patients with systemic sclerosis. Scand J Rheumatol. 2016;45:317–20.
18. Morgan ND, Shah AA, Mayes MD, et al. Clinical and serological features of systemic sclerosis in a multicenter African American cohort: analysis of the genome research in African American scleroderma patients clinical database. Medicine. 2017;96(51):e8980.
19. Pai S, Hsu V. Are there risk factors for scleroderma-related calcinosis? Mod Rheumatol. 2018;28:518–22.
20. Nishikai M, Itoh K, Sato A. Calcinosis and the anticentromere antibody: its clinical, radiological and immunogenetic aspects. Br J Rheumatol. 1992;31:9–12.
21. Jacobsen S, Halberg P, Ullman S, et al. Clinical features and serum antinuclear antibodies in 230 Danish patients with systemic sclerosis. Br J Rheumatol. 1998;37:39–45.
22. Vayssairat M, Hidouche D, Abdoucheli-Baudot N, Gaitz JP. Clinical significance of subcutaneous calcinosis in patients with systemic sclerosis. Does diltiazem induce its regression? Ann Rheum Dis. 1998;57:252–4.
23. Koschik RW, Fertig N, Lucas MR, Domsic RT, Medsger TA. Anti-PM-Scl antibody in patients with systemic sclerosis. Clin Exp Rheumatol. 2012;30(Suppl 71):S12–6.
24. D'Aoust J, Hudson M, Tatibouet S, et al. Clinical and serologic correlates of anti-PM/Scl antibodies in systemic sclerosis: a multicenter study of 763 patients. Arthritis Rheum. 2014;66:1608–15.
25. Wodkowski M, Hudson M, Proudman S, et al. Clinical correlates of monospecific anti-PM75 and anti-PM100 antibodies in a tri-

nation cohort of 1574 systemic sclerosis subjects. Autoimmunity. 2015;48:542–51.

26. Mouthon L, Mestre-Stanislas C, Berezne A, et al. Impact of digital ulcers on disability and health-related quality of life in systemic sclerosis. Ann Rheum Dis. 2010;69:214–7.
27. Koutaissoff S, Vanthuyne M, Smith V, et al. Hand radiological damage in systemic sclerosis: comparison with a control group and clinical and functional correlations. Sem Arthritis Rheum. 2011;40:455–60.
28. Johnstone EM, Hutchinson CE, Vail A, Chevance A, Herrick AL. Acro-osteolysis in systemic sclerosis is associated with digital ischaemia and with severe calcinosis. Rheumatology. 2012;51:2234–8.
29. Morardet L, Avouac J, Sammour M, et al. Late nailfold videocapillaroscopy pattern assocated with hand calcinosis and acro-osteolysis in systemic sclerosis. Arthritic Care Res. 2016;68:366–73.
30. Freire V, Bazeli R, Elhai M, et al. Hand and wrist involvement in systemic sclerosis: US features. Radiology. 2013;269:824–30.
31. Chung L, Valenzuela A, Fiorentino D, et al. Validation of a novel radiographic scoring system for calcinosis affecting the hands of patients with systemic sclerosis. Arthritis Care Res. 2015;67:425–30.
32. Hsu V, Bramwit M, Schlesinger N. Use of dual-energy computed tomography for the evaluation of calcinosis in patients with systemic sclerosis. Clin Rheumatol. 2015;34:1557–61.
33. Freire V, Becce F, Feydy A, et al. MDCT imaging of calcinosis in systemic sclerosis. Clin Radiol. 2013;68:302–9.
34. Hughes M, Hodgson R, Harris J, et al. Imaging calcinosis in patients with systemic sclerosis by radiography, computerised tomography and magnetic resonance imaging. Semin Arthritis Rheum. 2019;49:279–82.
35. Netsch D. Calcinosis cutis: WOC nurse management. J Wound Ostomy Continence Nursing. 2018;45:83–6.
36. Bogoch ER, Gross DK. Surgery of the hand in patients with systemic sclerosis: outcomes and considerations. J Rheumatol. 2005;32:642–8.
37. Muir L. Surgical management. In: Wigley FM, Herrick AL, Flavahan NA, editors. Raynaud's phenomenon. Berlin: Springer; 2015. p. 361–72.

38. Reiter N, El-Shabrawi L, Leinweber B, Berghold A, Aberer E. Calcinosis cutis. Part II. Treatment options. J Am Acad Dermatol. 2011;65:15–22.
39. Daoussis D, Antonopoulos I, Liossis SC, Yiannopoulos G, Andonopoulos AP. Treatment of systemic sclerosis-associated calcinosis: a case report of rituximab-induced regression of CREST-related calcinosis and review of the literature. Semin Arthritis Rheum. 2012;41:822–9.
40. Gutierrez A, Wetter DA. Calcinosis cutis in autoimmune connective tissue diseases. Dermatol Ther. 2012;25:195–206.
41. Bienvenu B. Traitement des calcinoses sous-cutanees des connectivites (treatment of calcinosis in systemic disorders). La Revue de Medecine Interne. 2014;35:444–52.
42. Dima A, Balanescu P, Baicus C. Pharmacological treatment in calcinosis cutis associated with connective-tissue diseases. Rom J Intern Med. 2014;52(2):55–67.
43. Valenzuela A, Chung L. Calcinosis: pathophysiology and management. Curr Opin Rheumatol. 2015;27:542–8.
44. Berger RG, Featherstone GL, Raasch RH, McCartney WH, Hadler NM. Treatment of calcinosis universalis with low-dose warfarin. Am J Med. 1987;83:72–6.
45. Cukierman T, Elinav E, Korem M, Chajek-Shaul T. Low dose warfarin treatment for calcinosis in patients with systemic sclerosis. Ann Rheum Dis. 2004;63:1341–3.
46. Balin SJ, Wetter DA, Andersen LK, Davis MD. Calcinosis cutis occurring in association with autoimmune connective tissue disease. Arch Dermatol. 2012;148:455–62.
47. Dolan AL, Kassimos D, Gibson T, Kingsley GH. Diltiazem induces remission of calcinosis in scleroderma. Br J Rheumatol. 1995;34:576–8.
48. Palmieri GM, Sebes JI, Aelion JA, et al. Treatment of calcinosis with diltiazem. Arthritis Rheum. 1995;38:1646–54.
49. Robertson LP, Marshall RW, Hickling P. Treatment of cutaneous calcinosis in limited systemic sclerosis with minocycline. Ann Rheum Dis. 2003;62:267–9.
50. Puche AM, Penades IC, Montesinos BL. Effectiveness of treatment with intravenous pamidronate for calcinosis in juvenile dermatomyositis. Clin Exp Rheumatol. 2010;28:135–40.
51. Martillotti J, Moote D, Zemel L. Improvement of calcinosis using pamidronate in a patient with juvenile dermatomyositis. Pediatr Radiol. 2014;44:115–8.

52. De Paula DR, Klem FB, Lorencetti PG, Muller C, Azevedo VF. Rituximab-induced regression of CREST-related calcinosis. Clin Rheumatol. 2013;32:281–3.
53. Giuggioli D, Lumetti, Colaci M, Fallahi P, Antonelli A, Ferri C. Rituximab in the treatment of patients with systemic sclerosis. Our experience and review of the literature. Autoimmun Rev. 2015;14:1072–8.
54. Hurabielle C, Allanore Y, Kahan A, Avouac J. Flare of calcinosis despite rituximab therapy. Sem Arthritis Rheum. 2014;44:e5–6.
55. Poormoghim H, Andalib E, Almasi AR, Hadibigi E. Systemic sclerosis and calcinosis cutis: response to rituximab. J Clin Pharm Ther. 2016;41:94–6.
56. Dubos M, Ly K, Martel C, Fauchais AL. Is rituximab an effective treatment of refractory calcinosis? BMJ Case Rep. 2016;31:2016.
57. Tosounidou, MacDonald H, Situnayake D. Successful treatment of calcinosis with infliximab in a patient with systemic sclerosis/myositis overlap syndrome. Rheumatology. 2014;53:960–1.
58. Malbos S, Urena-Torres P, Cohen-Solal M, et al. Sodium thiosulphate treatment of uraemic tumoral calcinosis. Rheumatology. 2014;53:547–51.
59. Thibodaux R, Miller B, Lindsey S. Intravenous sodium thiosulfate for treatment of refractory calcinosis in rheumatic disease. Arthritis Rheum. 2014;66(Suppl):S955.
60. Florestano MC, Alamo M. Successful therapy with intravenous sodium thiosulfate for adult dermatomyositis associated calcinosis. Arthritis Rheum. 2014;66(Suppl):S955–6.
61. Pelrine E, Gordon JK, Baron M, Spiera RF. Sodium thiosulfate in calcinosis. Arthritis Rheum. 2015;67(Suppl):Abstract 2960.
62. Ratsimbazafy V, Bahans C, Guigonis V. Clinical images: dramatic diminution of a large calcification treated with topical sodium thiosulfate. Arthritis Rheum. 2012;64:3826.
63. Pagnini I, Simonini G, Giani T, et al. Sodium thiosulphate for the treatment of calcinosis secondary to juvenile dermatomyositis. Clin Exp Rheumatol. 2014;32:408–9.
64. Bottomley WW, Goodfield MJ, Sheehan-Dare RA. Digital calcification in systemic sclerosis: effective treatment with good tissue preservation using the carbon dioxide laser. Br J Dermatol. 1996;135:302–4.
65. Chamberlain AJ, Walker NP. Successful palliation and significant remission of cutaneous calcinosis in CREST syndrome with carbon dioxide laser. Dermatol Surg. 2003;29:968–70.

66. Sparsa A, Lesaux N, Kessler E, et al. Treatment of cutaneous calcinosis in CREST syndrome by extracorporeal shock wave lithotripsy. J Am Acad Dermatol. 2005;53:S263–5.
67. Sultan-Bichat N, Menard J, Perceau G, Staerman F, Bernard P, Reguiai Z. Treatment of calcinosis cutis by extracorporeal shock-wave lithotripsy. J Am Acad Dermatol. 2012;66:424–9.
68. Blumhardt S, Frey DP, Toniolo M, Alkadhi H, Held U, Distler O. Safety and efficacy of extracorporeal shock wave therapy (ESWT) in calcinosis cutis associated with systemic sclerosis. Clin Exp Rheumatol. 2016;34(Suppl 100(5)):177–80.

Chapter 22
Pregnancy and Scleroderma

Jessica L. Sheingold and Virginia Steen

Case 1

A 32 year old female with diffuse systemic sclerosis presents for a preconception counseling appointment. She was diagnosed 9 months ago after she developed new onset Raynauds phenomenon and thickening of the skin in her hands and forearms. Laboratory evaluation revealed positive anti-nuclear antibody at 1:1280 in a speckled pattern, and a positive RNA polymerase III antibody. Her modified Rodnan Skin Score has increased to 21 from 18 at her visit 4 months ago, indicating progressively worsening skin disease. Pulmonary function tests 2 months ago were normal, as was a non-contrast CT scan of the chest and an echocardiogram. Her only medication is mycophenolate mofetil. She wants to start a family in the near future. How should she be advised?

J. L. Sheingold (✉)
MedStar Georgetown University Hospital, Washington, DC, USA
e-mail: Jessica.L.Sheingold@medstar.net

V. Steen
Georgetown University School of Medicine, Washington, DC, USA
e-mail: steenv@georgetown.edu

© Springer Nature Switzerland AG 2021
M. Matucci-Cerinic, C. P. Denton (eds.), *Practical Management of Systemic Sclerosis in Clinical Practice*, In Clinical Practice,
https://doi.org/10.1007/978-3-030-53736-4_22

Most women with scleroderma have normal pregnancies and deliver healthy babies. Women of childbearing age who have chronic diseases of any kind should be asked at each visit with their healthcare provider if they desire to have children in the near future so that they can be appropriately counseled. In scleroderma, there are certain situations in which pregnancy should be avoided or delayed due to the risks to mother and child. All women with scleroderma considering pregnancy should discuss their plans with a rheumatologist and a maternal-fetal medicine specialist to help determine their individual risk, and to make any necessary medication changes.

Pregnancies in scleroderma patients are generally uneventful, with similar rates of miscarriage, and only slightly increased rates of premature birth and small for gestational age newborns as compared to healthy women. Fertility does not appear to be affected by scleroderma. A study by Steen et al. demonstrated that 12–15% of women with scleroderma were unable to conceive after a year of trying, which was similar to healthy controls and patients with rheumatoid arthritis [1]. In the past, it was thought that miscarriages occurred more often in women with scleroderma, but many of these observational studies were not controlled for age, medication use, and access to care. More recent data has demonstrated that the rate is similar to the general population at about 12–13% of pregnancies [1]. This varies significantly by age, with rates as low as 9% in women under 30, and as high as 80% in women over 45 [2].

Premature births and small for gestational age newborns are seen more often in women with scleroderma. Premature birth has been observed in 15–28% of pregnancies [1, 3, 4]. Reassuringly, most of these premature births were near term. In one cohort, half of the observed premature births were between 36 and 37 weeks of gestation, and most of these were induced for “non-medical reasons” [3]. This number likely varies significantly by institution. An important observation is that women with early diffuse scleroderma have a markedly elevated risk of giving birth prematurely, at 65% of pregnancies [3]. It has been observed that women with severe lung or gastrointestinal involvement more commonly deliver early as well.

Several studies have noted a trend towards more small for gestational age newborns (below the tenth percentile for gestational age) born to women with scleroderma as compared to healthy controls, but this has not been universally observed. The Italian multi-center IMPRESS study followed women with scleroderma prospectively through their pregnancies and observed that although small for gestational age newborns were uncommon, 5% of newborns fell into the "very low birthweight" category, weighing less than 1500 grams [4]. This is in contrast to healthy controls who delivered very low birthweight newborns only 1% of the time.

Fortunately, studies agree that neonatal death is a rare phenomenon in scleroderma pregnancies. The IMPRESS study observed a rate of 2%, similar to the general population [4]. Similarly, in the Steen cohort, neonatal death occurred at comparable rates in scleroderma, rheumatoid arthritis, and healthy pregnancies [1].

Despite this reassuring data, there are several situations in scleroderma in which pregnancy should be avoided or delayed. Women with severe interstitial lung disease, pulmonary hypertension, and renal disease are underrepresented in the available observational studies. Scleroderma-specific pregnancy data is limited in such populations, and recommendations are extrapolated from studies of women with pulmonary and renal dysfunction of other etiology. Pulmonary hypertension in particular is associated with high rates of fetal and maternal death. While newer medications have allowed some women with mild disease to successfully deliver healthy babies, pulmonary hypertension is currently considered a contraindication to pregnancy [5]. Although not associated with the same high maternal mortality as pulmonary hypertension, pregnancy in interstitial lung disease is generally recommended against in women with a forced vital capacity less than 50% predicted, based on very limited data [2].

Scleroderma renal crisis is a situation unique to scleroderma that has serious implications for pregnancy. The primary treatment for renal crisis is prompt and continuous administration of ACE inhibitors, which are known teratogens. 10–20% of women with scleroderma will develop renal crisis during their disease course, and those with diffuse skin involvement are at highest risk during their first 5 years of disease [6]. RNA Polymerase III antibody positivity poses an additional risk factor for the development of renal crisis. In such women, and in the case above, pregnancy should be delayed until the disease stabilizes. After the 5 year mark, the risk of renal crisis drops significantly [6].

It is essential to discuss medication management prior to conception. Several medications are unsafe to take during early pregnancy as they are likely to cause miscarriage. Methotrexate is a commonly used anti-rheumatic medication that is associated with high miscarriage rates, and should be discontinued 3 months prior to conception. One prospective study found that women exposed to methotrexate during early pregnancy had a spontaneous abortion rate of 42.5%, but those exposed in the 12 weeks prior to conception had similar rates of miscarriage to healthy and disease matched controls [7]. Mycophenolate mofetil is commonly used in scleroderma, and is associated with high rates of major birth defects [8]. It should be stopped before conception, and alternative agents, such as azathioprine used as a maintenance therapy, if necessary. In women with interstitial lung disease, it may not be safe to abruptly stop mycophenolate. If pregnancy is desired, a rheumatologist should supervise the transition to a safer medication, such as azathioprine, prior to conception. See Table 22.1 for a summary of medication safety during pregnancy and lactation. It should be noted that this data is primarily based on observational studies, often with a limited number of patients.

Table 22.1 Commonly used medications in scleroderma and safety during pregnancy and lactation

Medication	Use in Pregnancy	Use in Lactation
NSAIDs	Recommended against throughout pregnancy, contraindicated in third trimester	Safe for use
Prednisone	Safe for use in low doses	Safe for use in low doses
Hydroxychloroquine	Safe for use	Safe for use
Azathioprine	Safe for use	Safe for use
Methotrexate	Contraindicated	Contraindicated
Leflunomide	Contraindicated	Safety unknown
Mycophenolate mofetil	Contraindicated	Contraindicated
Cyclophosphamide	Contraindicated	Contraindicated
Calcium Channel blockers	Safe for use	Safe for use
Phosphodiesterase type 5 inhibitors	Limited data suggests possible safety	Safety unknown
Endothelin receptor antagonists	Contraindicated	Safety unknown
Prostacyclin analogs	Limited data suggests safety	Safety unknown

Case 2

Two years later your patient, now 34 years old with persistent but stable diffuse scleroderma, is sent to the emergency room from clinic after her blood pressure is found to be 180/100 during a routine office visit. She is 34 weeks pregnant with her first child. There have been no complications through the pregnancy thus far, and she has always had normal blood pressure. She reports a mild frontal headache, but otherwise has no complains. Laboratory work up reveals new anemia, mild thrombocytopenia, creatinine of 2.3 mg/dL, and urinalysis with 3+ protein and 1+ blood. What diagnostic work up should be completed? What treatment should be recommended?

New blood pressure elevation in patients with scleroderma should always raise concern for scleroderma renal crisis, especially in those with diffuse skin involvement, disease duration of less than 5 years, and positive RNA polymerase III antibodies. Centromere antibody positivity is a negative risk factor [6]. In pregnancy, identifying renal crisis is complicated by the fact that pregnancy-related hypertensive disorders, such as preeclampsia, can present similarly. Both situations warrant emergent treatment. In renal crisis, the most worrisome complication is the rapid development of renal failure and need for dialysis. Early aggressive treatment with ACE inhibitors gives the best potential of a good outcome, and thus should be promptly administered if there is any evidence that hypertension might be relate to renal crisis, such as rising creatinine or hemolysis.

Preeclampsia is defined as new onset hypertension and proteinuria, or hypertension with evidence of end-organ damage after 20 weeks of gestation [9]. In the 2019 guidelines, preeclampsia is deemed severe if there is evidence of central nervous system dysfunction (vision changes, severe headache), liver dysfunction (right upper quadrant pain or liver enzymes elevated above two times the upper limit of normal), thrombocytopenia (platelets less than 100,000), renal insufficiency (creatinine >1.1 mg/dL or a doubling of the baseline creatinine), or pulmonary edema. Eclampsia is diagnosed when a woman with preeclampsia develops grand mal seizures [9]. HELLP syndrome (hemolysis, elevated liver enzymes, low platelets) is a subtype of severe preeclampsia which could be confused with renal crisis. Treatment of severe disease necessitates delivery of the baby as soon as reasonably possible. Alternatively, treatment of scleroderma renal crisis requires the immediate use of ACE inhibitors, and does not improve with delivery.

Differentiating scleroderma renal crisis from preeclampsia and related disorders is challenging, but treatment of both conditions may have life saving impacts on both mother and child. Preeclampsia is a major cause of maternal mortality, and thus the benefits of delivering a preterm child may be worth the associated risks [9]. On the other hand, renal crisis results in renal failure and death in the vast majority of patients without administration of ACE inhibitors, so there should be no delay in administration of these medications if there is any question of renal crisis [6]. Initial work up should include complete blood count, metabolic panel to assess creatinine and liver enzymes, and a spot urine protein:creatinine ratio. Elevated liver enzymes are seen more often in preeclampsia, although normal values do not rule it out. Assessing for thrombocytopenia and hemolysis is important, although this can be seen in both HELLP syndrome and renal crisis, which is associated with a microangiopathic hemolytic anemia. Uric acid can be checked, as elevations are associated with preeclampsia [10]. However, significant renal insufficiency and high cell turnover states such as hemolysis will also increase uric acid levels. Finally, serum renin levels are elevated in renal crisis, however, these test results are not usually available acutely [11].

The patient presented in the case above has multiple risk factors for renal crisis, and thus should receive an ACE inhibitor without delay. This class of medication is teratogenic if taken during the second or third trimester, and has been associated with IUGR, oligohydramnios, renal failure, and hypocalvaria [12]. Not all children will be negatively affected by exposure to ACE inhibitors. One review found that of 22 children exposed prenatally during the second and third trimester, two had end stage renal disease, 10 had mild impairments, and 10 had no long term issues [13]. Although use of calcium channel blockers and alpha blockers is safer in pregnancy, these agents are insufficient to manage the pathologic malignant hypertension of renal crisis [14]. Depending on the gestational age, it may be safest for the obstetrics team to deliver the baby, both in renal crisis and preeclampsia, with continuation of the ACE inhibitor after delivery.

References

1. Steen VD, Medsger TA. Fertility and pregnancy outcome in women with systemic sclerosis. Arthritis Rheum. 1999;42(4):763–8.
2. Sobanski V, Launay D, Depret S, et al. Special considerations in pregnant systemic sclerosis patients. Expert Rev Clin Immunol. 2016;12(11):1161–73.
3. Steen VD. Pregnancy in women with systemic sclerosis. Obstet Gynecol. 1999;94(1):15–20.
4. Taraborelli M, Ramoni V, Brucato A, et al. Successful pregnancies but a higher risk of preterm births in patients with systemic sclerosis: an Italian multicenter study. Arthritis Rheum. 2012;64(6):1970–7.
5. Jais X, Olsson KM, Barbera JA, et al. Pregnancy outcomes in pulmonary arterial hypertension in the modern management era. Eur Respir J. 2012;40(4):881–5.
6. Steen VD. Pregnancy in scleroderma. Rheum Dis Clin N Am. 2007;33(2):345–58.
7. Weber-schoendorfer C, Chambers C, Wacker E, et al. Pregnancy outcome after methotrexate treatment for rheumatic disease prior to or during early pregnancy: a prospective multicenter cohort study. Arthritis Rheumatol. 2014;66(5):1101–10.
8. Soh MC, Nelson-Piercy C. High-risk pregnancy and the rheumatologist. Rheumatology (Oxford). 2015;54(4):572–87.
9. Practice Bulletin No ACOG. 202: gestational hypertension and preeclampsia. Obstet Gynecol. 2019;133(1):e1.
10. Khalig OP, Konoshita T, Moodley J, et al. The role of uric acid in preeclampsia: is uric acid a causative factor or a sign of preeclampsia? Curr Hypertens Rep. 2018;20(9):80.
11. Lidar M, Langevitz P. Pregnancy issues in scleroderma. Autoimmun Rev. 2012;11(6–7):A515–9.

12. Al-Maawali A, Walfisch A, Koren G. Taking angiotensin-converting enzyme inhibitors during pregnancy: is it safe? Can Fam Physician. 2012;58(1):49–51.
13. Bullo M, Tschumi S, Bucher BS, et al. Pregnancy outcome following exposure to angiotensin-converting enzyme inhibitors or angiotensin receptor antagonists: a systematic review. Hypertension. 2012;60(2):444–50.
14. Zanatta E, Polito P, Favaro M, et al. Therapy of scleroderma renal crisis: state of the art. Autoimmun Rev. 2018;17(9):882–9.

Chapter 23
Sjogren's Syndrome (Ss) in Progressive Systemic Sclerosis (SSc)

Athanasios G. Tzioufas, Georgia Liantinioti, and Panayotis G. Vlachoyiannopoulos

Introduction

Sjogren syndrome (Ss) is a chronic autoimmune epithelitis that may occur as a distinct entity and it is classified as primary Sjogren syndrome (pSs) or in association with other autoimmune connective tissue diseases such as systemic lupus erythematosus (15%–36%), rheumatoid arthritis (20%–32%), systemic sclerosis (11%–24%), mixed connective tissue disease [1–4], thus classified as secondary SS [5]. It is characterized by a wide variety of manifestations, ranging from local involvement of exocrine glands with keratoconjuctivitis sicca and xerostomia which are the main symptoms of the disease, to systemic extraglandular manifestations includ-

A. G. Tzioufas (✉) · P. G. Vlachoyiannopoulos
Department of Pathophysiology, School of Medicine, University of Athens, Athens, Greece
e-mail: agtzi@med.uoa.gr; pvlah@med.uoa.g

G. Liantinioti
Department of Pathophysiology, General Hospital Laiko, Athens, Greece

© Springer Nature Switzerland AG 2021

M. Matucci-Cerinic, C. P. Denton (eds.), *Practical Management of Systemic Sclerosis in Clinical Practice*, In Clinical Practice,
https://doi.org/10.1007/978-3-030-53736-4_23

ing cutaneous, musculoskeletal, pulmonary, renal, hematological and neurological involvement [6]. Most patients are women, with a female-to-male ratio of 9:1, usually at age of 40–60 years. The onset is insidious and the wide variety of signs and symptoms, make often the diagnosis difficult or delayed for several years [7].

A Vignette Case of Co-Existence of pSs with SSc

A 60 years old lady presented with 6 years history of arthralgias but no arthritis, severe Raynaud's phenomenon, subjective muscle weakness, xerostomia and xerophthalmia, as well as a history of parotid gland enlargement which was spontaneously reduced 5 months later. Antinuclear antibodies were positive at a titer of 1: 2500 with a pattern compatible with anti-centromere antibodies (ACA), while she was also positive for anti-Ro/SSA autoantibodies by counterimmunoelectrophoresis (CIE). Minor salivary gland biopsy revealed dense periductal lymphocytic infiltrates compatible with a Tarpley 3+ score, having also germinal center formation. On clinical examination she presented xerostomia, xerophthalmia, severe Raynaud's phenomenon, crackles on auscultation in both lung bases and sclerodactyly. Laboratory evaluation except from ANA with an ACA pattern and anti-Ro/SSA by CIE, was remarkable for rheumatoid factor (RF) that was positive but at low titer, hypergammaglobulinemia and urine alkaline pH. She received calcium channel blockers in the era before the development of the endothelin receptor antagonists and methotrexate 12.5 mg per week for her arthralgias. She was well for one more year, when she developed dry cough, exertional dyspnea and 2+ edema in the legs. Pulmonary function tests were remarkable only for reduced $FEF_{25–75}$. Blood gases were as follows: PaO_2 = 75 mmHg, $PaCO_2$ = 29 mmHg, pH = 7.44 and HCO_3 = 20.2 mEq/L. Cardiac catheterization revealed a mean pulmonary artery pressure of 55 mmHg; 1+ insufficiency of mitral and 2+ insufficiency of tricuspid valve. Vasospasm of the right coronary artery during catheterization was resolved by immediate intracoronary infusion of nitrates and nifedipine.

The patient worsened month by month and 1 year later she died of accelerated pulmonary arterial hypertension.

Common Denominators in Pathogenesis of pSs and SSc

Apart from their obvious phenotypic differences, pSs and SSc share some common characteristics. For instance, the vignette case of coexistence of pSs and SSc presented above, underlines common pathogenic pathways between these diseases, at least in those SSc patients with Ss manifestations or the Ss patients with scleroderma changes. Although the pathogenic aspects of SSc will be presented in detail elsewhere in this book, a summary of pathogenesis of SSc and pSs in this chapter will make the coexistence of these diseases more understandable.

SSc pathogenesis relies upon three pylons: (a) extracellular matrix production by myofibroblasts, (b) severe vasculopathy as depicted by Raynaud's phenomenon, teleangiectasies and pulmonary arterial hypertension (PAH) and ((c) autoimmune reactivity, as depicted by production of numerous autoantibodies [8]. Raynaud's phenomenon occurs among 33% of Ss patients [9], while PAH, although it occurs also, is rare [10]. However in a small patient cohort of pSs a prevalence of PAH as high as 23.4% was recently reported [11]. On the other hand among 40 consecutive patients undergoing evaluation for PAH the prevalence of definite pSs was 8% and that of possible pSs 5%.

Autoimmune reactivity also occurs in both diseases, concerning both, innate and adaptive immunity, the later including both B and T cell immune responses; However the cohort studies focus mainly on B cell responses because their effects such as the production of autoantibodies are easily detected.

An initial observation by H.M.Moutsopoulos group in 1993 pointed out the presence of seven patients with pSs positive for anticentromere antibodies (ACA); the majority of them noticed Raynaud's phenomenon, while 4 out of 7 suffered of small airways disease as depicted by reduced FEF_{25-75}% predicted values and only one had sclerodactyly. Anti-Ro/SSA and anti-La/SSB antibodies were rather uncommon in this group as compared to pSs cohorts (4 and 1 out of 7 respectively) [12]. The patient with sclerodactyly (the vignette case presented above) developed full blown PAH and eventually died of PAH.

The Role of Epithelial Cell in pSs and SSc

Myofibroblasts contribute to tissue remodeling by synthesizing extracellular matrix (ECM) components, when these cells exert traction forces or sense other chemical stimuli. In normal situations, when tissue remodeling is completed, myofibroblasts die by apoptosis but this does not happen in SSc [13] . A major disturbance in tissue remodeling pathways seems to be initiated in SSc by the transition of endothelial cells to myofibroblasts [14]. However, another cell which is a common initiator in both diseases is probably the epithelial cell. This cell undergoes also a process called "epithelial to mesenchymal transition" especially in the lungs of patients with SSc [15], giving rise to more myofibroblasts independently of the initial trigger. In case of pSs, epithelial cell becomes a very effective antigen-presenting cell [16, 17]. Indeed, epithelial cells in patients with pSs express costimulatory molecules and innapropriatelly intracellular autoantigens Ro/SSA and La/SSB on their membranes providing thus, signals for lymphocyte activation; in addition they produce proinflammatory cytokines and lymphocyte-attracting chemokines important for sustaining the autoimmune lesion and allowing the formation of germinal centers, a finding predicting evolution to lymphoma, and express functional receptors of innate immunity such as toll-like receptors (TLRs) 3, 4 and

9, of which TLR-4 exists on the cell membrane [18, 19] and accounts for the initiation of innate immunity through NF-κB and AP-1 pathways. TLRs-3 and -9 in the endosome sensing viral and microbial constituents and give rise in interferon regulatory factors (IRFs) [20, 21]. It seems that an initial epithelial injury as depicted by IL-33 expression, plays some role in the pathogenesis of pSs [22] while an association of increased serum levels of the IL-33 neutralizing sST2 was also described in limited cutaneous SSc [23],both of the above findings suggesting that epithelial cells undergo and respond to various stresses.

Epigenetic Alterations in pSs and SSc

Systematic comparative studies of epigenctic changes in every cellular compartment of the tissues involved, between pSs and SSc are missing. SSc fibroblasts demonstrate hypomethylation of the following genes: integrin-α 9 (ITFA9) disintegrin and metalloproteinase domain-containing protein 12 (ADAM12), Collagen type XXIII alpha 1 chain (COL23A1), Collagen alpha-2(IV) chain (COL4A2), Myosin-Ie (MYO1E) and Runt-related transcription factors (RUNX) [24] Interestingly RUNX -1 to -3 transcription factors are over-expressed in lacrimal gland epithelium and are involved in regulation in gland morphogenesis and regeneration [25] . RUNX-1 and RUNX-3 genes are hypomethylated in labial salivary glands of patients with Ss [26], as depicted by a genome-wide DNA methylation study performed in human labial salivary gland biopsy samples. Hypomethylation and overexpression of CD70, Lymphotoxin alpha (LTA), forkhead box P3 (FOXP3) and interferon-inducible genes in CD4 + Tcells. In addition interferon regulatory factor 5 (IRF5) in T cells, B cells, monocytes and salivary gland epithelial cells, global DNA hypomethylation in minor salivary glands when are associated with lymphocytic infiltrates, hypomethylation and overexpression of long interspersed nuclear element-1 (LINE-1) in minor salivary glands, hypomethylation in CD19 + B cells and hypomethylation in interferon-induced genes in minor salivary epithelial cells [27] have been also found in pSs. The Wnt pathway related factors are hyper-methylated and hypo-expressed in minor salivary glands epithelial cells [27] but in this report authors underline the necessity to conduct pure cell analysis for future EWAS studies when analysing salivary glands from patients with pSS. On the contrary the genes of Wnt signaling associated factors are hypomethylated in SSc and this was attributed to silencing of Friend leukemia integration 1 (Fli1) and Kruppel-like factor 5 (KLF5) [28]. Active Wnt signaling was associated with fibrosis.

Activation of Interferon-I Pathway

Genome wide association studies have shown genetic polymorphisms in interferon regulatory factors (IRFs)—4,5,7 and 8 [29] . Similarly, polymorphism of Signal Transducer and Activator of Transcription (STAT)- 4, has been established as a genetic risk factor of SSc. IRFs and STAT4 proteins are key activators of type I IFN signaling pathways. An IFN signature (increased expression and activation of IFN-regulated genes) has been observed in the peripheral blood and skin biopsy samples of patients with SSc [30] . On the other hand Sjögren's syndrome (Ss) is characterized by chronic immune attacks against exocrine glands leading to exocrine dysfunction, plus strong up-regulated expressions of IFN regulated gene transcripts. Genome-wide transcriptome analyses indicate that differentially expressed interferon regulated genes are restricted during disease development and therefore define underlying etiopathological mechanisms [31]. All the above findings suggest that pSs and SSc share some common pathways in a manner of not being the same diseases but at the same time in a way co-exist [32] or to share some clinical features [33] in a minority of patients.

Clinical Manifestations of pSs

Sicca symptoms such as xerophthalmia (dry eyes) and xerostomia (dry mouth), are the most common manifestation of Sjögren's syndrome, with up to 98% of the cases. Dry eyes may be described as red, itchy, painfull and the most common complaint of the patients is that of a gritty or sandy sensation in the eyes. Symptoms typically worsen throughout the day. Oral symptoms include difficulty speaking, eating, or swallowing and the patients need frequent sips of water due to sensation of dry mouth [34]. The patient usually have an increased risk of dental caries and oral infections as a result of decreased salivary flow [34, 35].

Although dry eyes and dry mouth are the most common symptoms in patients with Sjögren's syndrome, most patients who report these symptoms may have other underlying causes. The incidence of sicca symptoms increases with age [36]. Common medications can cause sicca symptoms in any age group. Antidepressants, anticholinergics, beta blockers, diuretics, and antihistamines are some categories of drugs that can cause these symptoms [37]. Anxiety can also lead to sicca symptoms. Women who use hormone replacement therapy may be at increased risk of dry eye syndrome. Chronic viral infections such as HIV, HCV, HTLV-1 can also cause sicca symptoms [38].

Parotitis is another glandular manifestation of the disease. Up to 34% of patients with Sjögren's syndrome report episodic or chronic, typically bilateral swelling of the parotid glands [39]. Bilateral parotid gland enlargement is not always due to Sjogren, it may be the result of endocrine disorders (acromegaly or gonadal hypofunction), metabolic diseases (chronic pancreatitis, diabetes mellitus, hepatic cirrhosis, or hyperlipoproteinemias), sarcoidosis and viral infections (human immunodeficiency virus infection, hepatitis C). Rock-hard or unilateral parotid gland enlargement should prompt referral to an otolaryngologist for biopsy to exclude a tumor or lymphoma and especially malignant non-Hodgkin lymphoma (NHL) of B cell lineage which occurs in about 5% of patients with pSS [40].

Although the clinical manifestations of pSS patients are mainly those of an autoimmune exocrinopathy, almost half of the patients develop extraglandular disease. The most common are arthralgias and usually non-erosive polyarthritis which occur in approximately 50% of patients and due to this manifestation is often confused with RA [41].

Up to 30% of patients with SS have subclinical pulmonary disease. Pulmonary manifestations in SS typically develop late in the course of disease and are rarely the presenting feature. Cough is often the main respiratory symptom and is usually a symptom of xerotrachea. Other pulmonary manifestations are chronic interstitial lung disease (ILD) and lymphoinfiltrative or lymphoproliferative lung disease [42] .

Renal involvement is found in approximately 5% of patients. In pSS renal involvement is the result of two distinct pathophysiological processes: epithelial disease with a predominantly mononuclear lymphocytic infiltration resulting in tubulointerstitial nephritis (TIN) and non-epithelial disease with a secondary immune complex–mediated process resulting in glomerulopathy [43].

Neurological disorders are also common extraglandular manifestations of pSS. Available literature data estimate the prevalence of neurological symptoms as about 8.5–70% of patients diagnosed with pSS [44]. The most common neurological complication of SS is peripheral neuropathy, and in particular sensory polyneuropathy [45]. CNS involvement ranges from hemiparesis, transverse myelitis, and dystonia to encephalopathy and dementia. In 10–20% of patients there are lesions in the central nervous system analogous to those presented in the multiple sclerosis (multiple sclerosis-like lesions). Most often they concern the white matter of the brain (60%) and the spinal cord (40%), at these patients the differential diagnosis is challenging [46].

Cutaneous lesions of Sjogren's syndrome include dryness of the skin, annular erythema with scales, localized especially on the face and neck and nonpalpable or palpable, vasculitic purpura with lesions that are typically 2–3 mm in diameter and located on the lower extremities [47].

Patients with SS have an increased risk of lymphoma or lymphoproliferative disease compared to the general population [48]. Most lymphomas are of B-cell lineage and are of low- or intermediate-grade of malignancy. Persistent gland enlargement, purpura, low levels of C4 and monoclonal cryoglobulinemia, high levels of rheumatoid factor are the main risk factors.

Sjogren Syndrome in Scleroderma

Systemic sclerosis is a rare multisystem connective tissue disease which is characterized by excess collagen deposition resulting in skin thickening, fibrosis of the joint and tendon, as well as vasculopathy of the small vessels. Clinical manifestations of SSc varies with most of the patients presenting skin thickening and internal organ involvement such as interstitial lung disease, pulmonary hypertension, gastrointestinal dysmotility. SSc has two main types, the progressive systemic sclerosis and a milder form termed CREST. Published data about the true association between Sjogren's syndrome in scleroderma show a prevalence of Sjogren in 23.4% of patients with scleroderma. Sjogren's syndrome is found more frequently in the limited cutaneous form of SSc with positive ACA [49]. There are studies that emphasize that the overlap patients display a full blown SS phenotype while the manifestation of SSc are milder. In a study performed by Salliot et al. which compared patients with SSc alone and patients with SS—SSc, the most interesting finding was that SSc seems to be less serious when it is associated with SS. Lung fibrosis, one of the most severe complications of limited SSc, occurred in 29% of the patients with SSc alone and in only 11% of the patients with SS-SSc ($P = 0.05$). Also, this study showed a trend in favour of a reduced prevalence of PAH and of scleroderma renal crisis in the SS-SSc patients (7 vs. 15%) and (4 vs. 15%), respectively, while esophagus involvement was similar in the two groups. Moreover Baldini et al. showed that the "overlap patients" presented a higher prevalence of teleangectasia (43.7% vs. 3.4%, $p = 0.02$) but a lower prevalence of both digital necrosis and ulcers (12.2% vs. 49%). They also had a higher frequency of parotid swelling (31.7% vs. 1%), arthralgias (46.3% vs. 16.7%, $p < 0.0001$), purpura (14.6 vs. 0, $p = 0.0004$) and fatigue (39% vs. 2.9% $p < 0.0001$) comparing to the "SSc patients". As far as the frequency of lymphoma concern at the overlap patients Bournia et al. observed two lymphoma cases in patients with SSc and sicca manifestations and no cases in patients with SSc alone. The risk factors which associated with the development of lymphoma were salivary gland enlargement, purpura, leukocytopenia and hypergammaglobulinaemia similarly to pSS. Moreover Bournia et al. showed that the risk was higher in patients with ACA-positive limited cutaneous SSc and sicca symptoms and enlighted the necessity of these patients to be monitored tightly over the time. Serologically the overlap patients when compared to pSS patients had lower prevalence of hypergammaglobulinaemia, RF, anti-RoSSA and anti-LaSSB antibodies. Drosos et al. and Osial et al. found that anti-Ro/SSA antibodies were present in 33% (3 of 9) and 29% (5 of 17), respectively, of their patients with concurrent SSc and SS.

Common Problems in the DD?

Sicca symptoms are common in patients with systemic sclerosis (60%–70%) [50] the principal cause of sicca symptoms in SSc appears to be glandular fibrosis, rather than SS lymphocytic sialadenitis and it is explained by fibrosis of exocrine glands in patients with diffuse disease and extensive systemic involvement [50]. Fibrosis around capillaries and excretory ducts induce functional abnormalities leading to sicca symptoms. These abnormalities in collagen deposition are found usually in the minor salivary glands. In order to distinguise between sicca symptoms in SSc and secondary Sjogren, biopsy of minor salivary glands is necessary. At secondary Sjogren the biopsy reveals CD4-positive T-lymphocyte infiltration of the salivary glands and the presence of >50 lymphocytes/4 mm^2 on the biopsy is diagnostic [49].

Raynaud's phenomenon (RP) is seen at the majority of the patients with SSc as well as at 33% [49, 51]of the patients with SS, especially those who have ACA antibodies [52]. SS patients, and especially those with RP, present capillaroscopic abnormalities ranging from non-specific to more specific findings or, on some occasions, scleroderma-type findings. Crossed capillaries and pericapillary haemorrhages are the most common findings at the capillaroscopy and the mean capillary density is significantly lower at these patients [53]. There is a distinct entity of patients with pSS and anticentromere positivity, but without clinical features of SSc. The existence of this subgroup of SS patients who their predominant features are sicca manifestations and RP has raised the question of whether this group of patients constitutes an overlap between lSSc and SS [54]. Some investigators have proposed that these patients with RP, ACA and scleroderma pattern in capillaroscopy should be included in the spectrum of lSSc, although may not fulfill criteria for scleroderma.

Diagnosis and Treatment

It is difficult to distinguise between SSc with sicca symptoms and SSc—secondary Sjogren syndrome. Minor salivary gland biopsy is considered the "gold standard" for the diagnosis, although newer criteria permit classification of SS without necessarily performing this procedure. The American-European consensus committee recently modified and reapproved criteria that exhibit approximately 95% sensitivity and specificity for SS [55] (Table 23.1). These criteria

Table 23.1 ACR/EULAR criteria for Sjogren syndrome

Unstimulated salivary flow rate abnormal = 0.1 mL/min (1 point).
Abnormal Schirmer's test (<5 mm in 5 min) (1 point)
Abnormal findings with lissamine green or fluorescein staining (1 point)
Autoantibody detection: Anti-Ro/SSA (3 points)
Histology—Focal lymphocytic sialadenitis 1 focus = 50 lymphocytes/4 mm^2 (3 points)
Diagnosis is considered established if score = 4 points

encompass the presence of subjective and objective sicca manifestations, antibodies to Ro/SS-A and La/SS-B antigens, and characteristic histopathologic findings in minor salivary glands [56].

Because there is no known cure for Sjögren's syndrome, treatment focuses on relieving symptoms and preventing complications. Treatments can be grouped into regimens for xerophalmia, xerostomia, and systemic manifestations. Ocular dryness is treated with preservative-free teardrops or eye lubricants containing either sodium hyaluronate or hydroxypropyl methylcellulose. In cases of moderate to severe dry eye disease, anti-inflammatory treatment with cyclosporine A eye drops has gained significant importance [57]. To minimize xerostomia products that stimulating saliva secretion are used like pilocarpine [58]. Patients with SS should avoid diuretics, antihypertensive drugs, antidepressants, and antihistamines, all of which may worsen salivary hypofunction. For systemic symptoms in patients whom arthralgia or myalgia is the predominant symptom, hydroxychloroquine is used [59]. Anti-B–cell biologic agents, particularly rituximab, corticosteroids and cytotoxic drugs such as cyclophosphamide are reserved for severe extraglandular manifestations of sjogren's syndrome such as cutaneous vasculitis, glomerulonephritis and interstitial lung disease [60].

Conclusion

Sicca symptoms are common in systemic sclerosis patients due to fibrosis of salivary gland however true SS is present in only 22.3% of these patients and it is found more frequently in the limited form of SSc. Although we would expect that the coexistence of Sjögren's syndrome and systemic sclerosis would worsen the evolution and prognosis of these patients studies show the opposite. SSc seems to be less serious when it is associated with SS.

References

1. Salliot C, Gottenberg J-E, Sibilia J, et al. Sjögren's syndrome is associated with and not secondary to systemic sclerosis. Rheumatology. 2006;46:321–6.
2. Moerman R, Arends S, Kroese F, et al. AB0502 prevalence and clinical characteristics of secondary Sjögren's syndrome and Sicca symptoms in patients with rheumatoid arthritis in daily clinical practice. Ann Rheum Dis. 2016;75:1077.
3. Gilboe I-M, Kvien TK, Uhlig T, Husby G. Sicca symptoms and secondary Sjögren's syndrome in systemic lupus erythematosus: comparison with rheumatoid arthritis and correlation with disease variables. Ann Rheum Dis. 2001;60:1103–9.
4. Coll J, Rives A, Griñó MC, Setoain J, Vivancos J, Balcells A. Prevalence of Sjögren's syndrome in autoimmune diseases. Ann Rheum Dis. 1987;46:286–9.
5. Meyer D, Yanoff M, Hanno H. Differential diagnosis in Mikulicz's syndrome, Mikulicz's disease, and similar disease entities. Am J Ophthalmol. 1971;71:516–24.
6. Mavragani CP, Moutsopoulos HM. Sjögren syndrome. CMAJ. 2014;186:E579–E86.
7. Mavragani CP, Moutsopoulos HM. The geoepidemiology of Sjögren's syndrome. Autoimmun Rev. 2010;9:A305–A10.
8. Pattanaik D, Brown M, Postlethwaite BC, Postlethwaite AE. Pathogenesis of systemic sclerosis. Front Immunol. 2015;6:272.

9. Skopouli FN, Talal A, Galanopoulou V, Tsampoulas CG, Drosos AA, Moutsopoulos HM. Raynaud's phenomenon in primary Sjogren's syndrome. J Rheumatol. 1990;17:618–20.
10. Launay D, Hachulla E, Hatron PY, Jais X, Simonneau G, Humbert M. Pulmonary arterial hypertension: a rare complication of primary Sjogren syndrome: report of 9 new cases and review of the literature. Medicine. 2007;86:299–315.
11. Kobak S, Kalkan S, Kirilmaz B, et al. Pulmonary arterial hypertension in patients with primary syndrome. Autoimmune Diseases. 2014;2014:5.
12. Vlachoyiannopoulos PG, Drosos AA, Wiik A, Moutsopoulos HM. Patients with anticentromere antibodies, clinical features, diagnoses and evolution. Br J Rheumatol. 1993;32:297–301.
13. Korman B. Evolving insights into the cellular and molecular pathogenesis of fibrosis in systemic sclerosis. Transl Res. 2019;209:77–89.
14. Manetti M, Romano E, Rosa I, et al. Endothelial-to-mesenchymal transition contributes to endothelial dysfunction and dermal fibrosis in systemic sclerosis. Ann Rheum Dis. 2017;76:924–34.
15. Hinz B, Phan SH, Thannickal VJ, et al. Recent developments in myofibroblast biology: paradigms for connective tissue remodeling. Am J Pathol. 2012;180:1340–55.
16. Moutsopoulos HM. Sjogren's syndrome: autoimmune epithelitis. Clin Immunol Immunopathol. 1994;72:162–5.
17. Mitsias DI, Kapsogeorgou EK, Moutsopoulos HM. Sjögren's syndrome: why autoimmune epithelitis? Oral Dis. 2006;12:523–32.
18. Spachidou MP, Bourazopoulou E, Maratheftis CI, et al. Expression of functional toll-like receptors by salivary gland epithelial cells: increased mRNA expression in cells derived from patients with primary Sjögren's syndrome. Clin Exp Immunol. 2007;147:497–503.
19. Kapsogeorgou EK, Gourzi VC, Manoussakis MN, Moutsopoulos HM, Tzioufas AG. Cellular microRNAs (miRNAs) and Sjogren's syndrome: candidate regulators of autoimmune response and autoantigen expression. J Autoimmun. 2011;37:129–35.
20. Nezos A, Gkioka E, Koutsilieris M, Voulgarelis M, Tzioufas AG, Mavragani CP. TNFAIP3 F127C coding variation in Greek primary Sjogrens syndrome patients. J Immunol Res. 2018;2018:8.
21. Kiripolsky J, Kramer JM. Current and emerging evidence for toll-like receptor activation in Sjogrens syndrome. J Immunol Res. 2018;2018:12.

22. Awada A, Nicaise C, Ena S, et al. Potential involvement of the IL-33-ST2 axis in the pathogenesis of primary Sjogren's syndrome. Ann Rheum Dis. 2014;73:1259–63.
23. Wagner A, Kohm M, Nordin A, Svenungsson E, Pfeilschifter JM, Radeke HH. Increased serum levels of the IL-33 neutralizing sST2 in limited cutaneous systemic sclerosis. Scand J Immunol. 2015;82:269–74.
24. Altorok N, Tsou P-S, Coit P, Khanna D, Sawalha AH. Genome-wide DNA methylation analysis in dermal fibroblasts from patients with diffuse and limited systemic sclerosis reveals common and subset-specific DNA methylation aberrancies. Ann Rheum Dis. 2015;74:1612–20.
25. Li X, Hoeppner LH, Jensen ED, Gopalakrishnan R, Westendorf JJ. Co-activator activator (CoAA) prevents the transcriptional activity of runt domain transcription factors. J Cell Biochem. 2009;108:378–87.
26. Gupta B, Hawkins RD. Epigenomics of autoimmune diseases. Immunol Cell Biol. 2015;93:271–6.
27. Imgenberg-Kreuz J, Sandling JK, Nordmark G. Epigenetic alterations in primary Sjogren's syndrome - an overview. Clin Immunol. 2018;196:12–20.
28. Noda T, Murakami S, Nakatsu S, et al. Importance of the 1+7 configuration of ribonucleoprotein complexes for influenza a virus genome packaging. Nat Commun. 2018;9:54.
29. Skaug B, Assassi S. Type I interferon dysregulation in Systemic Sclerosis. Cytokine 2019.
30. Wu M, Assassi S. The role of type 1 interferon in systemic sclerosis. Front Immunol. 2013;4
31. Nguyen CQ, Peck AB. The interferon-signature of Sjögren's syndrome: how unique biomarkers can identify underlying inflammatory and Immunopathological mechanisms of specific diseases. Front Immunol. 2013;4:142.
32. Salliot C, Mouthon L, Ardizzone M, et al. Sjogren's syndrome is associated with and not secondary to systemic sclerosis. Rheumatology. 2007;46:321–6.
33. Bournia V-KK, Diamanti KD, Vlachoyiannopoulos PG, Moutsopoulos HM. Anticentromere antibody positive Sjögren's syndrome: a retrospective descriptive analysis. Arthritis Res Ther. 2010;12:R47.
34. Fox PC, Bowman SJ, Segal B, et al. Oral involvement in primary Sjögren syndrome. J Am Dent Assoc. 2008;139:1592–601.

35. Guggenheimer J, Moore PA. Xerostomia: etiology, recognition and treatment. J Am Dent Assoc. 2003;134:61–9.
36. Ship JA, Pillemer SR, Baum BJ. Xerostomia and the geriatric patient. J Am Geriatr Soc. 2002;50:535–43.
37. Shetty SR, Bhowmick S, Castelino R, Babu S. Drug induced xerostomia in elderly individuals: an institutional study. Contemp Clin Dent. 2012;3:173–5.
38. Mortazavi H, Baharvand M, Movahhedian A, Mohammadi M, Khodadoustan A. Xerostomia due to systemic disease: a review of 20 conditions and mechanisms. Ann Med Health Sci Res. 2014;4:503–10.
39. Baszis K, Toib D, Cooper M, French A, White A. Recurrent Parotitis as a presentation of primary pediatric Sjögren syndrome. Pediatrics. 2012;129:e179–e82.
40. Ioannidis JP, Vassiliou VA, Moutsopoulos HM. Long-term risk of mortality and lymphoproliferative disease and predictive classification of primary Sjogren's syndrome. Arthritis Rheum. 2002;46:741–7.
41. Amezcua-Guerra LM, Hofmann F, Vargas A, et al. Joint involvement in primary syndrome: an ultrasound target area approach to arthritis. Biomed Res Int. 2013;2013:9.
42. Argyropoulou OD, Gunti S, Kapsogeorgou EK, Notkins AL, Tzioufas AG. Decrease in the ratio of polyreactive IgG titers with IgG concentration is associated with long-term complications of primary Sjogren's syndrome. Clin Exp Rheumatol. 2018;36(Suppl 112):239–40.
43. Zdebik A, Evans R, Walsh SB, Ciurtin C. Renal involvement in primary Sjögren's syndrome. Rheumatology. 2015;54:1541–8.
44. Carvajal Alegria G, Guellec D, Mariette X, et al. Epidemiology of neurological manifestations in Sjögren's syndrome: data from the French ASSESS cohort. RMD Open. 2016;2:e000179.
45. Perzyńska-Mazan J, Maślińska M, Gasik R. Neurological manifestations of primary Sjögren's syndrome. Reumatologia. 2018;56:99–105.
46. Soliotis FC, Mavragani CP, Moutsopoulos HM. Central nervous system involvement in Sjögren's syndrome. Ann Rheum Dis. 2004;63:616–20.
47. Kittridge A, Routhouska SB, Korman NJ. Dermatologic manifestations of Sjögren syndrome. J Cutan Med Surg. 2011;15:8–14.
48. Fragkioudaki S, Mavragani CP, Moutsopoulos HM. Predicting the risk for lymphoma development in Sjogren syndrome: an easy tool for clinical use. Medicine. 2016;95:e3766-e.

49. Avouac J, Sordet C, Depinay C, et al. Systemic sclerosis-associated Sjogren's syndrome and relationship to the limited cutaneous subtype: results of a prospective study of sicca syndrome in 133 consecutive patients. Arthritis Rheum. 2006;54:2243–9.
50. Kobak S, Oksel F, Aksu K, Kabasakal Y. The frequency of sicca symptoms and Sjogren's syndrome in patients with systemic sclerosis. Int J Rheum Dis. 2013;16:88–92.
51. Katsikis P, Youinou P, Jouquan J, Pennec YL, Fauquert P, Goff PL. Raynaud's phenomenon in primary Sjogren's syndrome. Rheumatology. 1990;29:205–7.
52. Tsukamoto M, Suzuki K, Takeuchi T. Clinical and immunological features of anti-centromere antibody-positive primary Sjogren's syndrome. Rheumatol Ther. 2018;5:499–505.
53. Tektonidou M, Kaskani E, Skopouli FN, Moutsopoulos HM. Microvascular abnormalities in Sjogren's syndrome: nailfold capillaroscopy. Rheumatology. 1999;38:826–30.
54. Bournia V-KK, Diamanti KD, Vlachoyiannopoulos PG, Moutsopoulos HM. Anticentromere antibody positive Sjögren's syndrome: a retrospective descriptive analysis. Arthritis Res Ther. 2010;12:R47-R.
55. Vitali C, Bombardieri S, Jonsson R, et al. Classification criteria for Sjögren's syndrome: a revised version of the European criteria proposed by the American-European consensus group. Ann Rheum Dis. 2002;61:554–8.
56. Franceschini F, Cavazzana I, Andreoli L, Tincani A. The 2016 classification criteria for primary Sjogren's syndrome: what's new? BMC Med. 2017;15:69.
57. Leonardi A, Van Setten G, Amrane M, et al. Efficacy and safety of 0.1% cyclosporine a cationic emulsion in the treatment of severe dry eye disease: a multicenter randomized trial. Eur J Ophthalmol. 2016;26:287–96.
58. Saraux A, Pers JO, Devauchelle-Pensec V. Treatment of primary Sjogren syndrome. Nat Rev Rheumatol. 2016;12:456–71.
59. Gottenberg JE, Ravaud P, Puechal X, et al. Effects of hydroxychloroquine on symptomatic improvement in primary Sjogren syndrome: the JOQUER randomized clinical trial. JAMA. 2014;312:249–58.
60. Ramos-Casals M, Tzioufas AG, Font J. Primary Sjögren's syndrome: new clinical and therapeutic concepts. Ann Rheum Dis. 2005;64:347–54.

Chapter 24
Male Sexual Dysfunction in Systemic Sclerosis

Ulrich A. Walker

Case

A 35 year old man was diagnosed with secondary Raynaud's phenomenon in the year 2010. He was positive for ANA with anti-topoisomerase-1 specificity. At two annual visits in Feburary 2011 and February 2012, he had only slight scleredema, but no other signs of scleroderma skin involvement. Only 5 months later, in July 2012, he presented with diffuse skin sclerosis and a mRSS of 20. He noticed that he was less fit as a mountain biker and reported new erectile difficulties. His wife was 5 months pregnant. In March 2013, his mRSS had further increased to 35 and he had developed discrete ground-glass opacifications and a slightly depressed forced vital capacity (FVC, 79% of normal). At this time, his erectile function has declined further, his score on the International Index of Erectile Function (IIEF)-5 questionnaire had worsened to 15.

In March 2013, the patient underwent autologous hematopoietic stem cell transplantation as a treatment of systemic

U. A. Walker (✉)
Dept. of Rheumatology, Basel University, Basel, Switzerland
e-mail: ulrich.walker@usb.ch

© Springer Nature Switzerland AG 2021
M. Matucci-Cerinic, C. P. Denton (eds.), *Practical Management of Systemic Sclerosis in Clinical Practice*, In Clinical Practice,
https://doi.org/10.1007/978-3-030-53736-4_24

Table 24.1 Evolution of skin, lung and erectile function after autologous stem cell transplantation for systemic sclerosis in March 2013

Time of visit	Skin Score	Lung function	Erectile function
March 2013	mRSS 35	FVC: 79%	IIEF-5 15
August 2013	mRSS 13	FVC: 102%	IIEF-5 12
September 2014	mRSS 8	FVC: 107%	IIEF-5 22
Mai 2015	mRSS 8	FVC: 113%	IIEF-5 23

sclerosis. The skin score declined and lung function improved rapidly (Table 24.1), the erectile function normalized within the ensuing 18 months and the family has now a second baby. The patient is now not taking any medication.

Background

Erectile dysfunction (ED) is very common in men with systemic sclerosis (SSc) but frequently not addressed [1, 2]. The pathogenesis of ED in SSc involves a diminished arterial blood flow in the penis, and an excessive fibrosis of the penile corpora cavernosa due to an increased synthesis of collagen by local smooth muscle cells, and the accumulation of extracellular matrix [1]. The fibrotic processes are likely perpetuated by hypoxia, which fosters the local release of profibrotic cytokines such as transforming growth factor (TGF)-β_1, platelet derived growth factor (PDGF) and its receptors [1, 3]. Veno-occlusive dysfunction was also reported and may contribute to ED [4].

Even in the general population, the prevalence of ED is not negligible. About half of all men between 40 and 70 years of age have ED at some degree [4]. Cardiovascular risk factor such as diabetes mellitus, hyperlipidemia, arterial hypertension, tobacco exposure, lack of physical activity contribute to the risk of ED in the general population [5]. Other conditions associated with ED in men without SSc include prostatic disease, central nervous system disorders, hypogonadism and hyperprolactinemia [5]. Drugs that cause ED include thiazide

TABLE 24.2 Drugs associated with ED [5]

- Thiazides, spironolactone
- Antihypertensives (beta-blockers, clonidine)
- Digoxin
- Fenofibrate
- Antidepressants (tricyclics, monoamine oxidase inhibitors, lithium, selective serotonin reuptake inhibitors)
- Cimetidine, ranitidine
- Hormones (estrogens, progesterone, LH-RH agonists, cyproterone acetate)
- Corticosteroids
- 5-alpha reductase inhibitors
- Cytotoxic agents (cyclophosphamide and methotrexate)
- Anticholinergics
- Alcohol, cocaine, marihuana, opioids, tobacco

diuretics, spironolactone, beta-blockers, H2 antagonists, antidepressants, alcohol and cocaine (Table 24.2).

In SSc however, only about one fifth of all men have normal erectile function [2, 6, 7]. In SSc, the ED is generally also more severe than the ED in the general population as about 40% have severe impotence. The average IIEF-5 score in SSc was about 13 [8], in comparison to the IIEF-5 score in a non-SSc population of similar age (about 21) [9]. ED in SSc evolves quite rapidly after the first non-Raynaud's symptom of SSc, the delay of ED onset is on average as short as 3 to 4 years [2, 7]. An analysis by ED duration, revealed a negative correlation between the IIEF-5 score and time of ED [2], indicting that the severity of ED is progressive with time. Similar to the general population [4] the prevalence of ED in men with SSc also increases with age and with the degree of alcohol consumption but in SSc is additionally associated with severe cutaneous, muscular or renal involvement of SSc, elevated pulmonary pressures and restrictive lung disease [2].

No particular ANA specificity was found to be protective or conferring an elevated risk of ED development in SSc [2].

Management

In clinical practice, ED can be assessed easily with the International Index of Erectile Function (IIEF)-5, a self-administered sexual activity questionnaire that is linguistically validated in many languages, has high retest reliability, and has demonstrated sensitivity and specificity for detecting treatment-related changes [3]. It takes about 30 s of the patient's time to complete the IIEF-5 questionnaire. The IIEF-5 delivers a numerical score that is classified into five categories: severe ED (scores 5 to 7), moderate ED (scores 8 to 11), mild to moderate ED (scores 12 to 16), mild ED (scores 17 to 21), and no ED (scores 22 to 25).

Men with SSc should be routinely asked for symptoms of ED and issued an IIEF-5 score. When ED is diagnosed (IIEF-5 score below 22), the workup consists of excluding non-SSc causes by means of history, physical examination and a limited set of laboratory investigations (Table 24.2 and Fig. 24.1). One focus of the workup should focus be the search for modifiable cardiovascular risk factors.

Treatment guidelines of ED in the general population suggest that modifiable risk factors such as lifestyle, psychological and drug-related contributors to ED, be minimized prior to, or in conjunction with specific ED therapy [5, 10]. Patients with known cardiovascular diseases should be counselled appropriately, as ED could be the first sign of an underlying coronary artery disease.

A PDE-5 inhibitor is generally the recommended first line treatment modality in the non-SSc population [10]. In SSc however, the efficacy data of PDE-5 inhibitors for ED with on-demand sildenafil are disappointing [11] and the longer acting tadalafil is better evaluated [12, 13]. Different dosing regimens of tadalafil have been investigated: 20 mg of

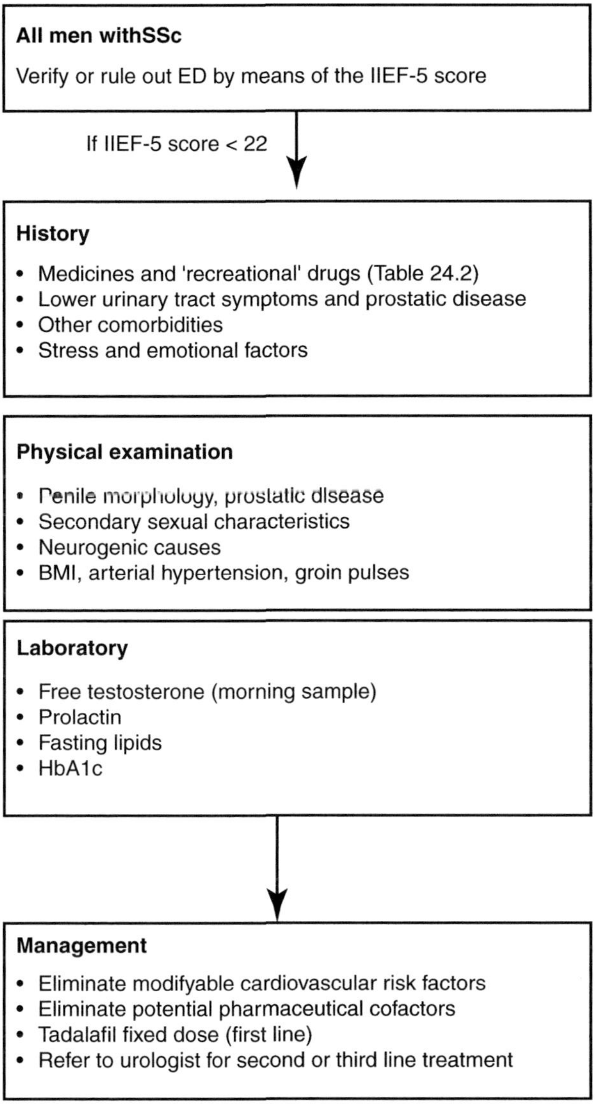

All men withSSc

Verify or rule out ED by means of the IIEF-5 score

↓ If IIEF-5 score < 22

History

- Medicines and 'recreational' drugs (Table 24.2)
- Lower urinary tract symptoms and prostatic disease
- Other comorbidities
- Stress and emotional factors

Physical examination

- Penile morphology, prostatic disease
- Secondary sexual characteristics
- Neurogenic causes
- BMI, arterial hypertension, groin pulses

Laboratory

- Free testosterone (morning sample)
- Prolactin
- Fasting lipids
- HbA1c

↓

Management

- Eliminate modifyable cardiovascular risk factors
- Eliminate potential pharmaceutical cofactors
- Tadalafil fixed dose (first line)
- Refer to urologist for second or third line treatment

FIGURE 24.1 Diagnosis and management of sexual dysfunction in men with SSc

tadalafil administered in a fixed alternate day regimen [26], and 10 mg of tadalafil given daily [27]. Both tadalafil dosing regimen were shown to have some efficacy, on demand tadalafil however was not [26]. Tadalafil must therefore be given in a fixed dose regimen. Tadalafil is also useful to alleviate Raynaud's phenomenon [14] and a licensed treatment for pulmonary arterial hypertension [15]. Tadalafil however must not be combined with riociguat and nitrates [16, 17]. Retinitis pigmentosa is another main contraindication [18].

Second line treatments of ED consist of intraurethral or intracavernous alprostadil (prostaglandin E1) applications [18]. In patients with SSc, however, a substantial percentage does not respond adequately to intracavernous alprostadil injections [8]. Vacuum devices are another second line option, but the experience is SSc is very limited. Penile prosthesis were used only very rarely in SSc, although successful implantations were reported [2]. In the non-SSc population, the satisfaction rate with penile prosthesis is high [18].

Although the case discussed above suggests a favorable course of erectile dysfunction after autologous hematopoietic stem cell transplantation, further data on the efficacy and mechanism of this treatment modality on ED in SSc is lacking. A study is however under way.

References

1. Walker UA, Tyndall A, Ruszat R. Erectile dysfunction in systemic sclerosis. Ann Rheum Dis. 2009;68:1083–5.
2. Foocharoen C, Tyndall A, Hachulla E, et al. Erectile dysfunction is frequent in systemic sclerosis and associated with severe disease: a study of the EULAR scleroderma trial and research group. Arthritis Res Ther. 2012;14:R37.
3. Aversa A, Basciani S, Visca P, et al. Platelet-derived growth factor (PDGF) and PDGF receptors in rat corpus cavernosum: changes in expression after transient in vivo hypoxia. J Endocrinol. 2001;170:395–402.
4. Nehra A, Hall SJ, Basile G, et al. Systemic sclerosis and impotence: a clinicopathological correlation. J Urol. 1995;153:1140–6.

5. McVary KT. Clinical practice. Erectile dysfunction. N Engl J Med. 2007;357:2472–81.
6. Nowlin NS, Brick JE, Weaver DJ, et al. Impotence in scleroderma. Ann Intern Med. 1986;104:794–8.
7. Hong P, Pope JE, Ouimet JM, et al. Erectile dysfunction associated with scleroderma: a case-control study of men with scleroderma and rheumatoid arthritis. J Rheumatol. 2004;31:508–13.
8. Aversa A, Proietti M, Bruzziches R, et al. The penile vasculature in systemic sclerosis: a duplex ultrasound study. J Sex Med. 2006;3:554–8.
9. Ponholzer A, Temml C, Mock K, et al. Prevalence and risk factors for erectile dysfunction in 2869 men using a validated questionnaire. Eur Urol. 2005;47:80–5.
10. Hatzimouratidis K, Amar E, Eardley I, et al. Guidelines on male sexual dysfunction: erectile dysfunction and premature ejaculation. Eur Urol. 2010;57:804–14.
11. Ostojic P, Damjanov N. The impact of depression, microvasculopathy, and fibrosis on development of erectile dysfunction in men with systemic sclerosis. Clin Rheumatol. 2007;26:1671–4.
12. Aversa A, Greco E, Bruzziches R, et al. Relationship between chronic tadalafil administration and improvement of endothelial function in men with erectile dysfunction: a pilot study. Int J Impot Res. 2007;19:200–7.
13. Proietti M, Aversa A, Letizia C, et al. Erectile dysfunction in systemic sclerosis: effects of longterm inhibition of phosphodiesterase type-5 on erectile function and plasma endothelin-1 levels. J Rheumatol. 2007;34:1712–7.
14. Roustit M, Blaise S, Allanore Y, et al. Phosphodiesterase-5 inhibitors for the treatment of secondary Raynaud's phenomenon: systematic review and meta-analysis of randomised trials. Ann Rheum Dis. 2013;72:1696–9.
15. Galie N, Brundage BH, Ghofrani HA, et al. Tadalafil therapy for pulmonary arterial hypertension. Circulation. 2009;119:2894–903.
16. Galie N, Muller K, Scalise AV, et al. PATENT PLUS: a blinded, randomised and extension study of riociguat plus sildenafil in pulmonary arterial hypertension. Eur Respir J. 2015;45:1314–22.
17. Kloner RA, Hutter AM, Emmick JT, et al. Time course of the interaction between tadalafil and nitrates. J Am Coll Cardiol. 2003;42:1855–60.
18. Wespes E, Amar E, Hatzichristou D, et al. EAU guidelines on erectile dysfunction: an update. Eur Urol. 2006;49:806–15.

Chapter 25
How to Assess a Patient for HSCT

J. M. van Laar, J. Spierings, and M. C. Vonk

The treatment of patients with diffuse cutaneous systemic sclerosis (dcSSc) poses the clinician with multiple challenges. When to start first-line immunosuppressive therapy and what to choose (mycophenolate mofetil or methotrexate)? When to switch to cyclophosphamide or dose-intensified cyclophosphamide with hematopoietic stem cell transplantation (HSCT)? The outcome of dcSSc has steadily improved over the decades due to early recognition and effective treatment of renal crisis, pulmonary arterial hypertension and interstitial lung disease, and prevention of malnutrition and deconditioning. Nevertheless a subset of dcSSc patients still develop progressive disease in spite of conventional treatment and such patients must be considered eligible for autologous HSCT, which has been employed in over 400 SSc patients in Europe and been proven superior in three controlled clinical

J. M. van Laar (✉) · J. Spierings
Department of Rheumatology and Clinical Immunology, University Medical Centre Utrecht, Utrecht, The Netherlands
e-mail: j.m.vanlaar@umcutrecht.nl; j.spierings@umcutrecht.nl

M. C. Vonk
Department of Rheumatology, Radboud University Medical Centre, Nijmegen, The Netherlands
e-mail: madelon.vonk@radboudumc.nl

© Springer Nature Switzerland AG 2021
M. Matucci-Cerinic, C. P. Denton (eds.), *Practical Management of Systemic Sclerosis in Clinical Practice*, In Clinical Practice,
https://doi.org/10.1007/978-3-030-53736-4_25

trials which together involved over 250 patients [1–4]. Selection criteria have shifted towards earlier disease to avoid toxicities from HSCT in advanced disease and to increase the probability of inducing sustained drug-free remission in early disease. Nevertheless, access to HSCT clinics with expertise in transplanting SSc is limited in most countries due to financial constraints, regulatory hurdles or lack of experience. In the absence of effective conventional therapies, progressive dcSSc will continue to be an area of unmet need for those not having access to HSCT.

HSCT is not a cure for all, however, and the potential risks and intended benefits need to be weighed carefully in each case. Comprehensive screening including assessment of visceral organ involvement is paramount before a go or no-go decision with respect to HSCT can be made. The dilemmas in clinical decision making are illustrated by two cases with early progressive dcSSc. These cases underscore the need for comprehensive cardiac screening, tight monitoring of disease course and repeated assessment of risk and outcome after HSCT, taking into account alternative treatment options and patient preference.

A 37-year-old male was referred to the Rheumatology outpatient clinic of a tertiary referral centre by his general practitioner because of recent onset fatigue and Raynaud's phenomenon. Puffy fingers and mild skin thickening (modified Rodnan Skin Score (mRSS 1/51)) were observed during his first visit. ANA and anti-topoisomerase antibodies were positive, nailfold capillaroscopy showed an active scleroderma pattern. He was diagnosed with early SSc. There were no signs of lung or renal involvement. In routine laboratory tests, a markedly elevated high-sensitivity cardiac troponin I (hs-cTnI) was detected (180 ng/L; normal range 0-18 ng/L). Creatine phosphokinase-MB and creatine phosphokinase levels were mildly increased as well. No cardiac symptoms were present. Electrocardiography was normal at rest and after ergometric stress testing. Cardiac ultrasound did not reveal any signs of peri- or myocarditis. Magnetic resonance imaging of the heart (CMR) showed an ejection fraction

(LVEF) of 64%, no acute ischemia (at rest and after adenosin stress testing). There was no delayed enhancement. T1 values were slightly increased (1100 ms) and disturbance of the extracellular volume fraction was seen in 35% of the assessed area, T2 values were higher than 2, indicating mild focal myocardial fibrosis. As the hs-cTnI was consistently raised in the presence of poor prognostic factors (male sex, anti-topoisomerase antibodies, early onset of non-Raynaud's symptoms), administration of oral mycophenolate (1.5 g bd) and an *angiotensin-converting-enzyme (ACE) inhibitor* was initiated. In the following months, however, both hs-cTnI and skin thickening increased (Fig. 25.1). Concomitantly, he developed pulmonary symptoms, which was attributed to new interstitial lung disease. The therapeutic options in this rapid progressive case, were discussed with the patient and multidisciplinary team. Cyclophosphamide (CYC) and rituximab was considered, but because of the fast deterioration and patient's preference, HSCT was opted for. Prior to HSCT, pulmonary hypertension was excluded with right heart catheterisation. 24-hour holter ECG was performed to exclude conduction disturbances. For HSCT, CYC (4 g/m^2) in

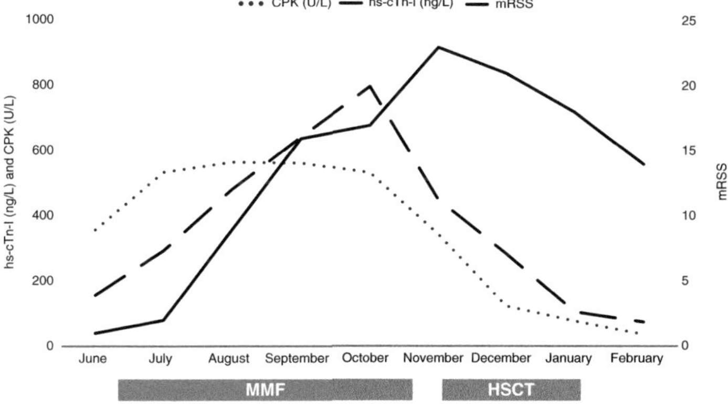

FIGURE 25.1 Changes in creatine phosphokinase (dotted line), high-sensitivity troponin (dashed line) and modified Rodnan skin score (uninterrupted line) in a patient following autologous stem cell transplantation

combination with granulocyte-colony stimulating factor (G-CSF) for mobilization and CYC 200 mg/kg and ATG 7.5 mg/kg for conditioning were used. No adverse events occurred. To date, 3 months after HSCT, he is recovering well without any cardiac events. hs-cTnI has decreased significantly.

A 50-year-old female patient was referred to the Rheumatology clinic of a tertiary referral centre by a local rheumatologist for possible systemic sclerosis. Her medical history consisted of bilateral carpal tunnel syndrome 6 months earlier. She reported edema of the legs with tightening since 3 months and a new onset Raynaud's phenomenon for 2 months but no other complaints. On examination she had a normal blood pressure, unremarkable examination of heart and lungs, arthralgia, a mRSS of 17 and no tendon friction rubs. Her laboratory workup was unremarkable apart from a positive result of antiRNApolymerase III. Pulmonary function showed a FVC 101% predicted and DLCO 60% predicted. On HRCT scan of the chest very mild ILD was present. Her echocardiography was unremarkable. Diagnosed with dcSSc, she was counselled on the different treatment options and she chose to start with cyclophosphamide iv pulses. ACE inhibition was started. After 3 pulses she was progressing with a decreased quality of life, fatigue, pruritis and a mRSS of 32. She was informed about HSCT and agreed to be evaluated and if eligible, treated with this option. A repeat echocardiography was normal, but pulmonary function tests showed deterioration of lung function (FVC 76% pred and DLCO 53% pred) upon which she was referred for left and right catheterisation with fluid challenge. Her coronaries were unremarkable, no pulmonary hypertension was present but her LVEDP increased from 12 to 16 during the fluid challenge with 500 cc normal saline, consistent with mild diastolic dysfunction. After multidisciplinary consultation with rheumatologists, pulmonologists, cardiologists and haematologists she was approved for HSCT. During the hyperhydration phase she experienced acute heart failure with elevated NT-proBNP of 5000 pg/mL (normal <250 pg/L) which was treated with diuretics. At day 18, during repopulation after successful apharesis, she again experienced dyspnea, chestpain, reduced saturation and fluid retention without parenteral fluid administration. At that time, her troponin was 248 ng/L (normal <14 ng/L), NT-proBNP 3900 pg/L and echocardiography showed a normal LV function, with EF of 61% and no diastolic dysfunction, but a pericardial effusion of 13 mm. The cause of her pericardiomyositis was considered to be progressive dcSSc or toxicity of cyclophosphamide. She was subsequently treated with diuretics, low dose betablockers and an increased dosage of ACE inhibition together with high dose corticosteroids. A new echocardiography after 10 days of treatment showed normal function of the left and right ventricle and a decrease in effusion to 1 mm.. Because of the cardiac event, the risk of HSCT was considered higher than normal in this patient, and she was again reviewed in the multidisciplinary team. The wish of our patient was to continue the HSCT and we decided to perform this on the ICU. The conditioning including ATG was unremarkable as well as the period to repopulation and she was discharged day +17. Her recovery has been unremarkable to date, and after 6 months she has an improved quality of life, a stable pulmonary, cardiac and renal function and her mRSS has decreased to 27.

In the first case, subclinical cardiac involvement was detected in early dcSSc by routine measurement of cardiac markers. Hs-cTnI is a highly specific marker for myocardiac involvement, in contrast to cTnT, which can also be elevated in skeletal muscle disease activity [5]. As cardiac disease in SSc can exist subclinically and may lead to severe complications, comprehensive cardiac screening in SSc patients eligible for HSCT is highly recommended. Elevated cardiac troponin levels are associated with heart failure, conduction disorders, extensive skin involvement and disease-related death [6, 7]. CMR can also be very helpful in the further work-up in patients with suspected cardiac SSc and rapidly progressive dcSSc [8, 9]. Close monitoring for disease progression is warranted in these patients, and although there is no robust evidence for the optimal treatment of patients with myocardial involvement, high intensity immunosuppressive therapies should be considered in case conventional therapies are not effective, if necessary in ICU as illustrated by the second case.Hyperhydration schemes may be adjusted in patients with cardiac involvement. Alternatively, as high dose cyclophosphamide is cardiotoxic, different transplant regimens have been propagated for patients with cardiac involvement although their risk/benefit have not yet been thoroughly evaluated in SSc-transplant settings. Prophylactic ICD (implantable cardioverter defibrillators) implantation has also been advocated in high-risk patients [10, 11]. More evidence on the optimal and safe management in this group may be provided by two ongoing studies (NCT03593902 and NCT01895244).

The pros and cons of HSCT in SSc patients with cardiac involvement should be discussed extensively with the patients and given the risks, HSCT in such patients is best performed by experienced multidisciplinary teams.

References

1. Snowden JA, Sharrack B, Ail M, Kiely DG, Lobo A, Kazmi M, Muraro PA, Lindsay JO. Autologous haematopoietic stem cell transplantation (aHSCT) for severe resistant autoimmune and inflammatory diseases - a guide to the generalist. Clin Med. 2018;18:329–34.
2. Sullivan KM, Goldmuntz EA, Keyes-Elstein L, McSweeney PA, Pinckney A, Welch B, et al. Myeloablative autologous stem-cell transplantation for severe scleroderma. N Engl J Med. 2018;378:35–47.
3. Burt RK, Shah SJ, Dill K, Grant T, Gheorghiade M, Schroeder J, et al. Autologous non-myeloablative haemopoietic stem-cell transplantation compared with pulse cyclophosphamide once per month for systemic sclerosis (ASSIST): an open-label, randomised phase 2 trial. Lancet. 2011;378:498–506.
4. van Laar JM, Farge D, Sont JK, Naraghi K, Marjanovic Z, Larghero J, et al. Autologous hematopoietic stem cell transplantation vs intravenous pulse cyclophosphamide in diffuse

cutaneous systemic sclerosis: a randomized clinical trial. JAMA. 2014;311:2490–8.

5. Hughes M, Lilleker JB, Herrick AL, Chinoy H. Cardiac troponin testing in idiopathic inflammatory myopathies and systemic sclerosis-spectrum disorders: biomarkers to distinguish between primary cardiac involvement and low-grade skeletal muscle disease activity. Ann Rheum Dis. 2015;74:795–8.
6. Bosello S, De Luca G, Berardi G, Canestrari G, de Waure C, Gabrielli FA, et al. Cardiac troponin T and NT-proBNP as diagnostic and prognostic biomarkers of primary cardiac involvement and disease severity in systemic sclerosis: a prospective study. Eur J Int Med. 2019;60:46–53.
7. Vasta B, Flower V, Bucciarelli-Ducci C, Brown S, Korendowych E, McHugh NJ, et al. Abnormal cardiac enzymes in systemic sclerosis: a report of four patients and review of the literature. Clinical Rheumatol. 2014;33:435–8.
8. Mavrogeni SI, Bratis K, Karabela G, Spiliotis G, Wijk K, Hautemann D, et al. Cardiovascular magnetic resonance imaging clarifies cardiac pathophysiology in early, asymptomatic diffuse systemic sclerosis. Inflamm Allergy Drug Targets. 2015;14:29–36.
9. Mavrogeni S, Schwitter J, van Rossum A, Nijveldt R, Aletras A, Kolovou G, et al. Cardiac magnetic resonance imaging in myocardial inflammation in autoimmune rheumatic diseases: an appraisal of the diagnostic strengths and limitations of the Lake Louise criteria. Int J Cardiol. 2018;252:216–9.
10. Farge D, Burt RK, Oliveira MC, Mousseaux E, Rovira M, Marjanovic Z, et al. Cardiopulmonary assessment of patients with systemic sclerosis for hematopoietic stem cell transplantation: recommendations from the European Society for Blood and Marrow Transplantation Autoimmune Diseases Working Party and collaborating partners. Bone Marrow Transplant. 2017;52:1495–503.
11. Henes JC, Koetter I, Horger M, Schmalzing M, Mueller K, Eick C, et al. Autologous stem cell transplantation with thiotepa-based conditioning in patients with systemic sclerosis and cardiac manifestations. Rheumatology (Oxford). 2014;53(5):919–22.

Chapter 26
Very Early Systemic Sclerosis: VEDOSS Type Case

Lepri Gemma, Tracy M. Frech, and Silvia Bellando-Randone

Background

Systemic sclerosis (SSc) is a chronic connective tissue disease characterized by a small-vessel vasculopathy, immune dysregulation with specific auto-antibodies (abs), and fibrosis of the skin and internal organs. The fact that SSc is heterogeneous and unpredictable makes the diagnosis more difficult in particular in the early phases of the disease. In addition, SSc patients present the highest mortality among rheumatic diseases because it is frequently resistant to immunosuppressive therapy [1].

Therefore, it is mandatory not to delay the diagnosis when organ involvement is evident in order to avoid the irrevers-

L. Gemma · S. Bellando-Randone (✉)
Dept of Experimental and Clinical Medicine, University of Florence, Florence, Italy

Dept of Geriatric Medicine, Div Rheumatology AOUC, Florence, Italy

T. M. Frech
Department of Internal Medicine, Division of Rheumatology, University of Utah, Salt Lake City, UT, USA

© Springer Nature Switzerland AG 2021

M. Matucci-Cerinic, C. P. Denton (eds.), *Practical Management of Systemic Sclerosis in Clinical Practice*, In Clinical Practice, https://doi.org/10.1007/978-3-030-53736-4_26

ible fibrotic damage [2–4]. The 1980 American College of Rheumatology (ACR) classification criteria requiring either the presence of skin fibrosis proximal to metacarpophalangeal (MCP) or metatarsophalangeal (MTP) joints or the presence of two items between sclerodactily, digital ulcers (DU) and lung fibrosis, have been shown to be not sensitive to diagnose early SSc [5]. In order to overcome this limitation, several different proposed classification criteria for SSc were proposed throughout the years [6]. The delay to diagnosis is calculated to be 6.1 years after the onset of Raynaud's phenomenon (RP) and 2.7 years after the onset of the first non-Raynaud's phenomenon symptom [7]. This large gap could be considered for the rheumatologist as the *windows of opportunity:* in fact, an early diagnosis may allow the choice of the treatment before SSc manifestations are still reversible.

A study conducted in more than 500 SSc patients demonstrated that RP, specific SSc-abs and/or typical abnormalities on nailfold videocapillaroscopy are sixty times more likely to develop definite SSc [8]. For this reason, in 2010, the EULAR (European League Against Rheumatism) Scleroderma Trials and Research Group (EUSTAR) identified preliminary criteria for very early diagnosis of SSc. The presence of RP, puffy fingers and ANA positivity are possible signs of a very early SSc. If patients also present SSc-specific abs (ACA or anti-TopoI abs) and/or abnormal capillaroscopic pattern (early, active, late) the diagnosis of very early SSc (VEDOSS) can be made [9]. The preliminary analysis of the VEDOSS database suggested puffy fingers together with RP and ANA positivity were the signs to raise suspicion of very early SSc [10]. When a patient fulfills VEDOSS criteria further investigations to assess internal organ involvement are mandatory. In particular esophageal manometry, B-mode echocardiography and lung function tests are recommended to detect preclinical alterations of internal organs in SSc. In fact, studies demonstrated that SSc organ internal involvement may be precocious and subclinical, emphasizing the importance of an early diagnosis [11, 12].

A breakthrough in the management of SSc is given by new ACR/EULAR 2013 classification criteria [13] that, considering seven items besides skin involvement allow a physician to identify patients in the early stages of disease (Table 26.1). In these classification criteria, vascular items (RP, DU and telangiectasia) together with puffy fingers and other instrumental and laboratory findings (nailfold videocapillaroscopy and

Table 26.1 2013 ACR/EULAR classification criteria (adapted from [17])

Item	Sub-item (s)	Score
Skin thickening of the fingers of both hands extending proximal to the metacarpophalangeal (MCP) joints (sufficient criterion)	–	9
Skin thickening of the fingers (only count the higher score)	Puffy fingers Sclerodactyly of the fingers (distal to MCP joints but proximal to the IP joints)	2 4
Fingertip lesions (*only count the higher score*)	Digital tip ulcers Fingertip pitting scars	2 3
Telangiectasia	–	2
Abnormal nailfold capillaries	–	2
Pulmonary arterial hypertension and/or interstitial lung disease (*maximum score is 2*)	Pulmonary arterial hypertension Interstitial lung disease	2 2
Raynaud's phenomenon	–	3
SSc-related autoantibodies	ACA Anti-TopoI Anti-RNA polymerase III	3

SSc-specific abs), are part of the score. In the literature, it is reported that DU could be present since the early phase of SSc and could be also be a sentinel sign for early internal organ involvement [14].

The fact that the scientific community is focusing on the need for early diagnosis of SSc remarks the importance to identify the *window of opportunity* for an early treatment of the disease. While not proven, some experts have suggested that aggressive therapy, despite drug toxicity, is warranted in early SSc to prevent disease progression. However, at present, no drug or combination of drugs has been studied adequately in the "very early" disease. It should be remarked that calcium channel blockers, phosphodiesterase inhibitors, prostanoids, endothelin receptor antagonists, angiotensin converting enzyme (ACE) inhibitors and immunosuppressive agents (as cyclophosphamide, mycophenolate mofetil, methotrexate) [15] have improved the survival of SSc patients in the last 25 years. This data highlights the importance of starting early treatment when it may be more effective and has the potential to induce durable remission.

Clinical Case 1

A 32-year female came to our attention for the first time in 2010 presenting a 3-year history of Raynaud phenomenon which worsened in the last year with associated paresthesias, puffy fingers, but without digital trophic lesions. Upper limbs arterial echocolordoppler and blood examinations were normal. ANA and ACA resulted positive. Nailfold videocapillaroscopy showed an early scleroderma pattern [16] (Fig. 26.1) with rare megacapillaries and microhaemorrhages. Lung function tests and echocardiography were normal. She also referred gastro-esophageal reflux and pirosis and the clinical examination revealed puffy fingers. Following the 2013 ACR/EULAR classification criteria patient was classified as SSc (score of 10). She was treated with proton pump inhibitor and calcium channel blockers: after 2 months, the

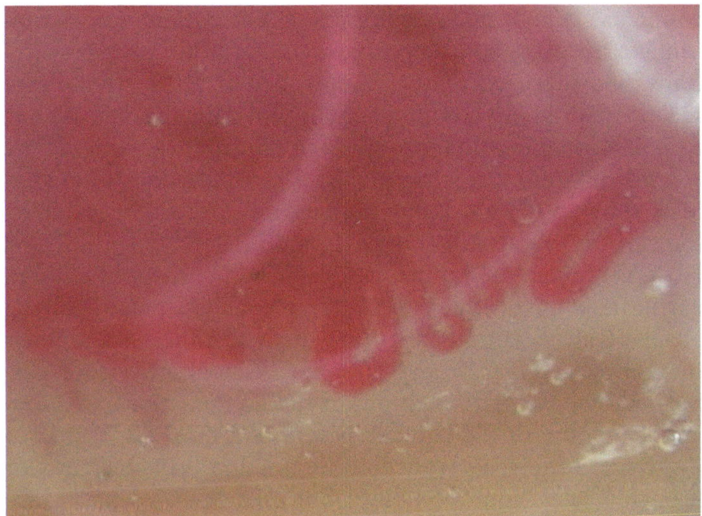

FIGURE 26.1 Early scleroderma pattern [16]

vasodilator was stopped due to severe headache. In order to avoid vascular complications, treatment with prostanoids was suggested but patient refused intravenous therapies and instead phosphodiesterase inhibitors were begun. Unfortunately, after 4 months the patient returned to clinic with a 2-week history of a DU and admitted to non-compliance with the phosphodiesterase inhibitor. The DU was treated with the endothelin antagonist (Bosentan) and local debridement: she maintained an adequate compliance with a rapid healing of DU documented in approximately a month.

Clinical Case 2

A 53-year old female that came to our attention in 2016 for the onset, 10 months earlier, of RP and puffy fingers. Nailfold videocapillaroscopy did not reveal SSc-specific abnormalities and the blood examinations showed ANA and anti-topoI positivity, a mild increase in C-reactive protein, normal blood count and hepatic and renal function. The patient was asymptomatic for dyspnoea, palpitations and gastrointestinal symptoms. She reported only rare episodes of RP in the winter season that did not limit her activities of daily life. The clinical examination did not reveal any sign of skin involvement. The echocardiography was normal and the pulmonary function tests showed normal lung volumes, but a diffusion capacity for carbon monoxyde (DLCO) value of 75% of predicted. However, given the known association of anti-topoI with an early organ involvement and the age of the patient at the onset of all symptoms also lung high resolution computed tomography (HRCT) and abdomen echography were performed. The two examinations excluded the presence of secondary nature of the clinical picture and the HRCT did not show sign of fibrosis (reticulation, traction bronchiectasis or bronchiectasis, honeycombing) but only bilateral basal limited areas of ground glass (Fig. 26.2a). These images were interpreted as an initial inflammatory lung involvement and i.v. cyclophosphamide was started. At follow-up at 9 months by mycophenolate mofetil. After 1 year, the HRCT chest (Fig. 26.2b) showed almost a complete disappearance of the ground glass areas. During this year and until today lung function tests were normal.

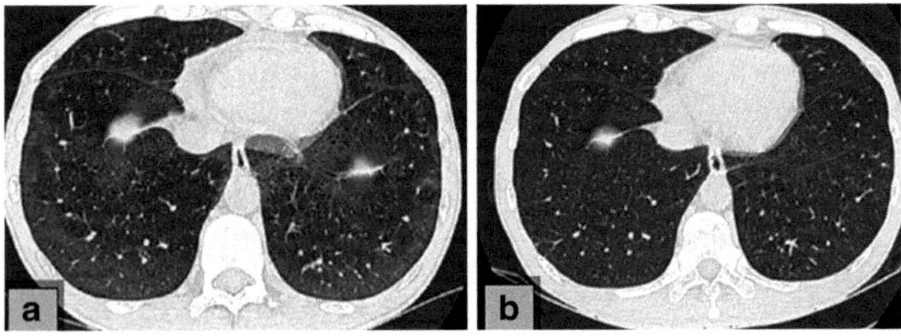

Figure 26.2 (**a**) the first HRCT with bilateral basal area of ground glass; (**b**) HRCT after 1 year shows the disappearance of ground glass

Discussion

These two cases show the importance of a careful evaluation of patients in the early stages of the disease. In fact, even in the absence of symptoms the involvement of internal organs may be already present. A comprehensive evaluation of organ involvement may identify the use of an effective treatment in a phase of the disease when damage is still reversible.

It is well known that in the early phase gastrointestinal involvement occurs in more than 80% of the patients and may predict disease progression [17]. In VEDOSS patients, Lepri et al. [12] showed that the lower oesophageal sphincter pressure and peristalsis resulted significantly abnormal, and oesophageal symptoms were detected in 49.1%. Also in patients without oesophageal symptoms, peristalsis speed was significantly lower. These data clearly show that the absence of symptoms does not exclude an oesophageal involvement and that in asymptomatic patients GI involvement should also be always suspected, and investigated. Additionally, lung involvement may be present in the early phase and should be assessed. In fact, if a DLCO reduction is identified by pulmonary function tests (PFTs), a subsequent assessment with HRCT chest for ground glass could be indicated. However, while HRCT is the gold standard examinationt in the assessment of SSs- ILD, it is characterized by high level of radiation exposure, for this reason modified protocols, PFTs [18] and lung ultrasound have been proposed in ILD screening and particularly for the patient follow-up n order to identify patients in which the repetition of HRCT may be justified. In conclusion, these two clinical cases show that the diagnosis of SSc must be early and a proactive approach for internal organ screening in SSc patients is important from the early stages. The possibility to use disease-modifying drugs in this stage is still debated, but is an important area of research.

Learning Key Messages

- The presence of RP, puffy fingers and ANA positivity are possible signs of a very early SSc. If patients also present SSc-specific abs (ACA or anti-TopoI abs) and/or abnormal capillaroscopic pattern (early, active, late) the diagnosis of very early SSc (VEDOSS) can be made.
- A careful evaluation of patients in the early stages of the SSc is recommended because organ involvement may be already present even in the absence of symptoms.
- Esophageal manometry, B-mode echocardiography and lung function tests are recommended to detect preclinical alterations of internal organs in SSc.

References

1. Varga J, Abraham D. Systemic sclerosis: a prototypic multisystem fibrotic disorder. J Clin Invest. 2007;117:557–67.
2. Hudson M, Taillefer S, Steel R, et al. Improving the sensitivity of the American College of Rheumatology classification criteria for systemic sclerosis. Clin Exp Rheumatol. 2007;25:754–7.
3. Czirjak L, Matucci-Cerinic M. Beyond Raynaud's phenomenon hides very early systemic sclerosis: the assessment of organ involvement is always mandatory. Rheumatology. 2011;50:250–1.
4. Avouac J, Fransen J, Walker UA, et al. Preliminary criteria for the very early diagnosis of systemic sclerosis (VEDOSS): results of a Delphi consensus study from EULAR scleroderma trials and research group (EUSTAR). Ann Rheum Dis. 2010;69(Suppl.3):128.
5. Subcommittee for scleroderma criteria of the American Rheumatism Association Diagnostic and Therapeutic Criteria Committee. Preliminary criteria for the classification of systemic sclerosis (scleroderma). Arthritis Rheum. 1980;23:581–90.
6. LeRoy EC, Medsger TA Jr. Criteria for the classification of early systemic sclerosis. J Rheumatol. 2001;28:1573–6.
7. Hudson M, Thombs B, Baron M. Time to diagnosis in systemic sclerosis: is gender a factor? Arthritis Rheum. 2007;56:487–9.

8. Koenig M, Joyal F, Fritzler MJ, et al. Autoantibodies and microvascular damage are independent predictive factors for the progression of Raynaud's phenomenon to systemic sclerosis: a twenty-year prospective study of 586 patients, with validation of proposed criteria for early systemic sclerosis. Arthritis Rheum. 2009;58:3902–12.
9. Matucci-Cerinic M, Allanore Y, Czirják L, et al. The challenge of early systemic sclerosis for the EULAR scleroderma trial and research group (EUSTAR) community. It is time to cut the Gordian knot and develop a prevention or rescue strategy. Ann Rheum Dis. 2009 Sep;68:1377–80.
10. Minier T, Guiducci S, Bellando-Randone S, et al. Preliminary analysis of the very early diagnosis of systemic sclerosis (VEDOSS) EUSTAR multicentre study: evidence for puffy fingers as a pivotal sign for suspicion of systemic sclerosis. Ann Rheum Dis. 2014 Dec;73(12):2087–93.
11. Valentini G, Cuomo G, Abignano G, et al. Early systemic sclerosis: assessment of clinical and preclinical organ involvement in patients with different disease features. Rheumatology. 2011;50:317–23.
12. Lepri G, Bellando-Randone S. Guiducci S, et al esophageal and anorectal involvement in patients with very early diagnosis of systemic sclerosis (VEDOSS): report from a single EUSTAR Centre. Ann Rheum Dis, Ann Rheum Dis. 2015 Jan;74(1):124–8.
13. van den Hoogen F, Khanna D, Fransen J, et al. Classification criteria for systemic sclerosis: an American college of rheumatology/European league against rheumatism collaborative initiative. Ann Rheum Dis. 2013;72(11):1747–55.
14. Bruni C, Guiducci S, Bellando-Randone S, Lepri G, Braschi F, Fiori G, Bartoli F, Peruzzi F, Blagojevic J, Matucci-Cerinic M. Digital ulcers as a sentinel sign for early internal organ involvement in very early systemic sclerosis. Rheumatology (Oxford). 2015;54(1):72–6.
15. Kowal-Bielecka O, Landewe R, Avouac J, Chwiesko S, Miniati I, Czirjak L, et al. EULAR/EUSTAR recommendations for the treatment of systemic sclerosis. Ann Rheum Dis. 2009;68:620–8.
16. Cutolo M, Pizzorni C, Tuccio M, Burroni A, Craviotto C, Basso M, et al. Nailfold videocapillaroscopic patterns and serum autoantibodies in systemic sclerosis. Rheumatology (Oxford). 2004 Jun;43(6):719–26.

17. Trapiella-Martínez L, Díaz-López JB, Caminal-Montero L, Tolosa-Vilella C, Guillén-Del Castillo A, Colunga-Argüelles D, et al. Very Early and Early Systemic Sclerosis in the Spanish Scleroderma Registry (RESCLE) Cohort. Autoimmun Rev. 2017 Aug;16(8):796–802.
18. Tashkin DP, Volkmann ER, Tseng CH, Kim HJ, Goldin J, Clements P, Furst D, Khanna D, Kleerup E, Roth MD, Elashoff R. Relationship between quantitative radiographic assessments of interstitial lung disease and physiological and clinical features of systemic sclerosis. Ann Rheum Dis. 2016 Feb;75(2):374–81. https://doi.org/10.1136/annrheumdis-2014-206076.

Chapter 27
Primary Biliary Cholangitis

Francesca Saffioti, Douglas Thorburn, and Massimo Pinzani

Hepatobiliary involvement is reported in about 7.5% of individuals affected by systemic sclerosis (SSc), with primary biliary cholangitis (PBC) diagnosed in about 60% of cases [1].

About 25% of patients affected by SSc show positivity for antimitocondrial antibody (AMA), the pathognomonic antibody of PBC, while 9–30% of PBC patients present a positive anticentromere antibody (ACA), the hallmark antibody of SSc [2]. It is estimated that 1.4–12.3% of PBC patients have concomitant SSc, in most cases represented by the limited cutaneous variant [3–5]. The pathogenesis of this association remains unclear but it has been suggested that common predisposing HLA alleles might exist [6].

Baseline biochemical values and overall survival rates are similar in patients with PBC alone and patients with PBC and SSc [1, 3, 7]. Pruritus and fatigue at diagnosis are more common in PBC alone, while patients with PBC-SSc appear to be more prone to develop septic complications [3].

F. Saffioti · D. Thorburn · M. Pinzani (✉)
UCL Institute for Liver and Digestive Health and Sheila Sherlock Liver Centre, Royal Free Hospital and UCL, London, UK
e-mail: francesca.saffioti@nhs.net; douglas.thorburn@nhs.net; m.pinzani@ucl.ac.uk

© Springer Nature Switzerland AG 2021
M. Matucci-Cerinic, C. P. Denton (eds.), *Practical Management of Systemic Sclerosis in Clinical Practice*, In Clinical Practice,
https://doi.org/10.1007/978-3-030-53736-4_27

Furthermore, patients with PBC alone seem to have a more rapid liver disease progression and a greater risk of liver transplantation (LT) and liver-related mortality, whereas PBC-SSc patients have higher rates of deaths from other causes [3].

Epidemiology of PBC

PBC is a chronic autoimmune cholestatic liver disease characterized by non-suppurative inflammation and subsequent destruction of the intrahepatic bile ducts. The disease is relatively rare, with a prevalence of 35–40/100,000 inhabitants.

and an estimate yearly incidence of 1–2 per 100,000 [8–10]; it is characterized by chronic cholestasis and typically affects middle-aged women (female to male ratio 9:1) [11, 12].

In about 95% of cases, PBC is characterised by the presence of AMA positivity [13]. Disease-specific antinuclear antibodies (ANA), anti-gp210 and anti-sp100, are also diagnostic and detected in up to 30% of AMA negative patients [14, 15].

PBC is likely the result of an interaction between environmental factors and genetic susceptibility, as confirmed by the identification of a large number of associated genetic loci in Genome-Wide Association Studies [16]. This explains why first-degree relatives, in particular females, carry a 10–35% increased risk of developing the disease compared to the general population [17]. Extrahepatic manifestations are seen in up to 73% of PBC patients, with SSc occurring in about 10% of cases within PBC cohorts [3, 7, 18].

Diagnosis

A diagnosis of PBC is established by the presence of persistent (>6 months) otherwise unexplained cholestasis [defined by an elevation of alkaline phosphatase (ALP) and/or gammaglutamyl-transpeptidase] associated with positive disease-specific autoantibodies (AMA>1:40 and/or PBC-specific ANA). A liver biopsy is required only in patients presenting with cholestatic serum biochemistry but negative diagnostic autoantibodies [11, 19] (Fig. 27.1). Typical histological features of PBC are florid bile duct lesions, mainly consisting of infiltrating T-lymphocytes, which affect interlobular and septal bile ducts and lead to the formation of non-suppurative epithelioid granulomas and progressive bile duct loss [20, 21]. In patients with SSc, the criteria for a diagnosis of PBC are not different. Similarly, in PBC patients a diagnosis of concomitant SSc is based on the standard diagnostic criteria [22, 23]. In the majority of PBC-SSc cases, the diagnosis of SSc predates that of PBC, and PBC is diagnosed at a younger age compared to individuals with PBC alone [3].

Natural History

The clinical course of PBC may be highly variable. The disease is generally slowly progressive, but can cause advanced liver fibrosis, cirrhosis and portal hypertension. Complications of portal hypertension include the development of ascites, oesophageal varices/variceal bleeding and hepatic encephalopathy. Cirrhotic patients are at risk of developing hepatocellular carcinoma, although its incidence in PBC is lower than in liver disease of other aetiologies [24]. The estimated mean survival in untreated patients is about 10 years from presentation [25].

Liver transplantation remains the definitive treatment for end-stage PBC but is also considered in patients with refractory pruritus. Post-transplant outcomes are generally better than for most of other chronic liver diseases, with a 5-year survival of up to 85% [26, 27]. Histological disease recurrence occurs in almost 70% of transplanted patients, at 15 years [28]. However, recurrent disease rarely leads to graft failure [29].

A lower rate of liver transplantation and, possibly, slower liver disease progression, have been described in PBC patients with concomitant SSc [3]. Despite this, cumulative

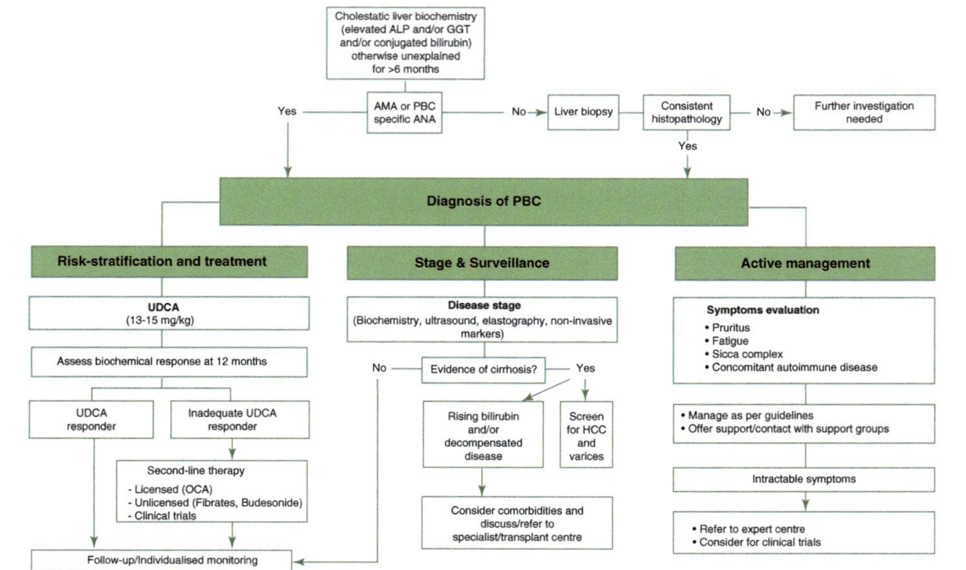

FIGURE 27.1 Diagnosis and treatment flowchart (according to EASL and BSG guidelines). Abbreviations: *EASL*, European Association for the Study of the Liver; *BSG*, British Society of Gastroenterology; *ALP*, alkaline phosphatase; *GGT*, gammaglutamyl-transpeptidase; *AMA*, antimitocondrial antibody; *PBC*, primary biliary cholangitis, *ANA*, antinuclear antibodies; *UDCA*, ursodeoxycholic acid; *OCA*, obethicholic acid; *HCC*, hepatocellular carcinoma

survival is not different in PBC patients with or without SSc, since in PBC-SSc patients the reduced liver-related mortality is disguised by an increased mortality due to other causes [3, 7]. Likely for the same reason, overall survival does not differ in patients with SSc with or without concomitant PBC [1].

Clinical Manifestations

PBC is frequently associated with symptoms such as fatigue, cholestatic pruritus, sicca syndrome and abdominal discomfort. These symptoms are not associated with prognosis but are often difficult to manage and can be debilitating [30]. Up to 60% of individuals are completely asymptomatic at diagnosis [31]. The overall prevalence of liver-associated symptoms is not significantly different between patients with PBC alone and patients with PBC-SSc, although pruritus and fatigue at diagnosis seem to be more frequent in PBC alone [3].

Hyperlipidemia is present in approximately 80% of patients, but there is no evidence for an increased cardiovascular risk, since the lipid elevation consists mainly of high-density lipoprotein (HDL) cholesterol and lipoprotein X [19].

Extrahepatic Autoimmune Conditions Associated with PBC

PBC patients have a higher prevalence of autoimmune diseases compared to the age and sex-matched population. Up to 10% of patients present features of autoimmune hepatitis ("AIH-PBC overlap syndrome") and may benefit from immunosuppressive treatment [32].

The most common concomitant extrahepatic autoimmune conditions are Sjögren's/sicca syndrome, Raynaud's disease, autoimmune thyroid disease, CREST syndrome (Calcinosis, Raynaud's, Esophageal dysfunction, Sclerodactyly, and Telangectasias) and scleroderma [7] (Table 27.1). Telangiectasia and calcinosis appear to be less frequent features in SSc patients with associated PBC [33].

Table 27.1 Typical features of primary biliary cholangitis

Characteristic of PBC patients	Prevalence
F:M rate	1:9
Mean age at diagnosis	55 years
AMA positivity	95%
Anti-sp100 and/or anti-gp210 positivity	In 30% of AMA negative patients
Elevated IgM	Very frequent
Hypercholesterolaemia (HDL), cutaneous xantomas and xantelasmas	Up to 80%
Frequently associated symptoms	
Chronic fatigue	80%
Cholestatic itch	40–80%
Dry eyes and mouth (sicca syndrome)	60–70%
Right upper quadrant pain	8–17%
Depression/cognitive dysfunction	30–45%
Autonomic dysfunction	60–100%
Restless leg syndrome	
Sleep disturbance	
Associated disease	
Autoimmune hepatitis	8–10%
Sjögren's/sicca syndrome	60–70%
CREST syndrome	3–4%
Autoimmune thyroid disease	Up to 25%
Raynaud's disease	25–30%
Cutaneous autoimmune disease	9–10%
Systemic sclerosis	8–12%
Osteopaenia/osteoporosis	30–44%

Table 27.1 (continued)

Characteristic of PBC patients	Prevalence
Systemic lupus erythematosus	3–4%
Rheumatoid arthritis	1.8–5.6%
Coeliac disease	6%
Autoimmune anaemia	Uncommon

Abbreviations: *PBC*, Primary biliary cholangitis; *AMA*, antimitocondrial antibody; *HDL*, High-density lipoprotein; *CREST*, Calcinosis, Raynaud's, Esophageal dysfunction, Sclerodactyly, and Telangectasias

Risk Stratification

Male gender, a younger age at presentation (<45 years) and the presence of symptoms are associated with poorer response to treatment, quicker progression and worse prognosis [34, 35].

The Mayo risk score [36], and the model for end-stage liver disease (MELD) score [37] are very good predictors of death but are not sensitive markers of progression in the early stages of the disease. ALP and bilirubin have been recently validated as robust pre-treatment predictors of response [38] and can be therefore used as surrogate markers of outcome in PBC [11].

Some histological characteristics and the direct measurement of the hepatic venous pressure gradient correlate with the probability of death or LT in PBC [39, 40]. Lately, the development of non-invasive methods (e.g. elastography) has considerably reduced the use of such invasive procedures in routine clinical practice [41].

The recently developed GLOBE score and UK-PBC score, which incorporate measures of treatment response and parameters of disease severity, seem to accurately predict death or LT in PBC [42, 43]. None of these tools to predict disease progression and outcomes has been evaluated in patients with PBC-SSc.

Treatment

Ursodeoxycholic acid (UDCA) at a daily dose of 13–15 mg/kg is the first-line treatment in PBC and leads to biochemical improvement in 60–70% of patients [44–46]. Histological improvement has also been reported [40]. A number of criteria assessed at 6–24 months after initiating treatment have been proposed as surrogate endpoints for clinical outcomes on treatment. The Toronto criteria (ALP <1.67 × ULN and/or bilirubin <2 ULN) are most widely used in clinical practice [19]. Patients who do not respond to UDCA have worse transplant-free survival, while responders have similar outcomes to age and sex-matched control patients without PBC [47].

PBC does not respond to the conventional immunosuppressive therapies [48]. Furthermore, a recent meta-analysis failed to demonstrate a clear beneficial effect on outcomes such as survival, LT, development of cirrhosis or decompensation, of any of the pharmacological treatments investigated until now [49].

Recently, obethicolic acid (OCA), a semi-synthetic hydrophobic bile acid analogue highly selective for the farnesoid X receptor (FXR), has been licensed, in addition to UDCA, for patients who have inadequate response or as a monotherapy in the small number of patients intolerant to UDCA [11]. OCA (initial dose 5 mg/day, titrating to 10 mg/day at 6 months, if tolerated) has been shown to be effective in improving liver biochemistry (ALP, bilirubin) in such cases, but its longer-term effects on clinical outcomes are still being evaluated. Furthermore, OCA therapy is associated with a dose-dependent exacerbation of pruritus, which leads to treatment discontinuation in up to 10% of patients. OCA should be used with caution at lower doses in patients with decompensated cirrhosis. An alteration of the serum lipids profile (in particular a reduction of the HDL levels) has also been described, although the impact on the general cardiovascular risk is still unknown [19].

Other treatment options include the off-label use of fibrates and budesonide (Fig. 27.1). However, confirmatory efficacy and safety data from phase III trials are awaited and survival benefit has yet to be demonstrated [11, 19].

Patients with SSc-PBC are more likely to receive immunosuppressive therapies, but these are known to be ineffective in PBC [48]. On the other hand, there is currently no evidence that SSc-PBC behaves differently to PBC alone in terms of treatment response, although specific data are lacking. Hence, the current recommendation is that SSc-PBC patients are treated, and their treatment response evaluated, similarly to patients with PBC alone.

Cholestatic pruritus is one of the most frequent symptoms experienced by PBC patients and may severely impact on quality of life. Cholestyramine, a non-absorbable bile-sequestrant resin, is the first-line of treatment, although often poorly tolerated due to the frequently associated side effects such as bloating and constipation.

Rifampicin is used as second-line agent, although there are some concerns regarding the safety profile (in particular hepatotoxicity), therefore liver function tests should be regularly monitored in treated patients. Naltrexone and Naloxone (opiate antagonists) are increasingly used as third-line therapy, but opiate withdrawal-like reactions or reduced threshold to pain may complicate long-term treatment. Finally, sertraline (a selective serotonin reuptake inhibitor) and gabapentin are used empirically in patients with pruritus not responsive to the above medical treatment [11, 19].

Chronic fatigue is reported by over 50% of PBC patients and is severe in up to 20% of cases. Severe fatigue is refractory to medical treatment and usually persists after LT. The current guidelines recommend seeking treatable causes of fatigue (e.g. hypothyroidism, anaemia, sleep disturbance, chronic co-morbidities). Managing concomitant symptoms such as nocturnal pruritus, dehydration, restless legs, autonomic dysfunction and depression may help reducing fatigue; structured exercise seems to have a positive effect [11, 19].

General Measures

Vitamin D levels and bone densitometry should be regularly assessed in patients with PBC, and the evidence of vitamin D deficiency, osteopaenia or osteoporosis treated with standard bone protective measures. PBC patients with concomitant metabolic syndrome and cardiovascular risk factors should be treated with cholesterol-lowering agents as per general practice [11, 19].

Patients with extrahepatic autoimmune conditions or associated symptoms resistant to medical treatment should be referred for specialist management (Fig. 27.1).

Conclusions

Screening for PBC amongst those affected by SSc is important to allow early diagnosis and treatment, which may improve patient outcomes.

While the natural history, risk stratification and need for second-line therapies in patients with PBC associated with SSc is poorly evaluated, currently a multidisciplinary approach to management is warranted in these complex cases.

References

1. Mari-Alfonso B, Simeon-Aznar CP, Guillen-Del Castillo A, et al. Hepatobiliary involvement in systemic sclerosis and the cutaneous subsets: Characteristics and survival of patients from the Spanish RESCLE Registry. Semin Arthritis Rheum. 2018;47:849–57.
2. Chou MJ, Lai MY, Lee SL, et al. Reactivity of anti-mitochondrial antibodies in primary biliary cirrhosis and systemic sclerosis. J Formos Med Assoc. 1992;91:1075–80.
3. Rigamonti C, Shand LM, Feudjo M, et al. Clinical features and prognosis of primary biliary cirrhosis associated with systemic sclerosis. Gut. 2006;55:388–94.

4. Chalifoux SL, Konyn PG, Choi G, et al. Extrahepatic manifestations of primary biliary cholangitis. Gut Liver. 2017;11:771–80.
5. Imura-Kumada S, Hasegawa M, Matsushita T, et al. High prevalence of primary biliary cirrhosis and disease-associated autoantibodies in Japanese patients with systemic sclerosis. Mod Rheumatol. 2012;22:892–8.
6. Bali G, Szilvasi A, Inotai D, et al. Comorbidity of localized scleroderma and primary biliary cholangitis. J Dtsch Dermatol Ges. 2018;16:1323–7.
7. Floreani A, Franceschet I, Cazzagon N, et al. Extrahepatic autoimmune conditions associated with primary biliary cirrhosis. Clin Rev Allergy Immunol. 2015;48:192–7.
8. Boonstra K, Beuers U, Ponsioen CY. Epidemiology of primary sclerosing cholangitis and primary biliary cirrhosis: a systematic review. J Hepatol. 2012;56:1181–8.
9. Boonstra K, Kunst AE, Stadhouders PH, et al. Rising incidence and prevalence of primary biliary cirrhosis: a large population based study. Liver Int. 2014;34:e31–8.
10. Griffiths L, Dyson JK, Jones DE. The new epidemiology of primary biliary cirrhosis. Semin Liver Dis. 2014;34:318–28.
11. European Association for the Study of the Liver. Electronic address: easloffice@easloffice.eu; European Association for the Study of the Liver. EASL Clinical Practice Guidelines: The diagnosis and management of patients with primary biliary cholangitis. J Hepatol. 2017;67:145–72.
12. Lleo A, Jepsen P, Morenghi E, et al. Evolving Trends in Female to Male Incidence and Male Mortality of Primary Biliary Cholangitis. Sci Rep. 2016;6:25906.
13. Kaplan MM, Gershwin ME. Primary biliary cirrhosis. N Engl J Med. 2005;353:1261–73.
14. Nakamura M, Kondo H, Mori T, et al. Anti-gp210 and anticentromere antibodies are different risk factors for the progression of primary biliary cirrhosis. Hepatology. 2007;45:118–27.
15. Invernizzi P, Podda M, Battezzati PM, et al. Autoantibodies against nuclear pore complexes are associated with more active and severe liver disease in primary biliary cirrhosis. J Hepatol. 2001;34:366–72.
16. Cordell HJ, Han Y, Mells GF, et al. International genomewide meta-analysis identifies new primary biliary cirrhosis risk loci and targetable pathogenic pathways. Nat Commun. 2015;6:8019.

17. Jones DE, Watt FE, Metcalf JV, et al. Familial primary biliary cirrhosis reassessed: a geographically-based population study. J Hepatol. 1999;30:402–7.
18. Watt FE, James OF, Jones DE. Patterns of autoimmunity in primary biliary cirrhosis patients and their families: a population-based cohort study. QJM. 2004;97:397–406.
19. Hirschfield GM, Dyson JK, Alexander GJM, et al. The British Society of Gastroenterology/UK-PBC primary biliary cholangitis treatment and management guidelines. Gut. 2018;67:1568–94.
20. Ludwig J, Dickson ER, McDonald GS. Staging of chronic nonsuppurative destructive cholangitis (syndrome of primary biliary cirrhosis). Virchows Arch A Pathol Anat Histol. 1978;379:103–12.
21. Scheuer P. Primary biliary cirrhosis. Proc R Soc Med. 1967;60:1257–60.
22. Hudson M, Fritzler MJ. Diagnostic criteria of systemic sclerosis. J Autoimmun. 2014;48-49:38–41.
23. van den Hoogen F, Khanna D, Fransen J, et al. 2013 classification criteria for systemic sclerosis: an American college of rheumatology/European league against rheumatism collaborative initiative. Ann Rheum Dis. 2013;72:1747–55.
24. Jones DE, Metcalf JV, Collier JD, et al. Hepatocellular carcinoma in primary biliary cirrhosis and its impact on outcomes. Hepatology. 1997;26:1138–42.
25. Prince M, Chetwynd A, Newman W, et al. Survival and symptom progression in a geographically based cohort of patients with primary biliary cirrhosis: follow-up for up to 28 years. Gastroenterology. 2002;123:1044–51.
26. Singal AK, Guturu P, Hmoud B, et al. Evolving frequency and outcomes of liver transplantation based on etiology of liver disease. Transplantation. 2013;95:755–60.
27. Carbone M, Neuberger JM. Autoimmune liver disease, autoimmunity and liver transplantation. J Hepatol. 2014;60:210–23.
28. Silveira MG, Talwalkar JA, Lindor KD, et al. Recurrent primary biliary cirrhosis after liver transplantation. Am J Transplant. 2010;10:720–6.
29. Nevens F. PBC-transplantation and disease recurrence. Best Pract Res Clin Gastroenterol. 2018;34-35:107–11.
30. Dyson JK, Wilkinson N, Jopson L, et al. The inter-relationship of symptom severity and quality of life in 2055 patients with primary biliary cholangitis. Aliment Pharmacol Ther. 2016;44:1039–50.
31. Inoue K, Hirohara J, Nakano T, et al. Prediction of prognosis of primary biliary cirrhosis in Japan. Liver. 1995;15:70–7.

32. Boberg KM, Chapman RW, Hirschfield GM, et al. Overlap syndromes: the International Autoimmune Hepatitis Group (IAIHG) position statement on a controversial issue. J Hepatol. 2011;54:374–85.
33. Cavazzana I, Ceribelli A, Taraborelli M, et al. Primary biliary cirrhosis-related autoantibodies in a large cohort of italian patients with systemic sclerosis. J Rheumatol. 2011;38:2180–5.
34. Carbone M, Mells GF, Pells G, et al. Sex and age are determinants of the clinical phenotype of primary biliary cirrhosis and response to ursodeoxycholic acid. Gastroenterology. 2013;144:560–e14.
35. Quarneti C, Muratori P, Lalanne C, et al. Fatigue and pruritus at onset identify a more aggressive subset of primary biliary cirrhosis. Liver Int. 2015;35:636–41.
36. Dickson ER, Grambsch PM, Fleming TR, et al. Prognosis in primary biliary cirrhosis: model for decision making. Hepatology. 1989;10:1–7.
37. Malinchoc M, Kamath PS, Gordon FD, et al. A model to predict poor survival in patients undergoing transjugular intrahepatic portosystemic shunts. Hepatology. 2000;31:864–71.
38. Carbone M, Nardi A, Flack S, et al. Pretreatment prediction of response to ursodeoxycholic acid in primary biliary cholangitis: development and validation of the UDCA Response Score. Lancet Gastroenterol Hepatol. 2018;3(9):626–34.
39. Huet PM, Vincent C, Deslaurier J, et al. Portal hypertension and primary biliary cirrhosis: effect of long-term ursodeoxycholic acid treatment. Gastroenterology. 2008;135:1552–60.
40. Kumagi T, Guindi M, Fischer SE, et al. Baseline ductopenia and treatment response predict long-term histological progression in primary biliary cirrhosis. Am J Gastroenterol. 2010;105:2186–94.
41. Corpechot C, El Naggar A, Poujol-Robert A, et al. Assessment of biliary fibrosis by transient elastography in patients with PBC and PSC. Hepatology. 2006;43:1118–24.
42. Carbone M, Sharp SJ, Flack S, et al. The UK-PBC risk scores: derivation and validation of a scoring system for long-term prediction of end-stage liver disease in primary biliary cholangitis. Hepatology. 2016;63:930–50.
43. Lammers WJ, Hirschfield GM, Corpechot C, et al. Development and Validation of a Scoring System to Predict Outcomes of Patients With Primary Biliary Cirrhosis Receiving Ursodeoxycholic Acid Therapy. Gastroenterology. 2015;149(7):1804–12.e4.

44. Tsochatzis EA, Gurusamy KS, Gluud C, Burroughs AK. Ursodeoxycholic acid and primary biliary cirrhosis: EASL and AASLD guidelines. J Hepatol. 2009;51(6):1084–6.
45. Lammert C, Juran BD, Schlicht E, et al. Biochemical response to ursodeoxycholic acid predicts survival in a north American cohort of primary biliary cirrhosis patients. J Gastroenterol. 2014;49:1414–20.
46. Corpechot C, Abenavoli L, Rabahi N, et al. Biochemical response to ursodeoxycholic acid and long-term prognosis in primary biliary cirrhosis. Hepatology. 2008;48:871–7.
47. Pares A, Caballeria L, Rodes J. Excellent long-term survival in patients with primary biliary cirrhosis and biochemical response to ursodeoxycholic acid. Gastroenterology. 2006;130:715–20.
48. Karlsen TH, Vesterhus M, Boberg KM. Review article: controversies in the management of primary biliary cirrhosis and primary sclerosing cholangitis. Aliment Pharmacol Ther. 2014;39:282–301.
49. Saffioti F, Gurusamy KS, Eusebi LH, et al. Pharmacological interventions for primary biliary cholangitis: an attempted network meta-analysis. Cochrane Database Syst Rev. 2017;3:CD011648.

Chapter 28
Arthritis in Systemic Sclerosis

Mikameh May Kazem and Janet E. Pope

Introduction

Systemic sclerosis or scleroderma is an autoimmune disorder hallmarked by autoantibodies, vasculopathy and pathologic collagen deposition and fibrosis which can affect many organs. The major subtypes of the disease include limited cutaneous (lcSSc), diffuse cutenaous systemic sclerosis (dcSSc), sine scleroderma, and systemic sclerosis overlap syndromes [1]. While the classic manifestation of most subtypes may be skin thickening, many can also have articular involvement of varying degrees [2]. Articular involvement can vary with manifestations such as arthralgias, inflammatory arthri-

M. M. Kazem
Schulich School of Medicine & Dentistry, University of Western Ontario, London, ON, Canada
e-mail: May.Kazem@lhsc.on.ca

J. E. Pope (✉)
Schulich School of Medicine & Dentistry, University of Western Ontario, London, ON, Canada

Division of Rheumatology, St. Joseph's Health Care, London, ON, Canada
e-mail: janet.pope@sjhc.london.on.ca

© Springer Nature Switzerland AG 2021
M. Matucci-Cerinic, C. P. Denton (eds.), *Practical Management of Systemic Sclerosis in Clinical Practice*, In Clinical Practice,
https://doi.org/10.1007/978-3-030-53736-4_28

tis, tendon friction rubs, tenosynovitis, flexion contractures, acro-osteolysis and erosive joint damage [3]. According to the "15% rule" of systemic sclerosis, defined by a 2013 systematic review, approximately 9–16% of patients with systemic sclerosis have concomitant inflammatory arthritis and far more with joint pain [4]. In some series, approximately half those patients need disease modifying drugs for their arthritis [4]. The presence of different subtypes of inflammatory arthritis has been previously described in the literature [2–4] however, there is currently no consensus on classification of inflammatory arthritis/joint involvement in SSc, or definitive management strategies depending on the musculoskeletal features seen in scleroderma patients. Other joint pain can occur from complications that are not part of inflammatory arthritis such as flexion contractures from ulcers at the proximal interphalangeal joints (PIPs).

Inflammatory arthritis can be present in all subsets of SSc (such as lcSSc and dcSSc). Some patients will have an overlap with rheumatoid arthritis (RA) and this occurs at a low frequency (approximately 3%) of those with SSc [2]. Some SSc patients have an overlap with systemic lupus erythematosus (SLE) and can manifest non-erosive inflammatory arthritis and even Jaccoud's arthropathy (with reducible subluxations). Even more rare is a mutilans type of inflammatory arthritis with severe periosteal resorption, contractures, foreshortening of digitals and large erosions [5, 6].

Prognostic Factors in Scleroderma Associated Inflammatory Arthritis

Inflammatory arthritis is one of the recognized musculoskeletal complications of SSc [1–4, 6–8] hence identification of poor prognostic factors could weigh into the decision of pursuing more aggressive therapies to prevent joint damage and disability. Studies from the European Scleroderma Trials and

Research group (EUSTAR) registry have demonstrated that findings of synovitis early on in SSc are associated with a higher chance of the disease progressing to diffuse SSc [9].

Seropositivity with rheumatoid factor (RF) and/or anti-cyclic citrullinated peptide antibody (ACPA) in addition to common SSc antibodies results in a worse prognosis. Kamalaksha et al. studied 132 SSc patients (with either lcSSc or dcSSc) and found a statistically and clinically significant association of double positivity with more arthralgias and erosive joint damage on radiographs (Xrays) [3]. Those with anti-CCP positive serology alone were also found to have more erosive disease on Xrays of the hands [3]. Others have studied ACPA positivity (measured by anti-cyclic citrullinated peptide; anti-CCP) in scleroderma and have found an association with higher frequency of arthritis as well as pulmonary, esophageal, and more skin involvement [10]. It is our impression that RA can overlap approximately equally in dcSSc and the lcSSc subsets whereas other forms of inflammatory arthritis (IA) are likely higher in dcSSc [2].

Socioeconomic status has been known to be associated inversely with many health outcomes. Mansour and colleagues specifically looked at this issue in SSc patients with from the Scleroderma Canadian Registry Group (CSRG) registry [11]. The group used level of education as a surrogate marker to assess outcomes in scleroderma patients. Interestingly, it was found that after adjusting for confounders associated with lower levels of education and controlling for other comorbid variables, lower level of education was not associated with worse prognosis [11]. They did find that mortality was higher with age, diffuse cutaneous disease, elevated pulmonary artery pressures, and lower diffusion capacity. However, inflammatory arthritis was not reported to be associated with higher mortality [11]. Thus, data are not fully consistent that positive RF is associated with a worse prognosis in SSc when adjusting for other variables.

Types of Arthritis

Historically, a few variants of arthritis have been described in patients with SSc. There are reports of overlap syndromes such as SSc and rheumatoid arthritis (RA), with erosive arthropathy and positive rheumatoid factor and/or anti-citrullinated protein antibody (ACPA) as hallmark of the arthritis type seen in these group of patients [2, 6, 8] . In a 1981 focused review, Blocka et al. identified several lcSSc patients with overlaying arthropathy and summarized several patterns of musculoskeletal manifestations including erosive arthritis of the hands with also ankylosis, juxta-articular demineralization, marginal and dorsal erosions, in addition to already described acro-osteolysis seen in many patients with SSc [2]. Basset and colleagues further described findings in SSc which included many similar features to rheumatoid arthritis (RA) such as metacarpophalangeal (MCP) and proximal interphalangeal (PIP) erosions while also displaying phenotypes of arthritis mutilans, arguing that this erosive arthropathy is in fact an independent clinical entity [8]. Furthermore, a review from a Hungarian registry with SSc-RA overlap patients found several allelic and phenotypic differences in patients with the overlap syndrome compared to the respective SSc-only, RA-only, and healthy controls [12]. American College of Rheumatology (ACR) criteria was used for diagnosis of RA and SSc and identified 22 cases of overlap syndrome (fulfilling both sets of criteria) out of a total of 447 patients in the registry. There were 17 patients with lcSSc and 5 with dcSSc. The genotypic comparators groups were 100 RA patients, 38 SSc patients, and 50 healthy controls. Of the patients with lcSSc 14 out of 17 had joint destruction and erosion, compared to 4 out of 5 patients with dcSSc. The authors did not comment on the particular type of inflammatory arthritis but mentioned that RF and ACPA positivity were observed at 73% and 82% respectively in their overlap cohort [12]. The authors also assessed a number of HLA-DR genotypes. They reported increased frequencies of HLA-DR3, DR7, DR11, and DRw53 in overlap patients compared to RA controls.

HLA-DR1 and DR4 were increased in both overlap patients and RA controls compared to SSc patients and healthy controls. The study demonstrated an increase in SSc associated as well as RA associated alleles in the overlap patients [12].

On the same spectrum, there are patients with clinical manifestations of other diseases such as inflammatory myositis or systemic lupus erythematosus (SLE) along with biochemical and phenotypic manifestations of SSc (both skin limited and diffuse) [13]. Some SSc patients with polyarthritis had features of SLE or inflammatory myositis (IM), while only a subgroup had erosive arthritis on imaging [4, 13].

Perhaps the inflammatory arthritis spectrum in SSc patients is linked to various genetics where a phenotype of non-erosive arthritis and features overlapping with SLE could be due to HLA DR2 or HLA DR3 whereas RA overlaps especially with RF and/or ACPA antibodies could have HLA DR4 and those with severe periosteal resorption and large erosions also have acro-osteolysis and are likely different genetically as the phenotype is very different from other subtypes. Joint, tendon and bone involvement in SSc may cluster but not necessarily. Acro-osteolysis is likely more associated with severe Raynaud's and vasculopathy and likely has a genetic component. Tendon friction rubs are more common in the dcSSc patients and especially in those with more active skin involvement.

SSc patients with inflammatory arthritis, joint contractures and/or tendon friction rubs have a more severe disease course and more systemic inflammation [9].

Diagnosis of Arthritis in SSc

Musculoskeletal involvement in scleroderma is common [14] but unfortunately often overlooked as internal organ involvement can overshadow other manifestations [1]. Concomitant immobility, skin fibrosis, soft tissue finger swelling and calcinosis of periarticular structures, seen in many patients with SSc poses a diagnostic challenge when assessing for arthritis [15].

Diagnosis of inflammatory arthritis relies on a thorough history to elucidate if there is any fusiform joint swelling, joint pain or stiffness, any limitation in range of motion (ROM), tendonitis, or any tendon friction rubs [16, 17]. Physical exam findings include synovial thickening, swelling at different joints in the hand (wrist, MCP, PIP, and rarely DIP involvement) super-imposed on skin findings. Some can progress to claw hand deformity as a result of flexion contractures even when no underlying inflammatory arthritis is present (Figure). Inflammatory arthritis may be difficult to diagnose and sometimes is confirmed on X-ray with joint damage, or joint ultrasound or MRI [8, 16]. Patients may also have concomitant osteoarthritis (OA), gout or chondrocalcinosis or pseudogout which need to be distinguished from SSc associated inflammatory arthritis. Pattern recognition for inflammatory arthritis vs. OA is important as well as looking for hints for gout (tophi which may be difficult to differentiate from calcinosis, high serum uric acid, acute transient joint erythema or a RA like pattern if from high uric acid from diuretics but involvement of atypical RA joints such as DIPs). Figure 28.1 shows the diagnostic algorithm for joint symptoms in someone with SSc. Table 28.1 lists types of inflammatory arthritis in scleroderma.

Serological investigations for the presence of RF or ACPA can be useful in determining prognosis (more likely to have erosive arthritis) vs. anti-DNA positive with SLE overlap (more likely to be non-erosive arthritis). The treatment may also be guided if initial disease modifying drugs are insufficient according to serology. ACPA and RF had been implicated in erosive SSc and possibly also in the presence of an overlap syndrome [3, 9, 16, 18]. Inflammatory markers such as C-reactive protein (CRP) and erythrocytes sedimentation rate (ESR) can be used to assess systemic inflammation in relation to presenting symptoms. The inflammatory markers may also be followed as assessment of disease activity. For instance, in RA outcome measurements are followed such as the tender joint count, swollen joint count, physician and patient global assessment of arthritis activity, pain, morning stiffness and CRP and/or ESR. Figures 28.2 and 28.3

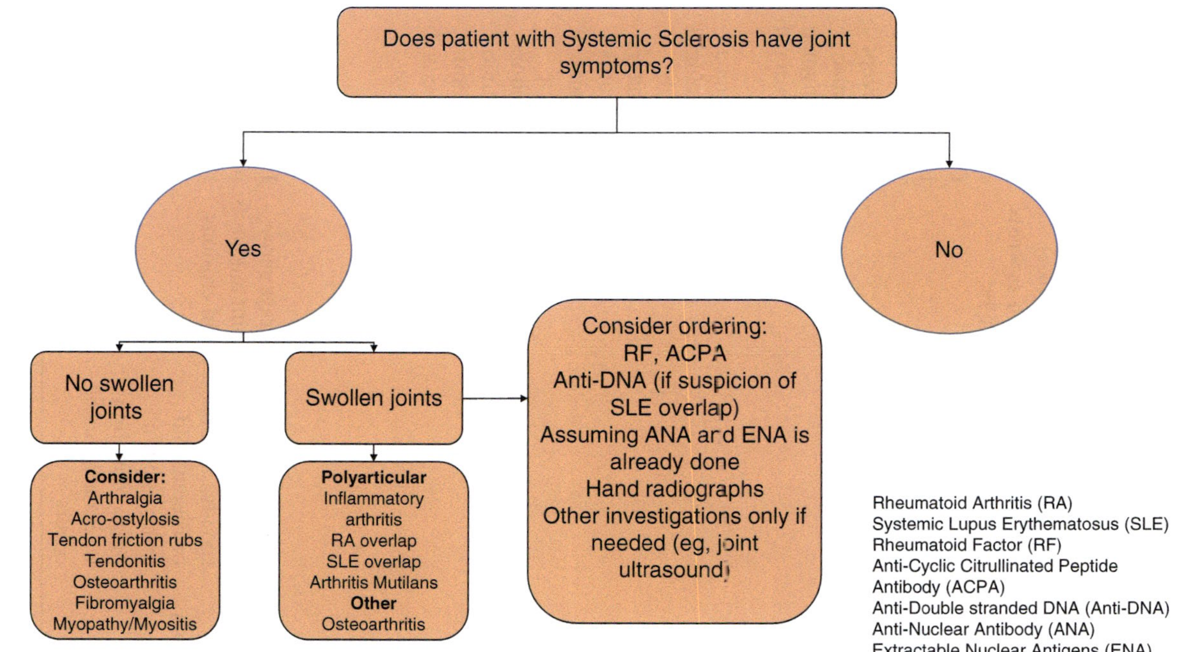

FIGURE 28.1 Diagnostic algorithm for joint pain in scleroderma

Table 28.1 Arthritis subtype patterns and associated features

Arthritis Subtype	**Signs & Symptoms on history**	**Radiologic findings**	**Treatment modalities**
Erosive polyarticular	Painful swollen joints, could be RA like Or patients with overlap syndromes	Erosive changes (RA like) such as wrists, MCPs	Treat like RA Methotrexate Other conventional synthetic DMARDs Leflunomide TNF inhibitors Etanercept Infliximab Adalimumab Certolizumab pegol Golimumab Other biologics Rituximab IL6 inhibitors Tocilizumab Sarilumab Abatacept Jak inhibitors Tofacitinib Baricitinib Upadacitinib Adjunctive NSAIDs Low dose glucocorticoids
Erosive arthritis with ankylosis	May look more like seronegative spondyloarthropathy or rheumatoid arthritis but no range of motion where ankylosing occurs	Xrays show joint ankylosis and erosions	Likely treat like polyarticular erosive arthritis

Table 28.1 (continued)

Arthritis Subtype	Signs & Symptoms on history	Radiologic findings	Treatment modalities
Non-erosive	Arthralgia, inflammatory arthritis	No erosions on Xrays	NSAIDs Low dose glucocorticoids Hydroxychloroquine Possibly if overlapping with SLE and uncontrolled arthritis Belimumab Rituximab
Mutilans	Inflammatory arthritis and rapid development of deformities, possibly shortening of the digits	Large erosions and periosteal resorption	Conventional synthetic DMARDs Methotrexate Leflunomide Rapid addition of TNF inhibitor If failing above treatments, follow the RA treatment algorithm Unknown if IL17 inhibitors IL12 inhibitors IL 12/23 inhibitor would be of benefit
Non arthritic bone abnormalities Acro-Osteolysis	Tuft resorption	Classic tuft resorption of digits on X-ray May or may not have inflammatory arthritis	Unknown if there is no inflammatory arthritis

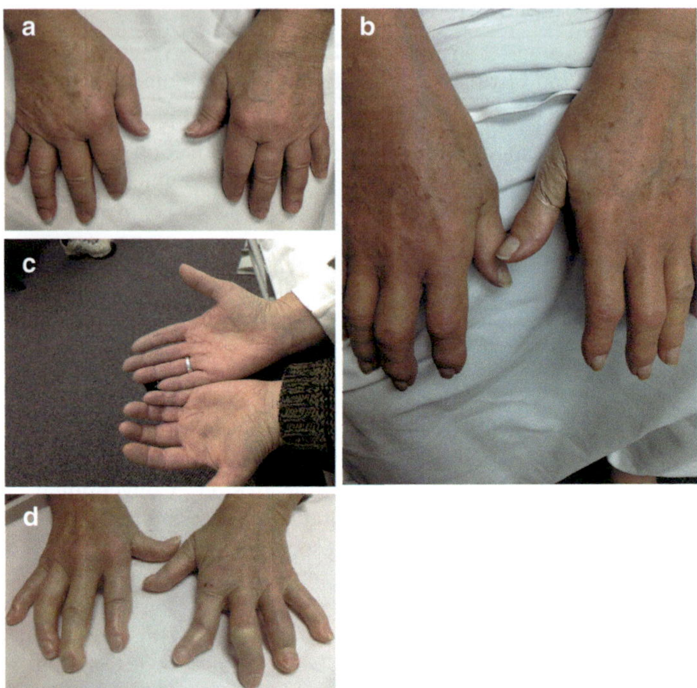

Figure 28.2 Photographs of joint changes in scleroderma. (**a**) Puffy fingers and synovitis in a patient with lcSSc, (**b**) SSc with polyarticular IA in dcSSc and PIP flexion changes, (**c**) SSc with tenosynovitis of palm and dactylitis, (**d**) Swelling and severe deformities

demonstrate joint and soft tissue changes seen in patients with scleroderma.

In addition to serology, radiographs have been used in identifying different phenotypes in patients with SSc. A radiographic survey from 1981 documented articular changes in patients with SSc [2]. Joint-specific radiological abnormalities were assessed in 55 patients with dcSSc and 10 with lcSSc and found to include joint-space narrowing, marginal erosions, juxta-articular demineralization, and ankylosis both at baseline and at 29-month follow-up, with a higher frequency in the dcSSc patients. These findings have been described in a

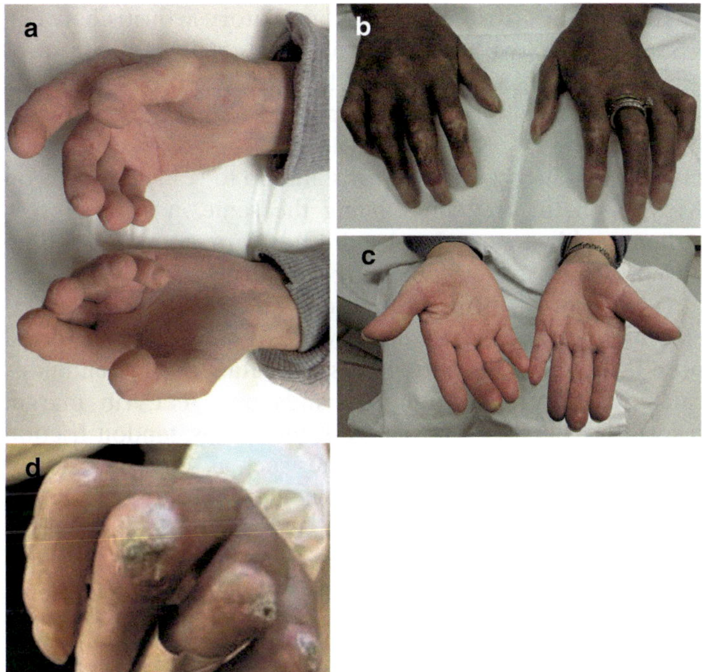

FIGURE 28.3 Other MSK changes in SSc, (**a**) Claw hands and tuft resorption, (**b**) Claw hands and PIP bony change, (**c**) Calcinosis right finger tip and right fourth flexor tendon, (**d**) Flexion contracture of PIPs with ulcers

number of other case series and database analyses [7, 16, 19, 20]. Ultrasound as well as magnetic resonance imaging (MRI) have also been used to better characterize joint and synovial involvement but are not necessarily routinely performed [21–23]. Ultrasound abnormalities observed include synovitis and tenosynovitis with layering appearance, calcinosis, and acro-osteolysis [21]. Comparisons between X-ray and ultrasound data, show more subtle inflammatory changes being detected by ultrasound [22] and other musculoskeletal manifestations may be more easily seen with ultrasound such periarticular calcinosis or acro-osteolysis [21].

In terms of distribution of inflammatory arthritis between lcSSc and dcSSc, Blocka and colleagues reported more progression of joint symptoms in the diffuse subset [2]. Others have reported similar occurrence of IA in dcSSc and lcSSc [24]. A series of 58 patients with SSc showed that approximately 19% had clinical arthritis and up to ¼ had arthritis on Xrays with the frequency being the same in both subsets. Patients with an overlap syndrome were also reported to have more erosive or deforming arthritis [12, 25].

Apart from arthritis, there are several other musculoskeletal manifestations of SSc. Several groups have reported presence of flexion contractures, subcutaneous or tendinous calcinosis, tuft resorption in hands and feet, rib margin resorption, bursitis, tenosynovitis, tendonitis, tendon friction rubs as well as shoulder syndromes such as adhesive capsulitis or synovitis of the acromioclavicular joint [2, 8, 13, 16, 21, 22, 26]. Others have presented cases of myositis-SSc overlap with elevated CK and serological profile (anti-PM Scl) in addition to scleroderma features [4, 13, 27]. Presence of fibromyalgia syndrome is also well described in patients with scleroderma, ranging from 18–30% [26, 28] depending on the publication and screening tool used.

Studies are lacking to clearly delineate and validate each type of arthritis in patients with concurrent SSc. Nonetheless, the features described in the literature, in combination with clinical findings can be utilized to create a tailored treatment plan for each subset of patients. Table 28.1 illustrates a summary of the subtypes observed and their respective proposed treatment modalities.

Who Gets Inflammatory Arthritis in SSc

Approximately 15% of patients with SSc have IA [4]. It may be more common in dcSSc than lcSSc (or equal) [2, 25]. The clinical presentation of IA, presence or absence of an overlap with RA or other connective tissue disease, serology and hand/feet Xrays may be helpful in determining the pattern/type of IA and potential treatment and prognosis.

Other MSK Features in SSc

The differential diagnosis of musculoskeletal (MSK) symptoms in SSc is broad. There may be IA related to SSc, other joint, bone, muscle or tendon problems that are due to SSc (calcinosis, contractures, tuft resorption, carpel tunnel, myopathy, myositis, tenosynovitis, tendon friction rubs, adhesive capsulitis, etc.) and other problems unrelated to scleroderma (osteoarthritis, gout, other crystal arthritis, tendonitis) or fibromyalgia which is increased in patients with connective tissue diseases.

Treatment

Non-pharmacological

Patient education around SSc is an important consideration given the day-to-day challenges that patients face as a result of multi-organ involvement of SSc. Educational gaps have been identified for SSc patients [29] and pilot educational interventions have reported improved patient-reported outcomes [30, 31]. To date, there are no specific studies looking at educational interventions as they pertain to inflammatory arthritis in patients with SSc.

Several physiotherapy (PT) or occupational therapy (OT) interventions have been assessed in patients with SSc with varying results. Landim et al. reported positive results on a home-based program designed to improve hand function, mobility, and pain [32]. Stafenantoni and colleagues also noted improved hand function with OT interventions [33] in their pilot study however, a larger randomized controlled trial did not reveal statistically significant differences in health assessment questionnaire (HAQ) scores in patients with a personalized PT program, though there were short-term improvements [34]. Other interventions for hand physiotherapy have been designed using an internet-based treatment of patients from multiple countries witin the Scleroderma Patient-centred Intervention Network (SPIN) but the studies have not been completed so results for this method of treatment using expertise over the internet for hand therapy in SSc are unknown [https://www.spinsclero.com].

Improving range of motion, resting and stretching joints to prevent/reduce contractures with exercises and hand splinting is common in SSc for arthritis or for skin/tendon involvement. Orthotics can be used for pain due to IA or loss of fascia in the feet which is seen in some patients with SSc.

Pharmacological Treatment

Analgesics and NSAIDs

Analgesics are considered adjunctive treatment in SSc such as acetaminophen/paracetamol, topical treatment (capsaicin cream) and possibly even weak narcotics (tramadol). However, many patients use nonsteroidal anti-inflammatory drugs (NSAIDs) to treat pain and inflammation from MSK pain in SSc.

NSAIDs can be used as topical (diclofenac) or oral. They increase the risk of ulcers and may be prescribed with a proton pump inhibitor for patients at risk of gastrointestinal (GI) bleeding (such as older patients, patients with past GI bleeds or gastric ulcers, erosive esophagitis, gastric antral vascular ectasia, etc). Often NSAIDs are prescribed on an as needed basis for joint pain, stiffness and swelling but they can be used chronically. Caution should be exercised if there is renal impairment, congestive heart failure, hypertension or significant anemia.

Low Dose Corticosteroids

Some patients with puffy hands and/or active inflammatory arthritis are prescribed low dose prednisone (prednisolone). The dose is often 10 mg daily of prednisone. Blood pressure monitoring is necessary when prescribing corticosteroids to patients with early active dcSSc as they can increase the risk of scleroderma renal crisis (SRC); especially if the patient is positive for RNA polymerase3 antibody, but this test is not readily available as part of the ENA. However, SRC is less likely to occur if using low dose prednisone compared to higher doses. This treatment could be considered adjunctive or bridging until a disease modifying drug is successful.

Disease Modifying Anti-Rheumatic Drugs (DMARDs)

There are no formal guidelines when it comes to treatment of SSc-associated inflammatory arthritis. The drugs prescribed are mostly from evidence in other types of inflammatory arthritis such as RA [7]. Synthetic conventional disease modifying antirheumatic drugs such as methotrexate have long been utilized as it helped both skin and joint symptoms [1, 7, 35]. Tradition or conventional synthetic DMARDs that could be considered for polyarticular IA include methotrexate, hydroxychloroquine, leflunomide, azathioprine and mycophenolate mofetil. The most recent attempt at unification of treatment algorithms was put forth by Fernández-Codina and colleagues. The authors included SSc experts from both Scleroderma Clinical Trials Consortium (CSTC) and the Canadian Scleroderma Research Group (CSRG) to determine treatment algorithms in SSc including inflammatory arthritis [36]. Experts were surveyed in three rounds: In round 1 they were asked about their agreement with the treatment strategy based on the previous 2012 algorithm and to make changes where appropriate [37]; then they were provided with frequencies of agreement with the previous algorithm and were again asked what they would add as second or switch to as the next line treatment. The third round of the survey was conducted to finalize the proposed algorithm and allow for modifications with respect to the line of therapy [36].

Regarding inflammatory arthritis in SSc, 45% of the experts responding to the survey agreed that conventional synthetic DMARDs were the first line of therapy. They varied on agreement of which DMARD but 59% did choose methotrexate, followed by 27% choosing hydroxychloroquine [36]. Low doses of glucocorticoids were added if needed and combination with methotrexate and hydroxychloroquine and then consideration of biologic treatment such as rituximab or tocilizumab [36]. Many others have suggested using low dose corticosteroids in conjunction with other csDMARDs in SSc associated inflammatory arthritis [1, 7] . The expert consensus also found an overwhelming 75% who reported they would consider low dose glucocorticoids if there were no safety concerns [36]. Most did however refer to this as a second line option, especially as corticosteroids in patients with dcSSc could precipitate scleroderma renal crisis and hence in those patients, the use of steroids should be evaluated judiciously and blood pressure carefully monitored if prescribed in dcSSc or early SSc [17].

With respect to biologic DMARDs (bDMARDs), anti-TNF agents have been used in refractory cases of inflammatory arthritis associated with SSc. Etanercept and infliximab were evaluated in previous observational studies [38, 39]. Some reports showed promising results with respect to improved signs (synovitis) and symptoms (pain, stiffness, Health Assessment Questionnaire (HAQ) scores) [38]. The etanercept study reported an 83% response rate (15 of 18 patients) in terms of improvement and/or resolution of joint symptoms as well as a decrease in HAQ and Rodnan skin score [40]. The infliximab study did not demonstrate any clear benefit in decreasing skin involvement using the modified Rodnan skin score (mRSS) but the study did not have inflammatory arthritis as an outcome [41].

Tocilizumab and abatacept have been evaluated and shown efficacy in treatment of polyarthritis in SSc in case series, though not as efficacious in addressing myositis symptoms [42]. Elhai et al. published on15 patients prescribed tocilizumab and 12 on abatacept; and of the 15 patients on tocilizumab, 10 were good responders and 4 were moderate responders for articular outcomes as per EULAR response criteria [42]. The abatacept group was also improved their inflammatory arthritis but in those with myopathy improvement was not statistically significant [42]. Other outcomes such as skin changes were not reported. Although experts commonly reported rituximab for inflammatory arthritis in SSc, most reports of rituximab in SSc have concentrated on skin and lung outcomes [36].

Cannabinoids

There are multiple cannabinoid receptors in various organs. Some patients with arthritis such as RA use medical cannabis that is mostly cannabidiol (CBD) to help for pain. There are drugs that affect the endocannabinoid pathway being studied in SSc and they may or may not alter inflammatory arthritis as the primary area of study is skin fibrosis [43, 44].

Proposed Outcome Measurements in SSc Clinical Trials for Inflammatory Arthritis

The heterogeneity of presentation of musculoskeletal symptoms in patients with scleroderma makes it challenging to outline unanimously agreed-upon metrics that are deemed appropriate surrogates or outcomes in clinical trials. Therefore, experts have put forth recommendations to consider in design of clinical trials when assessing efficacy of non-pharmacologic and pharmacologic interventions in SSc [14, 45].

Clements et al. proposed a trial design where validated outcome measures are included as primary endpoints in assessment of joint involvement [14]. The group further recommended trial length that should be conducive to detection of meaningful differences in the proposed primary outcomes represented by validated measures. Further recommendations on trial design included use of strong designs such as randomized controlled double-blind trials and inclusion patients with both limited and diffuse SSc with active inflammatory arthritis if testing a treatment for this purpose [14]. It would be difficult to have a study with several outcomes and multiple features of SSc being tested as hand function measurements may not change if there are flexion contractures and primary outcome measurements for inflammatory arthritis should be different than myositis (the latter having creatine kinase and muscle power as outcomes and the former having joint counts).

An alternative approach would be to use Disease Activity Score (DAS) responses to quantify inflammatory arthritis, as functional measures, though validated, could be affected by a number of other factors such as contractures and calcinosis [45]. Though tender and swollen joint counts are reported to be only partially validated in trials with SSc patients [46], inflammatory arthritis and its response to therapy is measured as a function of tender/swollen joint count [45].

Other indices such as physician global rating or acute phase reactants such as CRP/ESR may not strongly correlate or have utility pertaining to musculoskeletal manifestations in patients with SSc [46]. Some of the outcomes have not been validated in SSc as there are a paucity of randomized studies in SSc with inflammatory arthritis as the major organ studied. We suspect that core RA outcome measurements when used in SSc trials of active IA would likely perform appropriately.

System-specific outcome measures and patient reported outcome measures (PROMs) are often included in assessing patients in SSc trials. Several validated and emerging patient-reported outcome measures used in SSc have been validated [47]. Incorporation of these measures help to provide patient-centred care and can be reflective of quality of life nuances as they relate to day to day activities [48]. Of these measures, the Health Assessment Questionnaire (HAQ), the HAQ disability index (HAQ-DI), and the Scleroderma HAQ (SHAQ) which is a HAQ-DI and additional visual analogue scales, are some of the general measurement tools that can be reliably incorporated into periodic patient assessments as well as trials to better elucidate the patient experience [47]. Global assessments are also valuable as they are easy to use and can provide patient perspective and are sensitive to change [49]. There are differences in patient and physician global scores which inherently measure different aspects of disease. For instance, physicians may elect to provide a higher score when there is more/serious organ involvement whereas patients may rate their global assessment based on the symptom that is most disruptive to their daily life, whether it carries the same weight as the physician score or not [49].

Additionally, there are several organ-specific (i.e. hands) or symptom specific (i.e. pain) measures that are used in symptom assessment. Examples include Hand mobility in Scleroderma (HAMIS), Cochin Hand Function Scale and the Michigan Hand Questionnaire (MHQ) to name a few [49–51]. New and emerging tools are also currently in development. One example is the Combined Response Index for Systemic Sclerosis (CRISS) which aims to measure a comprehensive set of specific organ manifestations as well as patient reported outcomes [52]. Another innovative measure is adaptation of a measure that is not disease specific; the Patient Reported Outcome Measurement Information System (PROMIS) to SSc. PROMIS utilizes computerized adaptive tests and measures patient reported outcomes and has been standardized and is accessible [53].

Future Directions

For SSc associated arthritis, likely there will be immune modulation that can improve both skin and joints. However, properly designed trials are needed to assess appropriate treatment for IA in SSc. These studies may have to account for the various types/patterns of IA in SSc and use appropriate outcome measurements; possibly borrowing scales used in RA. There are many new classes of drugs that could be tested in SSc and may help arthritis such as JAK inhibitors and various biologics. Phenotypes of IA in SSc may be studied with respect to genomics, gene expression or proteomics which may lead to more precise treatment. Big data may be helpful for pattern recognition of SSc subsets and response to treatment which can only occur if patients are well characterized clinically, using other tests (labs, Xrays) and collecting and storing patient samples (most likely blood or serum). Research may enable the discovery of treatment options for SSc patients including joint manifestations.

Conflicts of Interest There are no conflicts of interest. There was no funding for this chapter. No copy righted material has been included.

References

1. Denton CP, Khanna D. Systemic sclerosis. Lancet. 2017;390(10103):1685–99.
2. Blocka KL, et al. The arthropathy of advanced progressive systemic sclerosis. A radiographic survey. Arthritis Rheum. 1981;24(7):874–84.
3. Kamalaksha S, White DHN, Solanki KK. Significance of combined anti-CCP antibodies and rheumatoid factor in a New Zealand cohort of patients with systemic sclerosis. Int J Rheum Dis. 2018;21(7):1430–5.
4. Muangchan C. The 15% rule in scleroderma: the frequency of severe organ complications in systemic sclerosis. Syst Rev. 2013;40(9):1545–56.
5. Pope JE, et al. Systemic sclerosis (scleroderma) and Raynaud's phenomenon. In: Stone JH, editor. A Clinician's pearls and myths in rheumatology, vol. 77-95. London: Springer; 2009.
6. Armstrong RD, Gibson T. Scleroderma and erosive polyarthritis: a disease entity? Ann Rheum Dis. 1982;41(2):141–6.
7. Avouac J, et al. Articular involvement in systemic sclerosis. Rheumatology (Oxford). 2012;51(8):1347–56.
8. Bassett LW, et al. Skeletal findings in progressive systemic sclerosis (scleroderma). AJR Am J Roentgenol. 1981;136(6):1121–6.
9. AVOUAC J, et al. Characteristics of joint involvement and relationships with systemic inflammation in systemic sclerosis:

results from the EULAR scleroderma trial and research group (EUSTAR). Database. 2010;37(7):1488–501.
10. Laustriat G, et al. Anti-citrullinated peptides antibodies in systemic sclerosis: meta-analysis of frequency and meaning. Joint Bone Spine. 2018;85(2):147–53.
11. Mansour S, et al. Low socioeconomic status (measured by education) and outcomes in systemic sclerosis: data from the Canadian scleroderma research group. J Rheumatol. 2013;40(4):447–54.
12. Kapitány A, et al. Systemic sclerosis–rheumatoid arthritis overlap syndrome: a unique combination of features suggests a distinct genetic, serological and clinical entity. Rheumatology. 2007;46(6):989–93.
13. Pope JE. Scleroderma overlap syndromes. Curr Opin Rheumatol. 2002;14(6):704–10.
14. Clements P, et al. Points to consider for designing trials in systemic sclerosis patients with arthritic involvement. Rheumatology (Oxford). 2017;56(suppl_5):v23–6.
15. Arslan Tas D, et al. Evaluating hand in systemic sclerosis. Rheumatol Int. 2012;32(11):3581–6.
16. Baron M, Lee P, Keystone EC. The articular manifestations of progressive systemic sclerosis (scleroderma). Ann Rheum Dis. 1982;41(2):147–52.
17. Young A, et al. Hand impairment in systemic sclerosis: various manifestations and currently available treatment. Curr Treatm Opt Rheumatol. 2016;2(3):252–69.
18. Ueda-Hayakawa I, et al. Usefulness of anti-cyclic citrullinated peptide antibody and rheumatoid factor to detect rheumatoid arthritis in patients with systemic sclerosis. Rheumatology (Oxford). 2010;49(11):2135–9.
19. Avouac J, et al. Radiological hand involvement in systemic sclerosis. Ann Rheum Dis. 2006;65(8):1088–92.
20. La Montagna G, et al. The arthropathy of systemic sclerosis: a 12 month prospective clinical and imaging study. Skelet Radiol. 2005;34(1):35–41.
21. Freire V, et al. Hand and wrist involvement in systemic sclerosis: US features. 2013;269(3):824–30.
22. Rotondo A, et al. Ultrasonographic features of the hand and wrist in systemic sclerosis. Rheumatology. 2009;48(11):1414–7.
23. Low AH, et al. Magnetic resonance imaging of the hand in systemic sclerosis. J Rheumatol. 2009;36(5):961–4.
24. Schmeiser T, et al. Arthritis in patients with systemic sclerosis. Eur J Intern Med. 2012;23(1):e25–9.

25. Misra R, et al. Arthritis in scleroderma. Br J Rheumatol. 1995;34(9):831–7.
26. Clements P. Management of Musculoskeletal Involvement in systemic sclerosis. Curr Treatm Opt Rheumatol. 2016;2(1):61–8.
27. Moinzadeh P, et al. Disease progression in systemic sclerosis-overlap syndrome is significantly different from limited and diffuse cutaneous systemic sclerosis. 2015;74(4):730–7.
28. Perrot S, et al. Patient phenotypes in fibromyalgia comorbid with systemic sclerosis or rheumatoid arthritis: influence of diagnostic and screening tests. Screening with the FiRST questionnaire, diagnosis with the ACR 1990 and revised ACR 2010 criteria. Clin Exp Rheumatol. 2017;35 Suppl 105(3):35–42.
29. Schouffoer A, et al. The educational needs of people with systemic sclerosis: a cross-sectional study using the Dutch version of the educational needs assessment tool (D-ENAT). Rheumatol Int. 2016;36(2):289–94.
30. Poole JL, et al. Taking charge of systemic sclerosis: a pilot study to assess the effectiveness of an internet self-management program. Arthritis Care Res (Hoboken). 2014;66(5):778–82.
31. Poole JL, Skipper B, Mendelson C. Evaluation of a mail-delivered, print-format, self-management program for persons with systemic sclerosis. Clin Rheumatol. 2013;32(9):1393–8.
32. Landim SF, et al. The evaluation of a home-based program for hands in patients with systemic sclerosis. J Hand Ther. 2017;
33. Stefanantoni K, et al. Occupational therapy integrated with a self-administered stretching program on systemic sclerosis patients with hand involvement. Clin Exp Rheumatol. 2016;34 Suppl 100(5):157–61.
34. Rannou F, et al. Personalized physical therapy versus usual Care for Patients with Systemic Sclerosis: a randomized controlled trial. Arthritis Care Res (Hoboken). 2017;69(7):1050–9.
35. Shah AA, Wigley FM. My approach to the treatment of scleroderma. Mayo Clin Proc. 2013;88(4):377–93.
36. Fernández-Codina A, Walker KM, Pope JE. Treatment algorithms for systemic sclerosis according to experts. 2018;70(11):1820–8.
37. Walker KM, Pope J. Treatment of systemic sclerosis complications: what to use when first-line treatment fails--a consensus of systemic sclerosis experts. Semin Arthritis Rheum. 2012;42(1):42–55.
38. Phumethum V, Jamal S, Johnson SR. Biologic therapy for systemic sclerosis: a systematic review. 2011;38(2):289–96.

39. Young A, Khanna D. Systemic sclerosis: a systematic review on therapeutic management from 2011 to 2014. 2015;27(3):241–8.
40. Lam GK, et al. Efficacy and safety of etanercept in the treatment of scleroderma-associated joint disease. J Rheumatol. 2007;34(7):1636–7.
41. Denton CP, et al. An open-label pilot study of infliximab therapy in diffuse cutaneous systemic sclerosis. Ann Rheum Dis. 2009;68(9):1433–9.
42. Elhai M, et al. Outcomes of patients with systemic sclerosis-associated polyarthritis and myopathy treated with tocilizumab or abatacept: a EUSTAR observational study. 2013;72(7):1217–20.
43. Gonzalez EG, et al. Synthetic cannabinoid ajulemic acid exerts potent antifibrotic effects in experimental models of systemic sclerosis. Ann Rheum Dis. 2012;71(9):1545–51.
44. Servettaz A, et al. Targeting the cannabinoid pathway limits the development of fibrosis and autoimmunity in a mouse model of systemic sclerosis. Am J Pathol. 2010;177(1):187–96.
45. Pope JE. Trial methodology in scleroderma: avoiding a shot in the dark. Rheumatology (Oxford). 2017;56(suppl_5):v1–3.
46. Clements PJ, et al. Arthritis in systemic sclerosis: systematic review of the literature and suggestions for the performance of future clinical trials in systemic sclerosis arthritis. Semin Arthritis Rheum. 2012;41(6):801–14.
47. Pellar RE, Tingey TM, Pope JE. Patient-reported outcome measures in systemic sclerosis (scleroderma). Rheum Dis Clin N Am. 2016;42(2):301–16.
48. Ndosi M, et al. Common measure of quality of life for people with systemic sclerosis across seven European countries: a cross-sectional study. 2018;77(7):1032–8.
49. Pope J. Measures of systemic sclerosis (scleroderma): health assessment questionnaire (HAQ) and scleroderma HAQ (SHAQ), physician- and patient-rated global assessments, symptom burden index (SBI), University of California, Los Angeles, scleroderma clinical trials consortium gastrointestinal scale (UCLA SCTC GIT) 2.0, baseline dyspnea index (BDI) and transition dyspnea index (TDI) (Mahler's index), Cambridge pulmonary hypertension outcome review (CAMPHOR), and Raynaud's condition score (RCS). Arthritis Care Res (Hoboken). 2011;63 Suppl 11:S98–111.
50. Chung KC, et al. Reliability and validity testing of the Michigan hand outcomes questionnaire. J Hand Surg Am. 1998;23(4):575–87.

51. Sandqvist G, Hesselstrand R, Eberhardt K. A longitudinal follow-up of hand involvement and activities of daily living in early systemic sclerosis. Scand J Rheumatol. 2009;38(4):304–10.
52. Khanna D, et al. Measures of response in clinical trials of systemic sclerosis: the combined response index for systemic sclerosis (CRISS) and outcome measures in pulmonary arterial hypertension related to systemic sclerosis (EPOSS). J Rheumatol. 2009;36(10):2356–61.
53. Khanna D, et al. The future of measuring patient-reported outcomes in rheumatology: patient-reported outcomes measurement information system (PROMIS). Arthritis Care Res (Hoboken). 2011;63(Suppl 11):S486–90.

Chapter 29
Systemic Sclerosis-Related Myopathy

Marco Sprecher, Carina Mihai, and Oliver Distler

Case

An 81-year-old female with known persistent atrial fibrillation was admitted to our hospital complaining of progressive difficulties rising from a chair, with the need to push herself out of the chair using her hands, and difficulties climbing stairs. She also reported a 10-month duration of Raynaud's phenomenon, diffuse swelling of her fingers and fatigue. Because of the muscle weakness, she had to move from her apartment on the third floor to a ground floor apartment. She later noticed difficulty to hang up the laundry and to comb

M. Sprecher · O. Distler (✉)
Department of Rheumatology, University Hospital Zurich, Zurich, Switzerland
e-mail: Marco.Sprecher@usz.ch; Oliver.Distler@usz.ch

C. Mihai
Department of Rheumatology, University Hospital Zurich, Zurich, Switzerland

Department of Internal Medicine and Rheumatology, Cantacuzino Hospital, Carol Davila University of Medicine and Pharmacy, Bucharest, Romania
e-mail: Carmen-Marina.Mihai@usz.ch

© Springer Nature Switzerland AG 2021
M. Matucci-Cerinic, C. P. Denton (eds.), *Practical Management of Systemic Sclerosis in Clinical Practice*, In Clinical Practice,
https://doi.org/10.1007/978-3-030-53736-4_29

her hair. She further suffered from mild dyspnea (NYHA II) without coughing or expectoration.

On physical examination, her skin revealed sclerodactyly with puffy fingers, and teleangiectasia over her face and chest, without any other skin lesions.

The manual muscle testing procedures (MMT-8) indicated a weakness of the neck flexors (M4) and hip abduction and extension (M3). The assessment for muscle endurance (Functioning index-2) showed a reduction for shoulder flexion (17%), shoulder abduction (18%), head lifting (5%) and hip flexion 15%). Reflexes and senses were intact.

Laboratory investigations showed a remarkable elevation of creatine kinase (CK, 1350 U/L), myoglobin (662 μg/L), cardiac troponin T (0.367 μg/L) and pro-BNP (3037 ng/L). ESR and CRP were not increased. Autoantibody testing was notable for positive ANA at a titer of 1:5120 with a nuclear fine speckled pattern (AC-4 pattern) and the presence of high-titer anti-Ku antibodies.

ECG revealed atrial fibrillation and left anterior fascicular block, both known for years. Transthoracic echocardiography showed a left ventricular ejection fraction of 55% and mild mitral regurgitation, but no signs of pulmonary hypertension, wall hypokinesia or pericardial effusion. Pulmonary function test revealed moderate restriction and mild reduction of diffusion capacity while the CT scan demonstrated moderate fibrosis of both basal lung lobes.

Magnetic resonance imaging showed evidence of symmetric edema of the gluteal and hamstring muscles, which were not easily accessible for a muscle biopsy.

Based on all these findings, the diagnosis of systemic sclerosis (SSc) with polymyositis was made, with involvement of the proximal muscles and the neck, as well as a probable cardiac involvement. A therapy with mycophenolate mofetil, rituximab and moderate dosage of prednisone (10 mg/d) was started.

During the next months, the patient noticed a reduction of muscle weakness. Clinically, there was an improvement of hip abduction and extension (M4), laboratory investigation revealed normal values for CK, myoglobin, pro-BNP and a

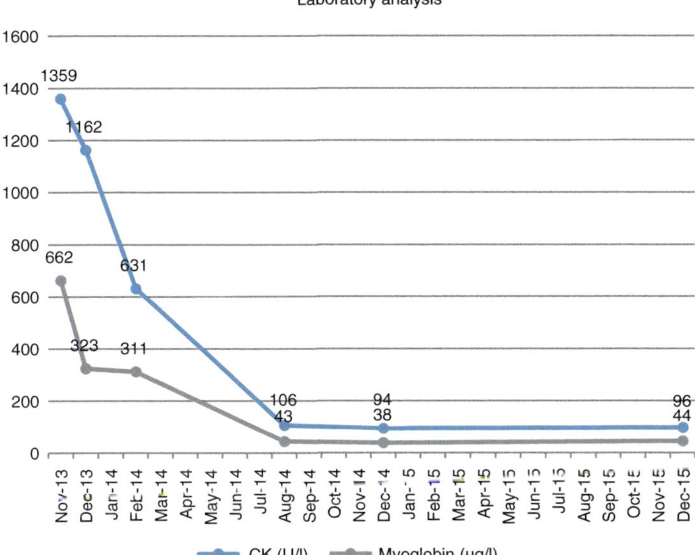

Figure 29.1 In November 2013, the patient was only treated with prednisone, 10 mg/day. Mycophenolate mofetil and rituximab were added in January 2014, while prednisone was stopped in May 2014. In August 2014, a normalization of CK und myoglobin was reached. The values remained stable over time by continuation of mycophenolate mofetil and rituximab

significant reduction of cardiac troponin T (0.042 µg/L). The interstitial lung changes remained stable. Over time, prednisone was stopped and mycophenolate mofetil and rituximab were continued as maintenance therapy. The course of serum CK and myoglobin over time is displayed in Fig. 29.1. Figure 29.2 shows the evolution of muscle strength and endurance on MMT-8 and respectively FI-2 testing.

Discussion

Muscle involvement in SSc has a wide variety of presentations. In mild cases, it can be indolent as a subclinical myopathy, presenting as a mild elevation of muscle enzymes on

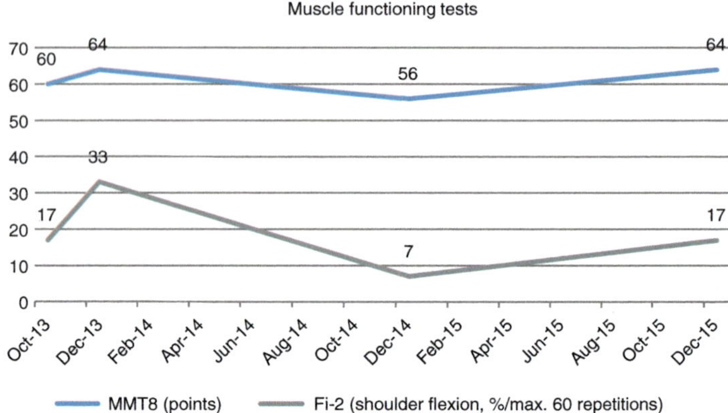

FIGURE 29.2 Muscle functioning tests over time, including the manual muscle testing procedure (MMT-8) for muscle strength and functioning index-2 (Fi-2) for muscle endurance

routine laboratory testing. It can also manifest as fibrosing myopathy, without evidence of inflammation, or more aggressively, as inflammatory myopathy/polymyositis [1]. There is no agreement among experts when such cases should be called overlap syndrome. In our clinical practice, we prefer to classify these patients as SSc-associated polymyositis and limit the term overlap to patients that present with polymyositis-defining autoantibodies, such as anti-synthetase antibodies.

Due to the lack of classification criteria for SSc-related myopathy, the prevalence of muscle involvement varies widely among different studies from 5 to 96% [2–7]. The typical clinical manifestation is symmetrical proximal muscle weakness. In some cases, also the head extensor muscles may be involved [5, 8]. Some patients report muscle pain, which is sometimes difficult to differentiate from myalgia of other causes, such as fibromyalgia, localized musculoskeletal pain or adverse drug reactions.

Involvement of extra-skeletal striate muscles is not infrequent in patients with an polymyositis associated with SSc. Vice-versa, several studies showed an increased prevalence of myositis in patients with SSc-associated myocardial involvement, who also had an increased mortality [9–11]. Esophageal dysmotility with dysphagia and respiratory dysfunction due to involvement of respiratory muscles are further aspects encountered in patients with SSc-associated polymyositis [12, 13]. Since 26% of SSc-related mortality is attributed to cardiac causes [14] and since myopathy in SSc may be associated with heart disease, all patients with SSc-associated polymyositis should be closely monitored because of late-stage complications.

Elevated levels of muscles enzymes such as creatine kinase (CK) or aldolase may help to confirm the suspicion of myositis, especially in patients with overlap of SSc and polymyositis [5, 12, 15], but these can also be normal. In the study by Paik et al. [16], histomyopathological findings such as inflammation and necrosis were associated with higher CK levels.

Immunologically, anti-Scl70 (anti-topoisomerase I) antibodies are considered to be associated with an increased risk of muscle involvement [17] along with anti-U1-RNP, anti-U3-RNP, anti-PM-Scl, anti-Ku, anti-Jo and anti-RuvBL1/2 antibodies. On the other hand, there is a negative association with anti-centromere and anti-RNA-polymerase III antibodies [6, 18]. Furthermore, SSc or myositis-specific antibodies can be completely absent in patients with SSc-related myopathy [19].

Similar to the approach of assessing disease activity in primary inflammatory myopathies, standardized muscle strength tests such as MMT-8 and muscle endurance tests such as FI-2 can also be used for SSc-related myopathy, even though they have not been evaluated in SSc and there are no international recommendations. Their validity depends on the experience and training of the examiners, as well as on patient-related variables such as motivation, test comprehension, general fitness level or motor skill impairment, for instance reduced range of motion because of skin fibrosis.

Electromyography findings resemble those of patients with primary inflammatory myopathies, with decrease of duration of single potentials, increased polyphasic potentials and increased insertional irritability [3].

MRI imaging has an important role in diagnosing inflammatory myopathy in patients with SSc. A myositis-specific protocol, consisting of coronal and axial short tau inversion recorvery (STIR) and coronal and axial T1-weighted sequences of proximal muscles, is supposed to be useful for confirming suspected muscle involvement and identifying a suitably biopsy site. However, there are only a few reports in the literature on this topic. Typical MRI findings are edema (increased T2 signal on STIR images), fatty replacement (on T1 weighted sequences) or muscle atrophy [16].

The rate of pathological muscle biopsies varies largely from 39% [4] to >90% [19, 20]. In a study by Ranque et al. from 2009, the main myopathological features were mononuclear inflammation (63%), muscle atrophy (60%), necrosis (59%), regeneration (44%), fibrosis (24%) or microangiopathy. On the other hand, a cohort study by Bhansing et al. from 2014 showed that 96% of patients diagnosed with SSc-associated-polymyositis had necrotic muscle fibers, which was significantly increased in comparison to the polymyositis-only control group (68%).

Along with the lack of international classification criteria, there are no published treatment recommendations regarding SSc-associated myopathy. This is of special concern as high-dose glucocorticoids are the mainstay of treatment for patients with idiopathic inflammatory myopathies, but are difficult to use in patients with SSc, due to the related risk of renal crisis. Therefore, high doses of glucocorticoids should be reserved only for severe cases of biopsy-proven myositis and severe forms of myocarditis, which are associated with increased mortality [11, 20, 21]. Immunosuppressive drugs such as methotrexate or mycophenolate mofetil [22, 23] addedare most frequently used. There are single reports of benefit using rituximab [22, 24] in refractory cases, but there are no clinical trials available. In a retrospective study in a small number of patients, abatacept did not show statistically significant benefit, but a trend toward in improvement in refractory cases of SSc-related myopathy was observed [25]. In moderately severe cases, low-dose glucocorticoids may be sufficient, while in mild cases with only slightly elevated CK levels, without evidence of inflammation on MRI or biopsy, myopathy may often remain untreated [2, 20].

Box: Proposed Checklist for the Work-up of Patients with Systemic Sclerosis with Myositis

- Physical examination including standardized muscle strength tests such as MMT-8 and muscle endurance tests such as FI-2
- Laboratory: ANA and autoantibody testing, creatin kinase, aldolase, myoglobin, cardiac troponin T, NT-pro-BNP
- Whole body MRI imaging
- Electromyography
- Muscle biopsy
- Heart MRI imaging and 24 h ECG (in selected cases)

MMT-8: manual muscle testing procedure 8; FI-2: functional index 2; ANA: anti-nuclear antibodies; NT-proBNP: N-terminal pro-B-type natriuretic polypeptide; MRI: magnetic resonance imaging; ECG: electrocardiography.

References

1. Javinani A, Kavosi H. Systemic sclerosis-related myopathy. Rheumatol Res. 2017;2(3):85–9. https://doi.org/10.22631/rr.2017.69997.1023.
2. Clements PJ, Furst DE, Campion DS, Bohan A, Harris R, Levy J, Paulus HE. Muscle disease in progressive systemic sclerosis. Diagnostic and therapeutic considerations. Arthritis Rheum. 1978;21:62–71. https://doi.org/10.1002/art.1780210111.
3. Hausmanowa-Petrusewicz I, Jabłońska S, Błaszczyk M, Matz B. Electromyographic findings in various forms of progressive

systemic sclerosis. Arthritis Rheum. 1982;25:61–5. https://doi.org/10.1002/art.1780250110.

4. Medsger TA, Rodnan GP, Moossy J, Vester JW. Skeletal muscle involvement in progressive systemic sclerosis (scleroderma). Arthritis Rheum. 1968;11:554–68. https://doi.org/10.1002/art.1780110405.
5. Mimori T. Scleroderma-polymyositis overlap syndrome. Int J Dermatol. 1987;26:419–25. https://doi.org/10.1111/j.1365-4362.1987.tb00580.x.
6. Ranque B, Bérezné A, Le-Guern V, Pagnoux C, Allanore Y, Launay D, Hachulla E, Authier F-J, Gherardi R, Kahan A, Cabane J, Guillevin L, Mouthon L. Myopathies related to systemic sclerosis: a case–control study of associated clinical and immunological features. Scand J Rheumatol. 2010;39(6):498–505. https://doi.org/10.3109/03009741003774626.
7. Tuffanelli D, Winkelmann R. Systemic scleroderma: a clinical study of 727 cases. Arch Dermatol. 1961;84(3):359–71. https://doi.org/10.1001/archderm.1961.01580150005001.
8. Garcin B, Lenglet T, Dubourg O, Mesnage V, Levy R. Dropped head syndrome as a presenting sign of scleromyositis. J Neurol Sci. 2010;292:101–3. https://doi.org/10.1016/j.jns.2010.02.015.
9. Follansbee WP, Zerbe TR, Medsger TA Jr. Cardiac and skeletal muscle disease in systemic sclerosis (scleroderma): a high risk association. Am Heart J. 1993;125:194–203. https://doi.org/10.1016/0002-8703(93)90075-K.
10. Hashimoto A, Tejima S, Tono T, Suzuki M, Tanaka S, Matsui T, Tohma S, Endo H, Hirohata S. Predictors of survival and causes of death in Japanese patients with systemic sclerosis. J Rheumatol. 2011;38:1931–9. https://doi.org/10.3899/jrheum.100298.
11. Pieroni M, DeSantis M, Gaetano Z, et al. Recognizing and treating myocarditis in recent-onset systemic sclerosis heart disease: potential utility of immunosuppressive therapy in cardiac damage progression. Semin Arthritis Rheum. 2014;43:526–35.
12. Marie I, Lahaxe L, Benveniste O, Delavigne K, Adoue D, Mouthon L, Hachulla E, Constans J, Tiev K, Diot E, Levesque H, Boyer O, Jouen F. Long-term outcome of patients with polymyositis/ dermatomyositis and anti-PM-Scl antibody. Br J Dermatol. 2010;162:337–44. https://doi.org/10.1111/j.1365-2133.2009.09484.x.
13. Walker UA. Imaging tools for the clinical assessment of idiopathic inflammatory myositis. Curr Opin Rheumatol. 2008;20:656–61.

14. Tyndall AJ, Bannert B, Vonk M, et al. Causes and risk factors for death in systemic sclerosis: a study from the EULAR scleroderma trials and research (EUSTAR) database. Ann Rheum Dis. 2010;69:1809–15. https://doi.org/10.1136/ard.2009.114264.
15. Troyanov Y, Targoff IN, Tremblay JL, Goulet J-R, Raymond Y, Senécal J-L. Novel classification of idiopathic inflammatory myopathies based on overlap syndrome features and autoantibodies: analysis of 100 French Canadian patients. Medicine (Baltimore). 2005;84:231–49. https://doi.org/10.1097/01.md.0000173991.74008.b0.
16. Paik JJ, Wigley FM, Lloyd TE, Corse AM, Casciola-Rosen L, Shah AA, Boin F, Hummers LK, Mammen AL. Spectrum of muscle histopathologic findings in forty-two scleroderma patients with weakness. Arthritis Care Res. 2015;67:1416–25. https://doi.org/10.1002/acr.22620.
17. Walker UA, Tyndall A, Czirják L, et al. Clinical risk assessment of organ manifestations in systemic sclerosis: a report from the EULAR scleroderma trials and research group database. Ann Rheum Dis. 2007;66:754–63. https://doi.org/10.1136/ard.2006.062901.
18. Steen VD. Autoantibodies in systemic sclerosis. Sem Arthr Rheum. 2005;35:35–42. https://doi.org/10.1016/j.semarthrit.2005.03.005.
19. Bhansing KJ, Lammens M, Knaapen HK, van Riel PL, van Engelen BG, Vonk MC. Scleroderma-polymyositis overlap syndrome versus idiopathic polymyositis and systemic sclerosis: a descriptive study on clinical features and myopathology. Arthritis Res Ther. 2014;16(3):R111. https://doi.org/10.1186/ar4562.
20. West SG, Killian PJ, Lawless OJ. Association of myositis and myocarditis in progressive systemic sclerosis. Arthritis Rheum. 1981;24:662–7. https://doi.org/10.1002/art.1780240506.
21. Ranque B, Authier F, Le-Guern V, et al. A descriptive and prognostic study of systemic sclerosis-associated myopathies. Ann Rheum Dis. 2009;68:1474–7. https://doi.org/10.1136/ard.2008.095919.
22. Bosello S, De Santis M, Lama G, Spanò C, Angelucci C, Tolusso B, Sica G, Ferraccioli G. B cell depletion in diffuse progressive systemic sclerosis: safety, skin score modification and IL-6 modulation in an up to thirty-six months follow-up open-label trial. Arthritis Res Ther. 2010;12(2):R54. https://doi.org/10.1186/ar2965.

23. Hietaharju A, Jaaskelainen S, Kalimo H, et al. Peripheral neuromuscular manifestations in systemic sclerosis (scleroderma). Muscle Nerve. 1993;16:1204–12. https://doi.org/10.1002/mus.880161110.
24. Akram Q, Roberts M, Oddis C, Herrick A, Chinoy H. Rituximab-induced neutropenia in a patient with inflammatory myopathy and systemic sclerosis overlap disease. Reumatologia. 2016;54(1):35–7. https://doi.org/10.5114/reum.2016.58760.
25. Elhai M, Meunier M, Matucci-Cerinic M, et al. Outcomes of patients with systemic sclerosis-associated polyarthritis and myopathy treated with tocilizumab or abatacept: a EUSTAR observational study. Ann Rheum Dis. 2013;72:1217–20. https://doi.org/10.1136/annrheumdis-2012-202657.

Chapter 30
Clinical Management of Tenosynovitis and Tendon Friction Rubs in Systemic Sclerosis

Bochra Jandali and Maureen D. Mayes

Introduction

Tenosynovitis

The presence of tenosynovitis has been described in SSc along with other musculoskeletal manifestations in both dcSSc and lcSSc. The use of advanced musculoskeletal imaging like ultrasound (US) and magnetic resonance imaging (MRI) showed a higher prevalence of tenosynovitis among SSc patients than reported by physical exam alone. In a cross-sectional observational study of 52 consecutive SSc patients, reported by Elhai et al. [1], the use of ultrasound of hands

B. Jandali (✉)
Division of Rheumatology and Clinical immunogenetics, University of Texas McGovern Medical School, Houston, TX, USA
e-mail: Bochra.Jandali@uth.tmc.edu

M. D. Mayes
Division of Rheumatology and Clinical Immunogenetics, University of Texas McGovern Medical School, Houston, Medical School Building (MSB) 5.270, Houston, TX, USA
e-mail: Maureen.D.Mayes@uth.tmc.edu

© Springer Nature Switzerland AG 2021

M. Matucci-Cerinic, C. P. Denton (eds.), *Practical Management of Systemic Sclerosis in Clinical Practice*, In Clinical Practice,
https://doi.org/10.1007/978-3-030-53736-4_30

showed tenosynovitis in 27% of SSc patients as compared to 6% using clinical observation. Tenosynovitis was considered inflammatory or fibrotic based on US features. Additionally, in a later study of 44 consecutive SSc patients by this group [2], US features of the hand and wrist demonstrated synovitis, tenosynovitis, calcinosis and acroosteolysis with high sensitivity and greater reliability than physical exam alone. In another study utilizing musculoskeletal (MSK) magnetic resonance imaging on the hand in 17 SSc patients [3], tenosynovitis was detected in 47% of these patients.

The early detection of tenosynovitis is not only important to understand sources of pain and hence to guide therapy, the presence of tenosynovitis was associated with higher skin scores and early, active or more severe disease [1].

Two types of tenosynovitis were identified in SSc patients using US imaging; the sclerosing type, which was only seen in SSc patients (compared to rheumatoid arthritis [RA] patients), and the inflammatory type, which was seen in both SSc and RA patients. To our knowledge, Elhai et al., was the first to describe patterns of tenosynovitis in SSc as compared to RA patients [1]. The findings of this one study, using US to assess tendon involvement in SSc and RA patients, showed that almost half of patients with tenosynovitis had a sclerosing pattern characterized by hyperechoic tendon sheath thickening. It also showed that tenosynovitis detected by US was more likely to be found in the presence of tendon friction rubs (TFRs) and in patients with more pronounced arthritis symptoms and signs.

Tendon Friction Rubs (TFRs)

Tendon friction rubs are a physical sign, which was first described in SSc by Westphal in 1876 in a 23 year old SSc patient as “coarse cracking and crepitus over fingers and knees” [4]. In a later report, they were contributed to fibrin deposition in the tendon structures [5]. They have also been described as leathery crepitus over moving joints [6].

TFRs are most commonly detected by clinical examination at the following sites (in order of decreasing frequency): hands, ankles, wrists, knees, elbows and shoulders (scapulae) [7]. The use of MSK US and MRI to assess tendon involvement in SSc patients offered alternative theories to explain the mechanism of TFRs. A study by Cuomo et al., suggested the presence of thickened retinaculum as the underlying etiology of TFRs [8]. The study included 55 dcSSc patients and 30 healthy controls. TFRs were detected in 12 dcSSc patients and 15 lcSSc patients. Ultrasound examination detected thickened retinaculum in dcSSc patients as compared to lcSSc and healthy controls in the following sites (wrist flexor and extensor tendons, patellar tendons and anterior ankle tendon). However, that would not possibly explain the TFRs in structures lack retinaculum like elbow and shoulder joints. Another study by Stoenoiu et al. [9] suggested the presence of deep infiltrates in the connective tissues surrounding the joint (wrists and ankles in 15 dcSSc patients) as a cause of impaired proper gliding of tendons during active motion.

Over the years, TFRs gained more attention in SSc registries, as researchers looked at the importance of identifying TFRs in SSc patients, which found a higher prevalence of TFRs among patients with dcSSc as compared to lcSSc.

Steen and Medsger [10] were the first to report the importance of TFRs prospectively in a large SSc cohort. Interestingly, TFRs were more frequently associated with the presence of dcSSc or later development of the diffuse form. TFRs were associated with more severe skin thickening, joint contractures, cardiac and renal disease, and more importantly, decreased survival.

Later, Khanna et al. [7] analyzed the data from a large randomized controlled trial of D-Penicillamine looking at the significance of TFRs in patients with early dcSSc. Their findings confirmed the presence of TFRs early at baseline and their association with worse skin involvement and disability scores. Moreover, detection of improvement (or worsening) in TFRs in the initial 6 months predicted improvement (or worsening) in MRSS and HAQ-DI over 12 months.

Furthermore, Dore et al. [11], showed in a case-control study including 287 cases with early dcSSc with TFRs matched to 287 early dcSSc patients without TFRs as controls, that having one or more TFR in early dcSSc was associated with a higher risk of developing cardiac, renal and gastrointestinal involvement and decreased survival.

Most recently, utilizing the large EUSTAR (European Scleroderma Trials and Research) database, Avouac et al. and colleagues [12] performed a prospective cohort study of 1301 SSc patients with disease duration $\leq$3 years and follow-up $\geq$2 years; these authors reported that both joint synovitis and TFRs (both assessed by clinical exam) are independent predictive factors for disease progression in patients with early SSc. These features are important when considering therapy as well as selecting subjects for clinical trials to identify patients at risk for skin progression.

Clinical Management

Evidence to guide management is meager at best.

Non-pharmacologic Management

Physical or Occupational Therapy (combined with home exercises):

Given the high prevalence of disability amongst SSc patients from skin and musculoskeletal involvement, it is reasonable to think that patients with the presence of tenosynovitis and TFRs would benefit from SSc oriented rehabilitation programs. There are no reported data to support this approach specifically in tendon involvement. However, recent reports showed encouraging data using non-pharmacological approaches in SSc patients with hand involvement focusing on hand contractures and function. Bongi et al. [13] reported results of a study combining joint manipulation and connective tissue massage with home exercises in SSc patients that had favorable outcomes on hand function and quality of life.

Other studies using home-based kinesiotherapy protocol or self-management program (using a book and DVD) showed beneficial results on hand function [14]. Landim et al. [15] also reported positive results of a home-based program for hands in SSc patients. However, large prospective clinical trials are lacking and SSc-specific programs are not readily available except in expert centers.

Pharmacologic Treatment

Data regarding pharmacologic treatment of tendon involvement in SSc are scarce. In patients with tenosynovitis with or without TFRs, nonsteroidal anti-inflammatory drugs (NSAIDs) or low dose steroids are frequently used. However, special caution should be paid to SSc patients given the potential toxicity of NSIADs in subjects with esophageal and/or gastric dysmotility and given the risk of renal crisis with the administration of higher dose steroids. It is worth mentioning that the 2017 EULAR updated recommendations for SSc treatment [16] did not include MSK management due to the lack of evidence-based studies.

Given the lack of robust evidence in management of tendon involvement in SSc, treatment decisions may be based on expert opinion and musculoskeletal manifestations of SSc are currently treated with therapies developed for related indications such as those for erosive or nonerosive synovitis. If first line therapy such as NSAIDs and low-dose prednisone prove inadequate, common recommendations include methotrexate, leflunomide, anti-malarials, azathioprine, mycophenolate, rituximab or other biologics [7, 17, 18].

References

1. Elhai M, Guerini H, Bazeli R, Avouac J, Freire V, et al. Ultrasonographic hand features in systemic sclerosis and correlates with clinical, biologic, and radiographic findings. Arthritis Care Res. 2012;64(8):1244–9.

2. Freire V, Bazeli R, Elhai M, Campagna R, Pessis E, et al. Hand and wrist involvement in systemic sclerosis: US features. Radiology. 2013;269(3):824–30.
3. Low AH, Lax M, Johnson SR, Lee P. Magnetic resonance imaging of the hand in systemic sclerosis. J Rheumatol. 2009;36(5):961–4.
4. Westphal C. Zwei Falle Von Schlerodermie. (translation of title: two cases of scleroderma). Charlete Annalen. 1876;3:341–60.
5. Shulman LE, Kurban AK, Harvey AM. Tendon friction rubs in progressive system sclerosis (scleroderma). Trans Asso Am Physicians. 1961;74:378–88.
6. Rodnan GP, Medsger TA. The rheumatic manifestations of progressive systemic sclerosis (scleroderma). Clin Orthop Relat Res. 1968;57:81–93.
7. Khanna PP, Furst DE, Clements PJ, Maranian P, Indulkar L. Tendon friction rubs in early diffuse systemic sclerosis: prevalence, characteristics and longitudinal changes in a randomized controlled trial. Rheumatology (Oxford). 2010;49(5):955–9.
8. Cuomo G, Zappia M, Iudici M, Abignano G, Rotondo A, et al. The origin of tendon friction rubs in patients with systemic sclerosis: a sonographic explanation. Arthritis Rheum. 2012;64(4):1291–3.
9. Stoenoiu MS, Houssiau FA, Lecouvet FE. Tendon friction rub in systemic sclerosis: a possible explanation--an ultrasound and magnetic resonance imaging study. Rheumatology (Oxford). 2013;52(3):529–33.
10. Steen VD, Medsger TA Jr. The palpable tendon friction rub: an important physical examination finding in patients with systemic sclerosis. Arthritis Rheum. 1997;40(6):1146–51.
11. Dore A, Lucas M, Ivanco D, Medsger TA Jr, Domsic RT. Significance of palpable tendon friction rubs in early diffuse cutaneous systemic sclerosis. Arthritis Care Res. 2013;65(8):1385–9.
12. Avouac J, Walker UA, Hachulla E, Riemekastan G, Cuomo G, et al. Joint and tendon involvement predict disease progression in systemic sclerosis: a EUSTAR prospective study. Ann Rheum Dis. 2016;75(1):103–9.
13. Bongi SM, Del Rosso A, Galluccio F, Sigismondi F, Miniati I, et al. Efficacy of connective tissue massage and mc Mennell joint manipulation in the rehabilitative treatment of the hands in systemic sclerosis. Clin Rheumatol. 2009;28(10):1167–73.
14. Piga M, Tradori I, Pani D, Barabino G, Dessi A, et al. Telemedicine applied to kinesiotherapy for hand dysfunction in patients

with systemic sclerosis and rheumatoid arthritis: recovery of movement and telemonitoring technology. J Rheumatol. 2014;41(7):1324–33.
15. Landim SF, Bertolo MB, Marcatto de Abreu MF, Del Rio AP, Mazon CC, et al. The evaluation of a home-based program for hands in patients with systemic sclerosis. J Hand Ther. 2017. [Epub ahead of print]
16. Kowal-Bielecka O, Fransen J, Avouac J, Becker M, Kulak A, et al. Update of EULAR recommendations for the treatment of systemic sclerosis. Ann Rheum Dis. 2017;76(8):1327–39.
17. Fernandez-Codina A, Walker KM, Pope JE, the Scleroderma Algorithm Group. Treatment algorighms for systemic sclerosis according to experts. Arthritis Rheum. 2018;70(11):1820–8.
18. Clements P. Management of musculoskeletal involvement in systemic sclerosis. Curr Treatm Opt Rheumatol. 2016;2(1):61–8.

Chapter 31
Management Challenges in the Early Systemic Sclerosis Population: Navigating Side Effects of Therapeutics and Approach to Diarrhea

Tracy M. Frech, Jeanmarie Mayer, and Silvia Bellando-Randone

Clinical Vignettes

A 49-year old female with an 11-month history of VEDOSS progressing to systemic sclerosis (SSc) complicated by diffuse skin involvement and nonspecific interstitial pneumonitis presents for her routine care visit. She was started on a CCB and PPI when she initially presented with VEDOSS criteria.

T. M. Frech (✉) · J. Mayer
Department of Internal Medicine, Division of Rheumatology, University of Utah, Salt Lake City, UT, USA
e-mail: tracy.frech@hsc.utah.edu; jeanmarie.mayer@hsc.utah.edu

S. Bellando-Randone
Department of Experimental and Clinical Medicine, University of Florence, Florence, Italy

Department of Geriatric Medicine, Division of Rheumatology and Scleroderma Unit AOUC, Florence, Italy

© Springer Nature Switzerland AG 2021

M. Matucci-Cerinic, C. P. Denton (eds.), *Practical Management of Systemic Sclerosis in Clinical Practice*, In Clinical Practice,
https://doi.org/10.1007/978-3-030-53736-4_31

She completed a Scleroderma Clinical Trials Consortium Gastrointestinal Tract 2.0 (SCTC GIT 2.0) questionnaire each visit per standard clinical practice. It was noted that her GIT 2.0 has progressively worsened in all categories with the exception of constipation over the past 9 months:

Month	Reflux	Distention/ Bloating	Soilage	Diarrhea	Constipation	Social	Emotional	Total
March	0.38	1	0	0.5	1.25	0	0.77	0.446
June	0.63	0.75	1	0.5	1.5	0	0.33	0.673
September	1.25	2	3	2	0	2	3.0	2.2

At her follow-up visit in June, even though her skin score had improved, a traumatic digital ulcer (DU) was noted to be painful with erythematous margins. At this appointment, she was treated for the ulcer with a seven-day course of amoxicillin/clavulanate. The ulcer was re-examined in wound clinic at the conclusion of the treatment course, the patient was without new complaints, and signs of infection had cleared. At her appointment in September, due to the worsening of soilage and diarrhea stool studies for *C. difficile* were ordered. The *C. difficile* toxin B gene was detected by nucleic acid amplification testing and presence of toxigenic *C. difficile* was confirmed by culture. She did not have leukocytosis nor fever, but her mycophenolate mofetil medication was discontinued to ensure there was an optimized response to treatment for *C. difficile*. After two courses of treatment for *C. difficile* infection and reoccurrence, it was decided in consultation with an Infectious Disease specialist to treat this patient with fecal microbiota transplant (FMT).

A 32 year-old female is referred for 6 months of Raynaud's phenomenon and puffy fingers with limited range of motion. She does not have skin thickening, digital ulcers, or telangiectases. She denies respiratory or gastrointestinal complaints. Nailfold capillaroscopy reveals early changes and her ANA and centromere autoantibody is positive. She is started on a CCB and methotrexate for hand complaints and is scheduled for follow-up in 2 months at which time her GIT 2.0 reveals:

Reflux	Distention/ Bloating	Soilage	Diarrhea	Constipation	Social	Emotional	Total
0.38	0.5	0	1	0	0	0	0.312

The patient asks whether her reflux, distention/bloating, and diarrhea are the result of medication side effect of therapeutics, an infection, or SSc. She reports the loose stools are occurring up to 4 times a day started after medication initiation, but do not correlate to dosing day.

Discussion

While use of patient reported outcomes can identify the frequency and severity of gastrointestinal tract symptoms [1], and best practice guidelines can direct the clinician to proper stepwise diagnostic pathways [2], the side effects of CCB, PPI, and immunosuppressant medications in VEDOSS patients warrant a thoughtful approach. These two vignettes of diarrhea detected by routine use of patient reported outcomes in early SSc patients highlight the concern for empiric PPI use in the VEDOSS population; the challenge of testing and treating for *Clostridium difficile* infection (CDI); and the importance of a thoughtful approach to medication side effects. Whether these patients would have benefited from a dose-reduction in CCB rather than addition of PPI (a risk factor for CDI) and whether immunosuppression should be held versus initiating a diarrhea work-up are important considerations. These medication choices highlight the potential management challenges in medication choices in this population.

Patients vary in their description of diarrhea, but terminology is important. Loose stool consistency, increased frequency, urgency of bowel movements, or incontinence can be key symptoms that are not adequately captured by use of PRO alone. Physicians need to distinguish acute diarrhea, which is self-limited and the result of acute infections, from chronic diarrhea, which has been present for more than 4 weeks and has a broader differential diagnosis. A common side effect of methotrexate and mycophenolate mofetil is diarrhea, thus it is important to review the timing of the onset of diarrhea related to medication dosing and indication for immunosuppression with VEDOSS patients.

Clostridium difficile is an obligate anaerobic, spore-forming, gram-positive rod that causes 25% of antibiotic-associated diarrhea and is the most commonly recognized cause of infectious diarrhea in healthcare settings [3]. The incubation period for CDI is unknown; however, symptoms can occur for up to 12-weeks after exposure to antibiotics. The risk of primary and recurrent CDI is greater in immunosuppressed individuals. CDI can vary in severity to mild diarrhea to fulminant colitis, and there is also a high prevalence of asymptomatic colonization found in up to 5–50% of hospitalized patients [4]. As such, the rheumatologist's ability to interpret results of diagnostic testing for *C. difficile* is imperative, as asymptomatic carriers require no treatment (with unnecessary antibiotics potentially increasing risk for CDI by disrupting the intestinal microbiota), while fulminant disease mandates treatment [5].

A panel of experts convened by the Infectious Diseases Society of America and Society for Healthcare Epidemiology of America recommend that the preferred target population for *C. difficile* testing for CDI are those patients with unexplained and new-onset ≥3 unformed stools in 24 hours. A diagnosis of CDI is defined by the presence of symptoms and diagnostic testing with either a stool positive for *C. difficile* toxin or detection of the toxin gene or colonoscopy or histopathologic findings revealing pseudomembranous colitis [6]. Both of the vignette patients diarrhea, but demonstrate some of the challenges in determining if there is new or worsening of diarrhea in individuals with baseline gastrointestinal symptoms to justify testing and in interpreting test results.

There are several methodologies for testing of *C. difficile* [6–8] that detect the organism or toxin in stool. The methods most often offered by clinical laboratories include testing for toxin using an enzyme immunoassay (EIA) or for the toxin B gene using a nucleic acid amplification test (NAAT). The

NAAT for the toxin B gene is highly sensitive, but should only be used as a stand-alone test to diagnose CDI in at risk individuals with new onset frequent loose stools without other explanation, such as laxatives. Combination EIA tests that include screening for the common antigen glutamate dehydrogenase (GDH) present in all toxigenic and non-toxigenic strains of *C. difficile*, as well as testing for toxin, can improve diagnostic accuracy and sensitivity. A diagnosis of CDI is supported when the toxin test is positive, or potentially when the toxin test is negative but GDH positive with reflex to NAAT with detection of the toxin gene. Laboratory assays cannot completely distinguish colonization from CDI, and normal leukocyte counts and failure to respond to treatment for CDI should prompt the clinician to question CDI as the etiology of diarrhea [3]. Repeat testing should not be performed within 7 days during the same episode of diarrhea, as the potential for false positives is high. Additionally, individuals treated for CDI should not have stool submitted for "test of cure", but instead be followed for resolution of the precipitating clinical symptoms. Recent guidelines provide updated recommendations on optimal treatment for CDI [3]. Recurrence of CDI can be found in 10–35% of patients following a first episode, nearly 40% after a first recurrence, and 60 to 100% after two or more recurrences [9]. For recurrence, the provider should avoid repeating the initial treatment regimen, and consider using tapering and pulsed regimens of vancomycin or following vancomycin with rifaximin. For patients that have failed at least two courses of antibiotic therapy for recurrent CDI, fecal microbiota transplantation (FMT) is strongly recommended [6, 10]. It is important to reduce modifiable risk factors for CDI. In the VEDOSS population, this includes dose reduction of CCB that is worsening GERD, rather than the empiric initiation of a PPI.

In summary, the assessment of diarrhea in a VEDOSS patient on PPI with recent antibiotic exposure requires an understanding of its chronicity and relation to therapeutics, as well as the diagnostics and treatment of *C. difficile* (Fig. 31.1). The vignettes highlight that recent expert guidelines recom-

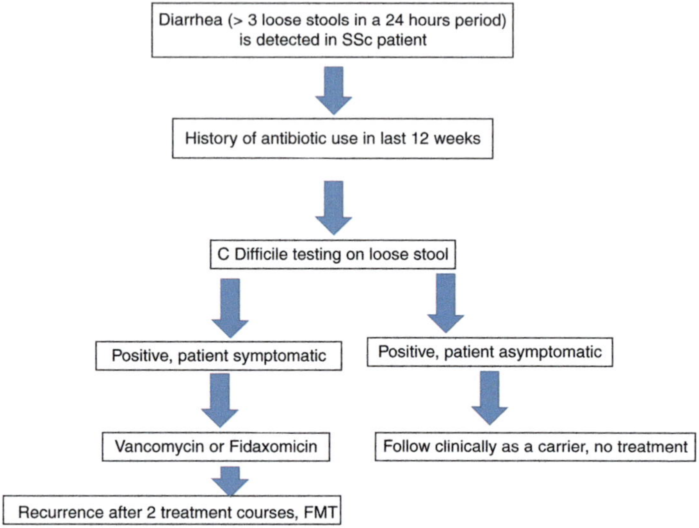

FIGURE 31.1 Stepwise management for *Clostridium Difficile* testing in early SSc patients with antibiotic exposure and diarrhea (adapted from references [2, 5, 6]

mend that only symptomatic patients, and not carriers, should receive treatment. It also highlights that recurrent CDI in SSc patients should be considered for FMT. The treating physician should ensure that CCB adverse drug effects are minimized, and that both PPI and immunosuppression are needed, especially during treatment of active CDI. Many treatments, including FMT, are part of ongoing research that are of particular interest for physicians evaluating VEDOSS and early SSc patients with diarrhea.

References

1. Khanna D, Nagaraja V, Gladue H, Chey W, Pimentel M, Frech T. Measuring response in the gastrointestinal tract in systemic sclerosis. Curr Opin Rheumatol. 2013;25(6):700–6.
2. Hansi N, Thoua N, Carulli M, Chakravarty K, Lal S, Smyth A, et al. Consensus best practice pathway of the UK scleroderma

study group: gastrointestinal manifestations of systemic sclerosis. Clin Exp Rheumatol. 2014;32(6 Suppl 86):S-214-21.
3. Curry SR. Clostridium difficile. Clin Lab Med. 2017;37(2):341–69.
4. Jawa RS, Mercer DW. Clostridium difficile-associated infection: a disease of varying severity. Am J Surg. 2012;204(6):836–42.
5. Surawicz CM, Brandt LJ, Binion DG, Ananthakrishnan AN, Curry SR, Gilligan PH, et al. Guidelines for diagnosis, treatment, and prevention of Clostridium difficile infections. Am J Gastroenterol. 2013;108(4):478–98.
6. Gupta A, Cifu AS, Khanna S. Diagnosis and treatment of Clostridium difficile infection. JAMA. 2018;320(10):1031–2.
7. Curry SR. Clostridium difficile. Clin Lab Med. 2017;37(2):341–69.
8. Pollock NR. Ultrasensitive detection and quantification of toxins for optimized diagnosis of Clostridium difficile infection. J Clin Microbiol. 2016;54(2):259–64.
9. McFarland LV, Surawicz CM, Rubin M, Fekety R, Elmer GW, Greenberg RN. Recurrent Clostridium difficile disease: epidemiology and clinical characteristics. Infect Control Hosp Epidemiol. 1999;20(1):43–50.
10. Kao D, Roach B, Silva M, Beck P, Rioux K, Kaplan GG, et al. Effect of Oral capsule- vs colonoscopy-delivered fecal microbiota transplantation on recurrent Clostridium difficile infection: a randomized clinical trial. JAMA. 2017;318(20):1985–93.

Suggested Reading

Avouac J, Fransen J, Walker UA, Riccieri V, Smith V, Muller C, et al. Preliminary criteria for the very early diagnosis of systemic sclerosis: results of a Delphi consensus study from EULAR scleroderma trials and research group. Ann Rheum Dis. 2011;70(3):476–81.

Valentini G, Cuomo G, Abignano G, Petrillo A, Vettori S, Capasso A, et al. Early systemic sclerosis: assessment of clinical and pre-clinical organ involvement in patients with different disease features. Rheumatology (Oxford). 2011;50(2):317–23.

Lepri G, Guiducci S, Bellando-Randone S, Giani I, Bruni C, Blagojevic J, et al. Evidence for oesophageal and anorectal involvement in very early systemic sclerosis (VEDOSS): report from a single VEDOSS/EUSTAR Centre. Ann Rheum Dis. 2015;74(1):124–8.

Bellando-Randone S, Matucci-Cerinic M. Very early systemic sclerosis and pre-systemic sclerosis: definition, recognition, clinical relevance and future directions. Curr Rheumatol Rep. 2017;19(10):65.

Hughes M, Herrick AL. Raynaud's phenomenon. Best Pract Res Clin Rheumatol. 2016;30(1):112–32.

Pope J, Harding S, Khimdas S, Bonner A, Baron M, Grp CSR. Agreement with guidelines from a large database for Management of Systemic Sclerosis: results from the Canadian scleroderma research group. J Rheumatol. 2012;39(3):524–31.

Frech TM, Shanmugam VK, Shah AA, Assassi S, Gordon JK, Hant FN, et al. Treatment of early diffuse systemic sclerosis skin disease. Clin Exp Rheumatol. 2013;31(2):S166–S71.

Index

© Springer Nature Switzerland AG 2021
M. Matucci-Cerinic, C. P. Denton (eds.), *Practical Management of Systemic Sclerosis in Clinical Practice*, In Clinical Practice,
https://doi.org/10.1007/978-3-030-53736-4

N

O

9783030537357